HERE'S WHAT REVIEWERS ARE SAYING ABOUT *A GUIDE TO ALTERNATIVE MEDICINE:*

Anyone interested in learning what alternative medicine is, how it works, what it is most useful for, how to use it, and where to find it would do well to get a copy of *A Guide to Alternative Medicine*. This is a comprehensive, readable, well-organized tour through the world of alternative approaches to health care.

Bill Thomson
Natural Health *Magazine*

It is the popularity and importance of alternative treatments that should make *A Guide to Alternative Medicine* an important part of people's health library.... Whether you experience an acute health problem or have a chronic condition, the information in *A Guide to Alternative Medicine* can be very beneficial.

Don R. Powell, Ph.D.
Founder and President
American Institute for Preventive Medicine

Throughout *A Guide to Alternative Medicine,* the information on alternative and complementary medicine is presented from an objective perspective....If your goal is to be an informed, educated consumer who has the right and the ability to make choices in your health care, then *A Guide to Alternative Medicine* is a book that you definitely want in your personal natural-health resource library.

Eric S. Jones, N.D.
Dean, Naturopathic Medicine Program
Bastyr University

A GUIDE TO
Alternative Medicine

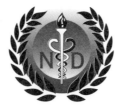

— IN CONSULTATION WITH —

THE AMERICAN ASSOCIATION OF

NATUROPATHIC PHYSICIANS

CONTRIBUTING WRITERS:

SUSANNE ALTHOFF

PATRICIA N. WILLIAMS

DIANNE MOLVIG

LARRY SCHUSTER

PUBLICATIONS INTERNATIONAL, LTD.

Consultants:
This publication was reviewed by the **American Association of Naturopathic Physicians**. The AANP's mission is to empower members of the association with the knowledge, tools, skills, and guidance to help them succeed in educating and guiding their communities and patients toward greater health and well-being and to transform the health care system from disease management to health promotion by incorporating the principles of naturopathic medicine.

Contributing Reviewers:
Kathi Head, N.D. (chief), Rita Bettenburg, N.D., Tim Birdsall, N.D., and Lori Kimatan, N.D., are all members of the American Association of Naturopathic Physicians.

Contributing Writers:
Susanne Althoff holds a masters degree in journalism with a focus on health and science reporting. Her writing has appeared in such magazines as *Vegetarian Times* and *Natural Health*.

Patricia N. Williams is a freelance health and science writer and editor. She has worked on projects and publications for the National Institutes of Health, the White House, and other government agencies and for a variety of consumer and professional publications.

Dianne Molvig is a freelance writer, researcher, and editor whose work has appeared in *Natural Health*, *Parents*, *Wellness*, and numerous other publications.

Larry Schuster is the science and technology editor at United Press International and has been a writer with the International Medical News Group and other publications.

Illustrations:
Yoshi Miyake

Contents

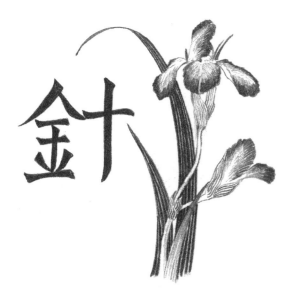

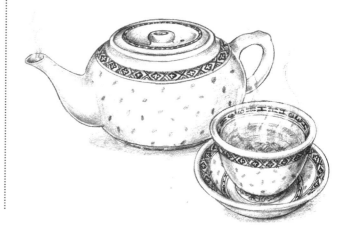

Contents

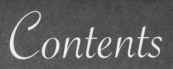

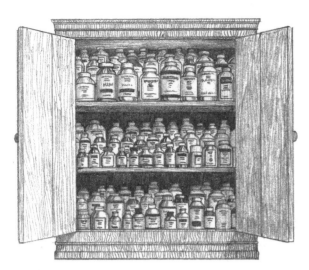

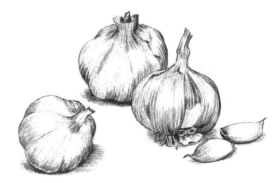

Contents

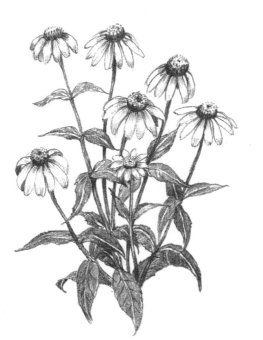

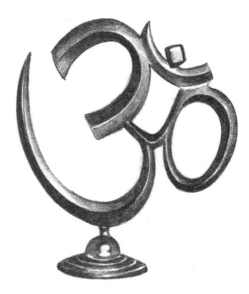

Introduction

IT SEEMS ALTERNATIVE MEDICINE IS SWEEPING THE COUNTRY. NEWSPAPERS, MAGAZINES, BOOKS, TV—IT'S STARTING TO LOOK LIKE A FAD. BUT THE TRUTH IS, ALTERNATIVE MEDICAL TREATMENTS HAVE BEEN AROUND IN THIS COUNTRY FOR CENTURIES AND PROMISE TO BE WITH US FOR AS LONG AS PEOPLE NEED HEALING.

There are so many traditions represented in the history of alternative therapies that to discuss a single line would not do justice to the others. There are traditions that go back millennia, and there are relatively new schools of thought based on recent discoveries. Some are still the primary health care systems in their native lands, and some have struggled to be recognized throughout their existence. The one thing they have in common, though, is that in this country, they have been relegated to the margins of medicine.

To understand what alternative medicine is, you have to know what it's an alternative to. In the United States, the medical establishment consists of a system of medical schools, hospitals, and M.D.s that many would call traditional medicine. But there is really nothing *traditional* about it. In fact, *traditional medicine* would be a better description of many of the alternative therapies described in this book—time-honored beliefs and practices relied on for generations. *Conventional* would be a better word to describe modern Western medicine, often called allopathic medicine. It is predominant in most of the Western world because it is the convention, the mode of thinking that is currently in vogue. That is not to say that allopathic medicine is just a fad. It is a valuable resource for health and healing, but it is not the only one. It is one system among many.

All of this may seem like a pointless discussion of words—allopathic, alternative, conventional, traditional—but the way we talk about them can mean a great deal. People's access to health care options—and even who will pay for what—depends on what people say about different modes of therapy. Many of the alternative therapies in this book are only now beginning to recover after veritable smear campaigns that threatened their very legality in this country.

THE RISE OF ALLOPATHY IN THE UNITED STATES

At the turn of the century, the medical landscape looked quite different from the way it does now. Medical practices varied widely across the country. In the American West especially, herbal medicine, which had been the predominant form of medicine since ancient times, was still very much in practice. And while allopathic medicine was beginning to dominate in the larger cities, practices such as homeopathy flourished especially in rural areas. In fact, 15 percent of the physicians practicing in the United States at that time were homeopathic physicians, and there were 22 medical schools teaching the practice. Osteopathic and chiropractic medicine were also beginning to receive recognition during this time, but all this was soon to end.

Rapid advances in chemistry, the discovery of "the miracle drugs" antibiotics, and sanitary improvements that allowed for safer surgical procedures caused allopathic medicine's reputation as the one true medicine to grow. In 1910, the Flexner report from the Carnegie Foundation for the Advancement of Teaching marked the beginning of the rise of allopathic medicine to dominance in the United States. It contained recommendations for codifying medical education along academic, and specifically, allopathic lines. In effect, allopathic medicine's successes were not lost on a public whose biggest health concerns—infectious disease and epidemic—seemed to have been resolved. As conventional medicine surged ahead, more and more alternatives such as homeopathy and herbal medicine waned.

CHINKS IN THE ARMOR

Certainly, allopathic medicine's accomplishments are formidable: The scourge of smallpox has been eradicated; polio and tuberculosis epidemics are no longer an ever-present danger; and procedures such as dialysis and transplantation have saved countless lives. No question that a big part of our lengthening life-expectancy can be attributed to the advances of the conventional medical community.

However, in recent years, allopathic medicine's shortcomings seem to be more prevalent than its successes. The miracles we've come to expect from conventional medicine don't seem to be forthcoming for chronic diseases such as heart disease and arthritis. New plagues such as AIDS are upon us. Cancer deaths are on the rise. And perhaps most disturbing of all, once-vanquished enemies such as tuberculosis are returning in more powerful strains brought about by the very drugs that combated them so successfully earlier in the century.

In addition to these alarming developments are the spiraling costs, caused in part by allopathic medicine's penchant for addressing health problems after they're well established. (It is much more expensive to treat a heart attack than it is to design a preventive diet and exercise program 15 years before it occurs.) Although the conventional medical community recognizes prevention and primary care as important, it is far from emphasized. After all, specialization is one of the hallmarks of allopathy, pushing expert care and intervention later and later along in the disease process.

ALTERNATIVE SOLUTIONS

It would be an overstatement to say that allopathic medicine has failed as a medical system, but certainly there are problems that need to be addressed. The alternative medical community has a surprising number of solutions.

To questions about chronic conditions such as arthritis that remain a stubborn mystery to conventional medicine, alternative therapists offer new innovative theories and approaches. To concerns about outrageous treatment costs, alternative therapists offer the common sense of prevention and wellness to head off problems before they need "fixing." To the public's dissatisfaction with allopathic physicians' growing detachment from their patients—seeing the patient as a case or instance of disease—alternative therapists offer healing to the whole person as a human being.

Although the traditions and practices that fall under the heading alternative medicine are diverse, most share a common principle that sets them apart from allopathic medicine: *health*. Conventional medicine concerns itself almost exclusively with treatment and defines health as the absence of disease, but alternative medicine recognizes our potential to be well instead of focusing on our potential to be sick. Health is as real as, or more real than, disease. Alternative therapists from acupuncturists to naturopaths to yogis understand the power of the human—body, mind, and spirit—to stay well and heal itself when necessary.

A ROLE FOR BOTH

It would seem from the history of medicine in the United States that conventional and alternative medicine are locked in a struggle to the death—M.D.s versus chiropractors and naturopaths; pharmaceutical companies versus herbalists—and only one will come out on top. However, the future will probably be a lot less black and white than that. And that's good news for our health.

More and more, patients, insurance companies, and even conventional doctors are recognizing the value of alternative therapies. Meditation managing high blood pressure without drugs, biofeedback treating bowel disorders without surgery, and mind/body medicine giving hope and quality of life to the terminally ill are just a few examples of the benefits of alternative medicine that conventional medicine simply cannot offer.

Likewise, one cannot ignore the power of allopathy's contribution to medical knowledge. For generations, conventional medicine has been the recipient of enormous resources; some of our most talented minds and certainly a great deal of money have gone into medicine. Because of these years of attention, conventional medicine is the smart place to look for health care in many instances.

The recognition that both types of medicine have a role to play in health has lead to a new term—one that, we hope, will eventually replace the title of this book and help break down the negative stereotypes that neither side deserves. The term is *complementary medicine*. In it is the idea that sometimes conventional approaches are warranted, other times alternative approaches are the better choice, and often using both is the best choice of all. Together, they complement each other to the great benefit of the patient. If we build on the strengths of both schools of thought, health care in this country and, indeed, the world has a very bright future.

USING THIS BOOK

There is a lot of information in this book on many different topics. Likewise, there are many ways to access that information, as well, depending on your interest and your aim.

If you're interested in the range of options for a particular condition, Part I: Illnesses & Conditions has profiles of many common ailments and the treatment options available. Within these profiles, you'll find specific suggestions from the different schools of thought, and you'll find references to the Part II: Therapies for where to find information on other therapies that can address the condition.

If you're interested in a type of alternative treatment or system, Part II: Therapies has chapters devoted to the most prevalent alternative therapies. Here you'll find a broader view of each alternative discipline, including its history, techniques, and notable successes. We've included reports on research where appropriate for your own edification, of course, but for another important reason, as well: Evidence is the cornerstone of scientific inquiry, and this documentation may help facilitate a discussion on alternatives with your doctor if you're interested.

Nothing can replace a well-informed health care consumer, and no one knows this better than doctors and practitioners. Knowing your options is part of being well informed, but so is communicating with your practitioner effectively. We've tried to make the information, suggestions, and ideas presented here immediately helpful to you in a practical way, but more often than not, good health care depends on the patient *and* the practitioner working together as a team.

A Guide to Alternative Medicine is your invitation to explore the wide range of medical possibilities available to you. Use it to access information and practitioners; use it to discuss options with your health care provider; share it with family and friends who might be looking for alternatives. Become well-informed and turn that power into good health.

Part I:

ILLNESSES & CONDITIONS

K nowing that there are alternatives out there is one thing, but knowing which ones are best for you in your situation is another. Part I is here to clear up some of that confusion. Fifty-seven common health conditions and discomforts are listed here with some of the alternative therapies that can offer relief.

Alternative therapists don't always have the same ideas and definitions of illness as conventional (or allopathic) physicians. A traditional Chinese therapist may have a vastly different concept from a medical doctor of what causes, say, influenza. And he or she may not even define a set of symptoms as the one disease named by allopathic doctors, but recognize several different imbalances appearing together. Other disciplines have their categories and definitions as well.

Therefore, the list of illnesses and conditions presented here in Part I is, from the beginning, flawed from the standpoint of many alternative therapists because we have used conventional medicine's categories and definitions. They are the most recognizable to most of us, and serve only as an organizing principle. Within each profile, alternative definitions are included when appropriate.

To help you use the information in this section, here are some of the features you'll find in a profile:

Definition and List of Symptoms—Allopathic medicine's understanding of a disease or condition and some of the signs that may help you recognize it.

Conventional Approach—Allopathic medicine's way of managing the condition from frequently prescribed medications to appropriate surgical procedures for the condition. You'll also frequently find lifestyle modifications recommended by conventional medicine. You can use this information to compare allopathic medicine's views and attitudes with the opinions and options presented by the various alternative therapies.

Alternative Approaches—A select few alternative therapies that can address the condition. Obviously, we can't list *every* therapy's approach to *every* condition, but those in the profile have been chosen because of their effectiveness or frequent use.

Prescription—After every alternative therapy in a profile, you'll find a section marked with a (⚗). This is where you'll find information on how you might be able to use that therapy's approach to treatment. In some cases it may be a prescription for herbs or supplements or a healing technique that you can implement yourself. For therapies that require a trained practitioner, you'll find a description of what that therapist might do or what you might expect as treatment in that discipline.

Other Therapies—Since not every approach to a given condition can get a thorough discussion, the list of other therapies found in every profile shows you other options that may be open to you. Use this list as a cross-reference; if a particular therapy sounds interesting, look for the chapter about it in Part II: Therapies.

Alternative therapists don't always have the same ideas and definitions of illness as conventional (or allopathic) physicians.

Acne

THE SKIN DISEASE ACNE STARTS WHEN HAIR FOLLICLES, THE SHAFTS THAT HAIRS GROW IN, BECOME CLOGGED WITH DEAD SKIN CELLS, BACTERIA, AND A MIXTURE OF OILS KNOWN AS SEBUM. THIS BACKED-UP MATERIAL CANNOT ESCAPE THROUGH THE PORES (THE OPENINGS AT THE TOP OF THE FOLLICLES), AND BLEMISHES APPEAR.

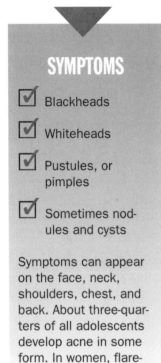

SYMPTOMS

- ☑ Blackheads
- ☑ Whiteheads
- ☑ Pustules, or pimples
- ☑ Sometimes nodules and cysts

Symptoms can appear on the face, neck, shoulders, chest, and back. About three-quarters of all adolescents develop acne in some form. In women, flare-ups can precede menstruation.

CONVENTIONAL APPROACH

Allopathic medicine offers medications, surgery, and basic skin care advice tailored to the different severities of acne. The focus is on easing or stopping the symptoms of acne and improving appearance.

DRUG TREATMENT

Topical and oral medications can fight current acne flare-ups and prevent new ones from starting. Some treatment regimens may take up to three months to work, though. Some of these treatments include

- peroxide, which works by killing bacteria. However, it can dry out and irritate the skin.
- sulfur, resorcinol, and salicylic acid, which help dry and heal existing blemishes. Excess drying and peeling may result.
- antibiotics (such as clindamycin, erythromycin, or tetracycline) that attack bacteria. They, too, can dry and irritate the skin, as well as cause side effects such as upset stomach and sun sensitivity. The long-term use of antibiotics can also lead to chronic yeast infection, decreased immunity, and future infections with antibiotic-resistant bacteria.
- retinoic acid (Retin-A), designed to lift dead skin cells from the follicles. Side effects include short-term worsening of the acne and some skin irritation.

- isotretinoin (Accutane), which halts oil production. The side effects—including liver disease and certain birth defects when given to pregnant women—can be dangerous, and patients must be closely monitored by a physician during treatment.

SURGICAL TREATMENT

Dermatologists can inject acne cysts with drugs or slice open and drain the cysts to reduce scarring.

Severe acne can lead to deep pits and other scars, which may be diminished by chemical peels, dermabrasion, or collagen injections. These therapies, however, do carry the risk of worsening the scars.

ALTERNATIVE APPROACHES

Alternative treatments work to strengthen the body's own defenses to prevent acne flare-ups in the first place, as well as to reduce the inflammation and scarring associated with the disease. Conventional medicine believes that dietary factors have little impact on acne, but many alternative practitioners disagree.

NUTRITIONAL THERAPY

Nutritional therapy holds that some foods may trigger the overproduction of oils in the skin and should, therefore, be avoided. Topping the list are refined carbohydrates (sugars) and foods loaded with saturated fat. Yes, that includes chocolate. Milk's fat and hormone content can also be a problem for some people. You should also avoid foods high in iodine such as seafood and iodized salt. A diet of whole grains, raw or steamed vegetables, fruits, and beans promote healthier skin.

A mineral or vitamin deficiency could also be putting the body in a weakened state, leaving it unable to fight off the factors, such as stress, that lead to acne flare-ups. But vitamin supplementation in acne treatment is not usually used to combat a deficiency. Rather, single nutrients are used for their therapeutic effect, such as their effect on hormone levels.

Supplements that are commonly prescribed to people with acne or who are prone to acne include

- zinc
- selenium
- vitamin A (usually in doses that require a doctor's supervision because of vitamin A's potential for serious toxicity)
- vitamin B_6 (especially in cases of premenstrual acne)
- vitamin E

Several studies conducted in the United States and Europe have reported a zinc deficiency in people who have acne and other skin disorders. In one French trial, acne patients were given daily doses of 200 mg of zinc gluconate capsules (approximately 24 mg of elemental zinc) or a placebo. After two months, those who took the zinc supplements had significantly fewer and significantly less severe pimples and cysts. Zinc is thought to have an anti-inflammatory effect, which would reduce the skin's reaction.

Whenever zinc supplementation is prescribed for an extended period, copper supplementation is also necessary because the two minerals compete in the body for absorption; when there is an abundance of zinc, the copper is less likely to be absorbed. Zinc used alone can cause a copper deficiency.

Depending on an acne patient's diet, a sample prescription for zinc might be 30 mg a day. Getting your body's requirement of zinc from whole foods rather than sup-

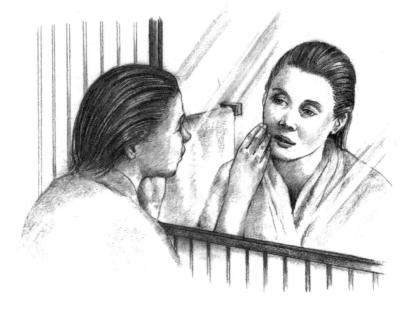

plements is also a good idea; a few of the foods rich in zinc are

- dried beans
- wheat germ
- oysters
- clams

HERBAL MEDICINE

Herbal medicine relies on certain plants that can eliminate the bacteria

OTHER THERAPIES

AROMATHERAPY—The essential oils of bergamot, chamomile, juniper, or lavender can be diluted with warm water and applied as a wash or spray.

DETOXIFICATION, FASTING, AND COLON THERAPY—Because acne can be a sign that the body's ability to eliminate waste and toxins has been compromised, detoxification treatments can be helpful.

HOMEOPATHY—Specific remedies must be tailored to the individual, but common prescriptions include kali bromatum, hepar sulphuris calcareum, and sulphur.

HYDROTHERAPY—Possible remedies include applying ice to skin sores, soaking in ocean water, and quickly rubbing the body (not the face) with a cold, damp washcloth.

MEDITATION—Regular meditation sessions can be effective for acne triggered by stress or nervous tension.

that contribute to acne flare-ups. These plants are also used to cleanse the body, righting its internal balance to prevent future flare-ups.

Tea tree oil, made from a shrub that grows mainly in eastern Australia, is used for its antibacterial properties. A group of Australian researchers showed that a gel made from five percent tea tree oil is just as effective in clearing up acne as five percent benzoyl peroxide lotion. The study volunteers found the tea tree oil took longer than the benzoyl peroxide to produce results, but the oil was significantly gentler on the face.

The herb calendula—more commonly known as marigold—can be used for its antibacterial and anti-inflammatory properties. The dried flowers are often steeped in hot water like tea and then used directly on the skin as a facial wash.

The herbs burdock and cleavers may be used in tincture form (prepared in an alcohol and water solution) for their cleansing action.

Several studies point to the effectiveness of vitex (chaste berry) for acne, especially in women. The herb seems to work internally by normalizing hormone levels.

Scan the aisles of your health food store and you'll find tea tree oil sold in many forms, including as an essential oil, shampoo, body lotion, lip balm, and even laundry detergent. Not all the forms necessarily contain enough tea tree oil to have antibacterial power, but because the herb is very potent, look for a form that has already been diluted for use as a body lotion or soap. The following is a sample herbal prescription for acne using tea tree oil:

- Test a drop of essential tea tree oil on the inner arm to see if it irritates your skin. (Leave it on for several hours to determine if there's a reaction.)
- If it does cause irritation, dilute one part of the oil with ten parts rosewater or almond oil, and test it again.
- When you have the right concentration, apply a very thin layer of tea tree oil on the acne blemishes with a cotton ball.
- Repeat the application daily.

ACQUIRED IMMUNODEFICIENCY SYNDROME (AIDS) IS A DISEASE THAT SEVERELY WEAKENS THE IMMUNE SYSTEM, MAKING THE BODY VULNERABLE TO CERTAIN INFECTIONS OR CANCERS, WHICH USUALLY PROVE FATAL. AIDS IS CAUSED BY THE HUMAN IMMUNODEFICIENCY VIRUS (HIV), WHICH CAN BE PASSED ALONG BY SEXUAL CONTACT, BY CONTACT WITH INFECTED BLOOD, AND FROM MOTHER TO FETUS.

CONVENTIONAL APPROACH

Because there is no cure for AIDS, allopathic medicine focuses on two aspects of treatment: 1) slowing the progression from HIV infection to AIDS and 2) fighting or weakening the accompanying infections or cancers. Drugs are the main weapon in the arsenal. The side effects of these medications are often severe, and the effects of their long-term use are often unknown. The treatments commonly used include

- antiviral drugs to slow the multiplication of HIV
- antibiotics to fight opportunistic bacterial infections
- anticancer drugs or radiation therapy for treatment of some cancers

ALTERNATIVE APPROACHES

The goal of many alternative treatments is to treat HIV infection and AIDS as a chronic disease that one may live with for a long time. Patients often combine alternative medicine with conventional HIV and AIDS drugs in the hope of making fewer of the allopathic drugs necessary and minimizing their toxic side effects.

A Seattle study combined several alternative therapies into one naturopathic treatment program for HIV infection. The men who followed the program for one year experienced a decline in their HIV-related complications and an improved sense of well-being. Their treatments included

- nutritional therapy
- herbal medicine
- hyperthermia
- mind/body medicine
- homeopathy

NUTRITIONAL THERAPY

In nutritional therapy, a certain diet and nutritional supplements are used to strengthen a frail immune system. Supplements can also make up for the frequent nutrient deficiencies found in people with HIV infection and AIDS, which are often caused by chronic diarrhea, the body's reduced ability to absorb nutrients, or an eating disorder.

Naturopathic physicians, in particular, recommend a diet with plenty of fresh and organic vegetables, beans, and whole grains and low in sugar, animal fats, alcohol, and caffeine. This diet doesn't tax the body's defense system. More nutrients may be absorbed by the body if meals are small and eaten frequently. Nutritional supplements, many with antioxidant properties, that can be helpful to people with HIV infection and AIDS include

- vitamin A (beta-carotene)
- vitamin C
- vitamin B_6
- vitamin B_{12}

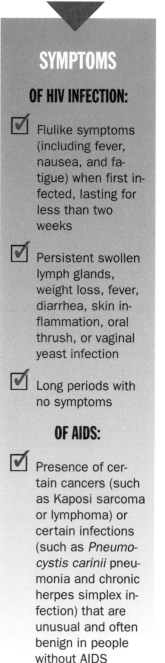

SYMPTOMS

OF HIV INFECTION:

☑ Flulike symptoms (including fever, nausea, and fatigue) when first infected, lasting for less than two weeks

☑ Persistent swollen lymph glands, weight loss, fever, diarrhea, skin inflammation, oral thrush, or vaginal yeast infection

☑ Long periods with no symptoms

OF AIDS:

☑ Presence of certain cancers (such as Kaposi sarcoma or lymphoma) or certain infections (such as *Pneumocystis carinii* pneumonia and chronic herpes simplex infection) that are unusual and often benign in people without AIDS

- folate
- selenium and vitamin E
- zinc
- *N*-acetyl-L-cysteine (NAC)
- quercetin
- L-carnitine

Several small-scale trials have shown the effectiveness of nutritional supplements for people with HIV infection and AIDS. In one study, 29 patients took over a six-month period: (1) vitamin, mineral, and amino acid supplements; (2) essential fatty acids (such as linoleic and eicosapentaenoic acids); and (3) aloe vera juice. They maintained their regular diet and continued taking conventional drugs. At the end of the trial, all of the participants reported fewer symptoms and a weight gain. None complained of adverse effects from the treatment.

There are many dietary suggestions that people with HIV infection and AIDS can follow to minimize contact with food additives, preservatives, pesticides, bacteria, and parasites. Here are some tips concerning fruits and vegetables:

- Buy fresh instead of frozen and canned.
- Choose organic whenever possible.
- Thoroughly wash and scrub foods.
- At the minimum, lightly steam all vegetables.

HERBAL MEDICINE

Herbs can provide several benefits for people with HIV infection and AIDS. Some may improve the performance of the immune system. Others can weaken the AIDS virus and prevent its spread. Still others offer relief from the symptoms associated with AIDS.

Those herbs commonly prescribed include

- astragalus (often taken as part of a combination from traditional Chinese medicine)
- goldenseal
- isatis (often taken as part of a combination from traditional Chinese medicine)
- licorice root
- St.-John's-wort
- curcumin (a constituent of turmeric)

For patients using conventional drugs, herbs may also lessen some of the negative side effects. For example, antibiotics can severely disrupt the healthy balance of flora (bacteria) in the intestines. *Lactobacillus acidophilus* and *Lactobacillis bifidus* bacteria (found in live-culture yogurt) and garlic can offset these effects.

Acemannan (from aloe vera), in addition to being a potent immune system stimulator and antiviral substance,

---

CLOSER LOOK AT ALTERNATIVE MEDICINE FOR AIDS

The study of alternative therapies for HIV infection and AIDS got a recent boost from the federal government. In 1994, the Office of Alternative Medicine, part of the National Institutes of Health, granted an $840,000 three-year award to Bastyr University of Seattle to set up a center that would research alternative treatments for HIV and AIDS. Bastyr offers degree programs in naturopathic medicine, acupuncture, Oriental botanical medicine, and nutrition.

also seems to boost the effects of the conventional anti-AIDS drug zidovudine. The effects can be so dramatic that some researchers say the dosage of zidovudine can be reduced by as much as 90 percent when acemannan is used as an adjunct. Zidovudine has serious side effects, so anything that allows for a decrease in the dosage is welcome.

A sample prescription for licorice root *(Glycyrrhiza glabra)* might be three capsules taken three times a day, between meals. Licorice is thought to assist the workings of the immune system. It also has antiviral properties, which can be useful against herpesvirus (a common problem for AIDS patients). A word of caution, though: People with high blood pressure should not use this herb.

HYPERTHERMIA

Because the AIDS virus is unstable when exposed to heat, hyperthermia offers some promise. The therapy aims to raise the body temperature, creating an artificial fever. This is thought to weaken HIV and affect the makeup of the blood, in particular increasing the number of white blood cells (which fight off invading organisms).

The common way to apply hyperthermia treatments is to submerge the body (up to the head) in heated water. Layers of clothes and blankets can also be used to keep the body temperature high for a period of time.

A more controversial form of hyperthermia therapy—one that has not been approved for use in the United States—involves filtering a person's blood through a machine that heats the blood to temperatures above which HIV cannot survive. Unconfirmed reports have indicated that this type of treatment can make HIV-positive patients revert to HIV-negative status.

A typical hyperthermia treatment for someone with HIV infection or AIDS would be to soak in a tub of water warmed to about 104°F (enough to raise the body temperature to 102°F). The treatment should last about 40 minutes and would be repeated over the course of several months.

OTHER THERAPIES

TRADITONAL CHINESE MEDICINE—Acupuncture, acupressure, and Chinese herbal therapy may help restore the flow of energy in the body and boost the immune system. A person whose energy flow is in harmony has a better chance of warding off other infections or cancers.

OSTEOPATHY—This works to manipulate parts of the body to remove built-up tension in an effort to strengthen the overall health of someone with AIDS. Osteopathic physicians are also qualified to give conventional treatments.

BODYWORK—Massage, in particular, relieves muscle tightness and tension, leaving the body free to focus on healing other AIDS-related ailments.

MIND/BODY MEDICINE—Techniques such as guided imagery, support groups, spirituality, and neurolinguistic programming, to reduce stress, enhance the immune system, and perhaps slow the progression of AIDS.

Alcoholism & Drug Addiction

ADDICTION TO ALCOHOL OR OTHER DRUGS (FROM BARBITURATES TO COCAINE) IS A PHYSICAL AND EMOTIONAL DEPENDENCE ON THAT SUBSTANCE AND THE EFFECTS IT PRODUCES. IT INVOLVES A LOSS OF CONTROL, OFTEN CAUSING DEVASTATING EFFECTS ON ALL ASPECTS OF THE INDIVIDUAL'S LIFE INCLUDING WORK, FAMILY, AND HEALTH.

SYMPTOMS

- ☑ Higher and higher doses are needed to achieve effects that were once attained at lower doses (called increased tolerance)

- ☑ Intense cravings

- ☑ Avoiding the substance for a period of time leads to withdrawal symptoms, which can include anxiety, agitation, pronounced heartbeat, insomnia, hallucinations, and seizures

CONVENTIONAL APPROACH

For allopathic medicine's treatment program for drug and alcohol addiction to be successful, drinking or taking drugs must stop completely and, usually, voluntarily. This can be attempted through counseling, support groups, and drug therapy. Treatment can be intensive, as in a residential facility, or informal, with meetings with a therapist or support group.

PSYCHOLOGICAL TREATMENT

Counseling is the main thrust of conventional medicine's treatment program. A trained therapist can help pinpoint what emotions and behaviors led to the onset of addiction. It can also address problems such as low self-esteem or depression that precipitate continued use. The counseling sessions can be done on a one-to-one or group basis. Self-help groups such as Alcoholics Anonymous and Narcotics Anonymous provide much-needed support and encouragement.

DRUG TREATMENT

In most cases of addiction treatment, drugs are used sparingly. Some examples are

- disulfiram, which acts as a deterrent by producing undesirable and potentially dangerous side effects (such as vomiting and blurred vision) whenever alcohol is consumed

- tranquilizers, which relieve the anxiety that often accompanies withdrawal (Extreme caution should be exercised because these drugs can be habit-forming.)

- methadone, which can reduce the symptoms of heroin withdrawal (This drug is also addictive and may have to be taken for years before success is achieved.)

ALTERNATIVE APPROACHES

Many alternative therapists assert that conventional medicine's treatment program for addiction fails to support the body adequately as it withdraws from the once-steady presence of alcohol or other drugs. The following therapies attempt to offer that support. They are often used in combination with counseling and other support programs that address any underlying psychological causes of addiction.

NUTRITIONAL THERAPY

People with alcohol or drug addiction are usually malnourished and have suffered some damage to the body, such as liver damage. Nutritional therapy attempts to correct any nutritional shortcomings and to help the body eliminate toxins.

Several supplements can aid in the detoxification process, including zinc and vitamin C. People with alcohol addiction are often deficient in these nutrients anyway, as alcoholism can severely affect a person's judgement about diet and can limit the body's ability to absorb certain nutrients.

Alcohol and drug use may increase the body's load of free radicals, compounds that can damage tissues. Antioxidants are, therefore, recommended for their ability to neutralize free radicals. Nutrients that are antioxidants include

- beta-carotene
- vitamins C and E
- zinc
- selenium

Alcoholics are almost always deficient in the B vitamins, particularly vitamin B_1 (thiamine). In fact, this deficiency is responsible for many of the behaviors exhibited by severe alcoholics. Thiamine levels need to be restored during rehabilitation, which often requires injections of the vitamin at least initially.

Other helpful supplements are quite numerous, including calcium and magnesium.

The majority of people with alcohol addiction have a state of low blood sugar (hypoglycemia). Unanswered is which came first: Did the addiction and resulting malnutrition bring on hypoglycemia? Or did a previous state of hypoglycemia set up a type of craving for alcohol? Either way, to remedy low blood sugar:

- Significantly increase the intake of unrefined complex carbohydrates, including whole grains and fresh vegetables and fruits.
- Avoid all sugars, from corn syrup to fruit juices.
- Reduce the intake of refined carbohydrates, such as white bread.

As these dietary changes are made, many practitioners of nutritional therapy recommend adding more protein and supplement with the B complex. Chromium supplementation (200 µg twice a day) is also appropriate.

Here's a sample high-dose vitamin C prescription for alcohol or drug addiction treatment: Begin by taking 3 grams a day and increase the dose by 1 gram every day until you reach your bowel tolerence (that is, until you get mild diarrhea), then back down a little. Maintain that dose until abstinence has been maintained for several months.

HERBAL MEDICINE

Herbs can ease some alcohol or drug withdrawal symptoms (from anxiety to insomnia) and help detoxify the body. They also may be used to reduce the addicted person's craving for alcohol and other drugs.

Especially helpful are herbs that influence the nervous system, gently encouraging a relaxed and sedated state. These include catnip, chamomile, peppermint, and skullcap, which can be

---

TRIED AND TRUE

Joining the well-known self-help group Alcoholics Anonymous, which offers support and advice on how to live without alcohol, is often thought by both conventional and alternative medicine to be one of the most effective ways to maintain sobriety. Started in 1935, the group counts an estimated half-million members worldwide.

---

used together as a tea. To replace mild depression with a state of calmness, St.-John's-wort is often prescribed.

For detoxification, several herbs contribute to cleansing the blood. They include burdock root and echinacea (purple coneflower). Others such as milk thistle, which contains silymarin, support the liver—the main toxin-filtering organ—and may help prevent drug-induced damage to this organ. (For suggestions on how to use purple coneflower, see Appendix 3.)

Kudzu root, often prescribed as a bitter tea, has long been used by traditional Chinese doctors to reduce the appetite for alcohol. Recent research confirmed that alcohol-free kudzu root extract can cut the consumption of alcohol in half. The patients in this study, however, were not humans but a breed of hamsters.

An herbalist may prescribe the following remedy to someone with alcohol addiction to treat or prevent serious liver damage: Take 100 to 200 mg of milk thistle extract (standardized to 80 percent silymarin content) three times daily.

THE BENEFITS OF WORKING OUT

Adopting a regular exercise program is an important part of addiction treatment. Not only does it improve overall health, but exercising can cut down stress and anxiety, which may have provoked the addiction in the first place. Exercise also stimulates the production of endorphins—the body's own natural opiates.

ACUPUNCTURE

The ancient Chinese science of acupuncture has earned widespread regard in America as an effective treatment for alcohol and drug addiction. Success rates can be as high as 50 percent of patients treated, and various municipalities offer it as part of their health care and criminal justice programs.

Acupuncture looks at addictions as imbalances in the flow of the body's vital life energy, or qi, particularly on the kidney, liver, or nervous system meridians (channels). Using tiny needles inserted in particular acupuncture points on the body, this therapy works to correct the qi imbalances. Not only does this ease or eliminate withdrawal symptoms, but the patient's mind is then prepared to tackle some of the factors that led to the addiction.

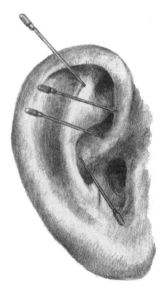

Auriculotherapy, a form of acupuncture that treats the entire body through points on the ears, is particularly recommended for addiction treatment. Treatment usually consists of several months of acupuncture sessions coupled with counseling and lifestyle modifications.

One clinical study done in Minneapolis tested acupuncture therapy on the ear on people with severe alcoholism. Patients who received fake acupuncture therapy had more than two times the number of relapses into drinking compared with those who received real acupuncture therapy.

Acupuncturists, traditional Chinese physicians, some naturopathic and osteopathic physicians, and even a few medical doctors are trained to give acupuncture treatments.

GUIDED IMAGERY AND CREATIVE VISUALIZATION

Many people who are addicted to alcohol or other drugs started using these substances as a way to relax, ease tension, or improve self-esteem and confidence. Guided imagery and creative visualization can teach people to reach these ideals without the assistance of harmful toxins.

For example, a treatment session can consist of a patient picturing the positive results of a drug-free state (from the concrete, such as clear, shiny pink breathing airways, to the abstract, beams of light radiating from the lungs), as well as the negative aspects of a drug-induced state.

Breathing exercises and other relaxation techniques are used to clear the mind as a way to maximize these imagery exercises. The mental exercises can also give the mind negative suggestions about the particular alcohol or drug so that the next time the sub-

stance is consumed the body produces unpleasant effects. (This is similar to conventional medicine's drugs that produce unwanted side effects whenever alcohol is consumed.)

Progressive muscle relaxation is often performed before a guided imagery exercise as a way of "warming up." It involves letting go of tension in small, isolated steps until you are relaxed.

After you're relaxed, imagine and revel in the positive aspects of sobriety—healthy liver, clear mind, proud loved ones—and picture the degrading, unhealthy aspects of addiction. These exercises, which can be scripted more precisely by a practitioner, can reinforce the will to sobriety.

OTHER THERAPIES

BIOFEEDBACK TRAINING—The training, together with relaxation techniques, can help bring relaxation and reduce withdrawal symptoms and cravings.

CHIROPRACTIC—Adjustments and manipulations can correct any disturbances that may be contributing to physical withdrawal symptoms.

HOMEOPATHY—There are several common remedies for different addictions and different types of addicts.

HYPNOTHERAPY—Hypnotic trances can give the subconscious mind suggestions of new ways to behave—important in maintaining abstinence.

MEDITATION—Regular meditation can encourage relaxation and lessen some withdrawal symptoms.

Allergies

AN ALLERGY IS A SUPER-SENSITIVITY OF THE BODY'S IMMUNE SYSTEM TO CERTAIN SUBSTANCES SUCH AS FOODS, CHEMICALS, DUST MITES, POLLEN, OR ANIMAL DANDER. EXPOSURE TO THE ALLERGEN (THE MATERIAL THAT CAUSES THE ALLERGY) CAN RESULT IN UNCOMFORTABLE, DEBILITATING, OR POSSIBLY EVEN LIFE-THREATENING REACTIONS.

SYMPTOMS

☑ Runny nose and sneezing

☑ Itchy, watery eyes

☑ Dry, red, itchy skin

☑ Welts (hives) on the skin

☑ In severe reactions, swollen body tissue, difficulty breathing, vomiting, cramps, and a sudden drop in blood pressure (known collectively as *anaphylactic shock*)

CONVENTIONAL APPROACH

Allopathic medicine offers two basic treatment approaches to allergy sufferers: avoiding the allergen, whenever possible, and taking drugs to relieve the symptoms. The medications include

- over-the-counter antihistamines (such as chlorpheniramine and diphenhydramine)
- over-the-counter nasal decongestants (such as phenylephrine and phenylpropanolomine)
- prescription antihistamines (such as terfenadine and astemizole)
- injections of epinephrine (a synthetic hormone), an emergency measure that may be used during anaphylactic shock

In stubborn cases of allergies, physicians sometimes use immunotherapy. The patient receives shots containing larger and larger doses of the offending allergen to build up an immunity to it.

ALTERNATIVE APPROACHES
HOMEOPATHY

Homeopathy, like conventional medicine's immunotherapy, holds that the body's ability to tolerate allergens can be stimulated by diluted, nontoxic doses of certain natural substances (which, if given to a healthy person in full, toxic strength, would produce the same symptoms as the allergy patient's). The difference between homeopathy and immunotherapy (allergy shots) is that homeopathy uses extremely diluted doses. Homeopathic remedies should also produce results faster than immunotherapy and without the annoying and possibly dangerous side effects.

In addition to bolstering the body against future allergy attacks, homeopathic treatments can relieve symptoms such as runny nose and watery and irritated eyes. Here's how the therapy is administered:

- A homeopath begins by assessing the patient's symptoms and overall health and lifestyle.
- Then, a preparation is prescribed in the form of tablets or liquid drops. Depending on which school of thought the practitioner adheres to—from classical homeopathy to isopathy—the remedy may be a single substance (such as an herb, animal product, or mineral), a cocktail of several substances, or the actual allergen.
- The patient may experience aggravated symptoms for the first week or so, but this soon subsides.
- If there's no improvement, the practitioner may try another remedy.

Homeopathic treatments are also available as over-the-counter products designed for groups of allergies. Because these preparations are not tailored to individual symptoms, they are considered less effective.

For sufferers of seasonal allergic rhinitis (commonly known as hay fever), this therapy is especially promising; at least four scientific studies have shown the effectiveness of a homeopathic treatment for hay fever. In one Scottish trial, patients who were given a homeopathic preparation of mixed grass pollens for two weeks had dramatically reduced symptoms. The symptoms of the patients who received the placebo remained the same.

Together with diet and lifestyle changes, a homeopath might instruct a hay fever sufferer to take a tablet containing grass pollen, 30c, twice a day (the *30c* describes the potency of the substance, or how many times it has been diluted). Homeopathic treatment should be supervised by a trained practitioner.

HERBAL MEDICINE

Several herbs hold hope for allergy sufferers. Although the precise prescription for an individual patient may require professional consultation, urtica (stinging nettles) can generally provide relief from acute attacks of hay fever. Eyebright can be useful for the symptoms of runny nose and watery eyes. Siberian ginseng, elder, and licorice can also reduce symptoms associated with hay fever.

Teas of Siberian ginseng can help reduce inflammation in the sinus area. A possible occasional treatment might be the following:

- Heat one cup of water to a simmer.
- Add a teaspoon of chopped ginseng root and steep.
- Drink about three cups a day.

ENVIRONMENTAL MEDICINE

Environmental medicine recognizes that there may be more to blame for an allergy attack than a specific allergen. Poor diet, previous exposure to pollutants or pesticides, stress, infections—almost anything in the environment—can predispose people to allergies. What's more, environmental medicine holds that the symptoms of allergies go beyond runny nose and itchy skin: Allergies may also be responsible for ailments such as hyperactivity in children, mental fuzziness, and irritable bowel syndrome.

When treating a patient, an environmental physician first performs a physical exam and takes a detailed history, noting diet, home and work environments, emotional state, family members' allergies, and other factors. Skin tests, blood tests, elimination diets, and other testing procedures can help pinpoint the allergens. One procedure, for example, checks for allergens by placing drops of certain substances under the tongue. If symptoms develop, drops of a "neutralizing dose" ease the symptoms and build up the body's tolerance for that allergen.

Perhaps the simplest way to find relief from allergies is to create a supportive environment by

- removing chemicals or pollutants from the home and office (such as using water filters or negative ion generators)
- altering the diet (avoiding the offending food, eliminating processed foods, or switching to a whole-foods vegetarian diet)
- changing lifestyle (such as reducing stress)

The steps toward healing an environmental illness involve careful examination of your home. Some general measures to remove environmental irritants may also help:

- If your house has wall-to-wall carpeting, replace it with wooden or tile flooring. Then, use scatter rugs that can be washed periodically in hot water. If you can't revamp the entire house, at least do your bedroom (where you regularly spend a third of your day!).
- Move electronic equipment (alarm clocks, stereos, etc.) at least six feet away from your bed. This reduces your chances of exposure to the potentially harmful the electromagnetic radiation that these devices genrate. Likewise, use an electric blanket only to warm up the bed, not while you are underneath it.

NUTRITIONAL THERAPY

An elimination diet can rout out food allergies. Foods are cut from the diet for a couple of weeks to see if symptoms disappear. If the condition has improved, foods can be added back one at a time, with careful monitoring. Food additives can also bring on allergy symptoms.

In one London study, three patients completely recovered from chronic hives (urticaria) after they stripped ingredients such as azo dyes and sulphur dioxide from their diets.

Diet recommendations for hay fever sufferers could include increasing the intake of nutrients that have an antihistimine effect, including

- vitamin C (Bufferered supplement preparations are usually best because regular ascorbic acid can aggravate some allergy patients.)
- bioflavonoids
- pantothenic acid

Avoiding dairy products, which stimulate the production of mucus, can also be useful.

OTHER THERAPIES

ACUPUNCTURE—Treatments can correct any imbalances in vital life energy that may be weakening or oversensitizing the immune system.

DETOXIFICATION, FASTING, AND COLON THERAPY—Short, supervised fasts and juice diets can be helpful in eliminating allergens.

HYPNOTHERAPY—Hypnotic trances can give the subconscious mind healing suggestions, such as that the immune system is able to tolerate a certain allergen.

MIND/BODY MEDICINE—Because allergies can be learned, the mind can play an active role in treating them as well.

Alzheimer Disease

ALZHEIMER DISEASE IS A PROGRESSIVE DETERIORATION OF THE BRAIN, RESULTING IN DECREASED MENTAL POWERS. IT MOST OFTEN STRIKES AFTER AGE 65 AND IS THE FOURTH LEADING CAUSE OF DEATH AMONG ADULTS IN THIS AGE GROUP. ITS CAUSE IS UNKNOWN, BUT SLOW VIRUSES, GENETIC TRAITS, ENVIRONMENTAL FACTORS (SUCH AS ALUMINUM AND PESTICIDES), AND OTHER POSSIBILITIES MAY BE CONTRIBUTING FACTORS.

CONVENTIONAL APPROACH

Because no cure or effective treatment for Alzheimer disease is available, allopathic medicine focuses on helping the person with the disease function as well as possible and on easing the other conditions that often appear with the disease (ranging from depression to insomnia).

The home environment of someone with Alzheimer disease should be well structured and largely free from stress. Identification bracelets and other safeguards are needed in case the person wanders away from home. Regular exercise, good nutrition, and social interaction should be maintained.

The drug tacrine hydrochloride was approved by the Food and Drug Administration to treat Alzheimer disease, but it can only provide short-term reductions in symptoms for just a small percentage of patients and carries the risk of severe liver damage.

Other medications are available to relieve some of the "problem behaviors" that often accompany the disease. For example, the tranquilizer haloperidol can induce calm feelings when the patient is aggitated.

ALTERNATIVE APPROACHES

Several alternative therapies offer ways to slow the onset and progression of Alzheimer disease in some patients. Various treatments can be used as preventive measures for people whose families have a history of the disease.

NUTRITIONAL THERAPY

Nutritional therapists use diet to deter Alzheimer disease in susceptible people. Many practitioners now believe that certain nutritional deficiencies or excesses may actually trigger the disease.

For example, free radicals, compounds in the body that can damage tissues and quicken the aging process, have been linked to the progression of the disease. Antioxidants have the ability to neutralize free radicals and are, therefore, typically recommended as preventive measures. Nutrients that are antioxidants or help in the antioxidant process include

- beta-carotene
- vitamins C and E
- selenium

Good food sources of beta-carotene include apricots, carrots, spinach, and sweet potatoes. Vitamin C is found in broccoli, grapefruits, oranges, and strawberries, and vitamin E is available from nuts and vegetable oils. Selenium is found in brewer's yeast, cabbage, fish, liver, and whole-grain cereals. Supplements may also be prescribed to

SYMPTOMS

- ☑ Gradual loss of memory
- ☑ Disorientation
- ☑ Change in personality
- ☑ Difficulty with routine tasks
- ☑ Decline of learning, communicating, judgement, and planning skills

WHO USES ALTERNATIVE THERAPIES?

Fifty-five percent of people with Alzheimer disease have tried at least one unconventional therapy to improve memory, according to a 1994 survey by the University of North Carolina School of Medicine. The most commonly used therapies included vitamins, health foods, and herbal medicines. The patients' caregivers, who answered the surveys, reported some memory gains in one third of the patients.

supply antioxidants, especially in the case of vitamin E, which has high-fat food sources.

Some supplements may actually be useful for slowing the progression of the disease. Phosphatidyl choline (10 to 20 grams daily) enhances the production of the neurotransmitter acetylcholine. Acetylcholine-transmitting neurons and their target nerve cells are the most frequently affected part of the brain in Alzheimer disease. N-Acetyl-L-carnitine also appears to protect neurons in a similar manner. Phosphatidyl serine can enhance neural functioning significantly by normalizing cell membrane fluidity.

People with Alzheimer disease are frequently deficient in vitamin B_{12}, vitamin B_6, and folate. Adding these can also be preventive measures. Vitamin B_{12} deficiency is often associated with depression, confusion, neurologic problems, and memory loss. Folate deficiency can also cause these symptoms, and deficiency of vitamin B_6 is associated with a decline in the number of re-

ceptors in the brain for the neurotransmitter dopamine. All of these symptoms of deficiency seem to parallel the major symptoms of Alzheimer-related brain disfunction.

Other helpful supplements include
- zinc
- niacin
- coenzyme Q_{10}

Because high concentrations of aluminum may contribute to Alzheimer disease—autopsies have revealed high levels of aluminum in the brains of people with the disease—cookware and utensils made from this metal should not be used when preparing food. Avoiding aluminum requires detective work; it can be found in drinking water, processed foods, toothpaste, deodorants and antipersprirants, antacid tablets, and other everyday products.

A nutritional preventive strategy may call for taking the following supplements each day:
- vitamin E (400 IU)
- vitamin C (1,000 mg)
- beta-carotene (25,000 IU)
- phosphatidyl serine (300 mg)

CHELATION THERAPY

Whether or not Alzheimer disease is triggered by the presence of heavy metals in the body is the subject of much debate. The usual metal suspect is aluminum, although mercury and manganese have also been implicated. Amid this debate, practitioners of chelation therapy have reported that their patients who are in the early stages of the disease have found relief from their symptoms after these metals are removed from the body.

To treat Alzheimer disease, chelation therapy involves intravenous injections of disodium ethylenediaminetetraacetic acid (EDTA)—an amino acid that binds to metallic ions in the body and renders them chemically inactive. These joined-together substances are then excreted by the kidneys in the urine. Clinical studies have shown that this process also improves the flow of blood in the brain.

The treatments are often combined with a supplemental regimen of vitamins, minerals, and trace elements to replace any lost during the chelation process. Reported side effects have included nausea and vomiting and, if high doses of a chelating agent are used in the therapy, some damage to the kidneys.

Only a licensed physician is qualified to perform chelation therapy. Look for someone who has been well trained in this treatment area and has experience specifically with Alzheimer disease.

WAVE THERAPY

Sound therapy offers several benefits during the many stages of Alzheimer disease. Sound and music are very useful in treating the "problem behaviors" that often accompany the disease, such as agitation, anxiety, and insomnia. Sound therapy can be used
- to induce feelings of calmness and relaxation
- to lower blood pressure
- to improve the overall sense of well-being

Music from the patients' earlier days may be used to give them some sense of place and time and reminders of their lives. This is especially helpful in the early and middle stages of Alzheimer disease. Hearing music they know and remember may also encourage people to dance, offering much-needed exercise. Finally, music can replace forms of communication that are lost as Alzheimer disease progresses.

In the home, familiar music can be played to provide stimulation to the person with Alzheimer. Making tapes of music from different periods in the individual's life can also be helpful in calming and orienting the person with the disease.

OTHER THERAPIES

BODYWORK—Massage, dance therapy, and other bodywork therapies can boost mood and relieve anxiety and agitation.

ENVIRONMENTAL MEDICINE—Some believe that mercury amalgam tooth fillings, aluminum in antiperspirants, certain allergenic foods, and several other factors in the environment may trigger Alzheimer disease in susceptible people. Treatment involves avoidance and removal (in the case of fillings).

HERBAL MEDICINE—Ginkgo extract is often prescribed to boost mental function. Another herb with promise is evening primrose oil.

HOMEOPATHY—Several remedies may be effective in the early stages of the disease.

HYDROTHERAPY—Treatment such as a neutral bath (98°F to 99°F) can ease agitation and other accompanying symptoms.

Anemia

ANEMIA IS A PROBLEM WITH THE OXYGEN-CARRYING CAPACITY OF THE BLOOD. A PERSON WITH ANEMIA HAS EITHER TOO FEW OXYGEN-CARRYING RED BLOOD CELLS OR NOT ENOUGH HEMOGLOBIN IN THE RED BLOOD CELLS. ANEMIA RESULTS WHEN, FOR ANY NUMBER OF REASONS, THE BONE MARROW MAKES DEFECTIVE RED BLOOD CELLS OR NOT ENOUGH NORMAL ONES, OR IF RED BLOOD CELLS ARE DESTROYED BEFORE THEY HAVE COMPLETED THEIR JOB. THERE ARE SEVERAL FORMS OF ANEMIA, BUT THE MOST COMMON TYPE IS CAUSED BY A LACK OF IRON—AN IMPORTANT COMPONENT OF THE HEMOGLOBIN IN RED BLOOD CELLS.

SYMPTOMS

- ☑ Headaches
- ☑ Fatigue, lack of energy, drowsiness
- ☑ Unusually pale skin, especially on the face
- ☑ Sore mouth and tongue (occasionally)
- ☑ Brittle and ridged nails (occasionally)
- ☑ Dizziness, shortness of breath during heavy activity, chest pains, and heart palpitations (occasionally)
- ☑ Jaundice, a yellowing of the skin (rarely)
- ☑ Tinnitus
- ☑ Seeing spots

CONVENTIONAL APPROACH

Allopathic medicine's treatment program for anemia greatly depends on the type of anemia and any underlying disorders (such as nutrient deficiency, ulcer, or colon cancer) that are causing the anemia.

Iron-deficiency anemia can often be helped by injections of iron, taking iron tablets, or simply eating an iron-rich diet.

Anemia caused by deficiencies in vitamin B_{12} is treated with vitamin injections in the muscles. Anemia resulting from deficiencies in folate (one of the B vitamins) requires taking oral tablets or injections (often in the form of folic acid). Dietary changes are also effective for both conditions.

If a person's sensitivity to certain drugs (such as antibiotics or antimalarials given for another condition) or foods (such as fava beans) is triggering the anemia, then these precipitating factors should be avoided.

If the anemia is related to a malfunctioning immune system, then immunosuppressant drugs are often used. These medications may increase the risk of infection or the risk of getting certain cancers.

Depending on the form of the disorder, several procedures are available for serious anemia, including
- blood transfusions
- bone marrow transplantation, which requires a donor who is a close genetic match
- removal of the spleen, the organ where used-up red blood cells are normally destroyed

ALTERNATIVE APPROACHES

The majority of anemia cases are caused by nutritional deficiencies. Several alternative therapies offer ways to boost the body's use of nutrients.

NUTRITIONAL THERAPY

Three types of anemia are caused by a lack of one of three nutrients—iron, folate, or vitamin B_{12}. The deficiency can result from
- a lack of the nutrient in the diet
- an inability to absorb that nutrient (Certain hereditary conditions and deficiencies of other nutrients can keep the body from absorbing iron, folate, or vitamin B_{12} regardless of the amount present in the diet. Alcoholism can prevent proper absorption of folate in particular.)

an excessive loss of that nutrient (For women, heavy blood loss during menstruation or pregnancy can lead to problems with iron-deficiency anemia.)

Nutritional therapy offers several ways to satisfy the body's need for these nutrients. (Of course, any underlying causes of the anemia need to be treated before these guidelines can be helpful.)

Increasing your intake of iron, folate, and vitamin B_{12} can be accomplished with supplements, but including more whole foods rich in these nutrients in your diet is generally a more healthful idea for mild cases.

Iron-rich foods include

- liver
- dried beans (especially kidney, garbanzo, and pinto)
- prunes
- raisins
- dried apricots

Vitamin C, although not a direct factor in the development of anemia, helps the body absorb iron, so foods high in this vitamin (including citrus fruits and juices, broccoli, cauliflower, and sweet peppers) should accompany meals with iron-rich foods. On the other hand, certain foods limit the absorption of iron. Foods on this list include black tea, coffee, dairy products consumed in large amounts, and wheat bran.

Hydrochloric acid, normally produced by the stomach, is needed for the body to use iron and may be low in some people. Supplementation with hydrochloric acid at mealtimes may be helpful for people with this problem. Another helpful supplement can be vitamin E.

Some whole foods that are good dietary sources of folate, or folic acid, include

- dried beans
- dark-green leafy vegetables (such as spinach and kale)
- asparagus
- oranges

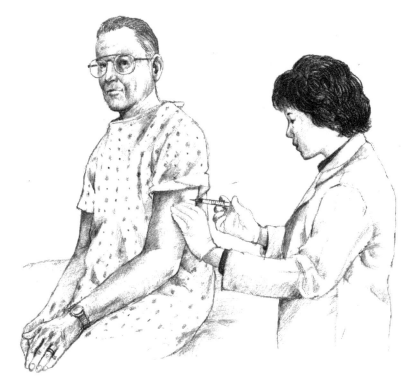

Common food sources of vitamin B_{12} include

- tuna
- nutritional yeast
- dairy products
- beef
- eggs
- liver

Fortified cereals and less known items, such as some seaweed varieties, spirulina, chlorella, and wild blue-green algae, are other vegetarian sources. People who cannot adequately absorb this vitamin require muscular injections.

Some people are unable to absorb vitamin B_{12} from food. These people may require injections of the nutrient.

OTHER THERAPIES

ACUPRESSURE—Pressure applied to specific points, such as along the liver and kidney meridians, can stimulate blood circulation and the production of energy, or qi.

DETOXIFICATION, FASTING, AND COLON THERAPY—Fasting may be helpful in a few cases to encourage better nutrient absorption.

HYDROTHERAPY—Various treatments can improve circulation.

For a woman with iron-deficiency anemia (who is still menstruating), a naturopathic physician may prescribe eating foods containing approximately 15 mg of iron per day. Pair up each iron-rich food with a vitamin C–dense food.

HERBAL MEDICINE

Herbs can help the body maximize the use of the nutrients in food and provide some useful nutrients on their own as well.

The group of herbs known as bitters signal the stomach to produce more digestive juices to help in the break-down process. The herbs' bitter taste on the tongue is probably responsible for sending these messages to the brain and stomach. Gentian root and wormwood are two examples of bitters.

Several herbs are rich in iron and other minerals and vitamins. For example, the leaves and stalks of stinging nettle pack both iron and vitamin C. Dandelion root is also helpful. Certain Chinese herbs such as dong quai and rehmannia are also used to build the blood.

An herbalist may prescribe 10 drops of stinging nettle extract, mixed in a cup of warm water, once a day.

HOMEOPATHY

Homeopathic treatment can ease some of the symptoms of anemia and stimulate the body to use certain nutrients from food more efficiently. Homeopathy uses highly diluted doses of natural substances that would produce the symptoms of anemia if given in full strength to a healthy person. A classical homeopath goes about tailoring a remedy for a patient by studying the anemia symptoms and the general state of physical and emotional health. Every patient receives an individualized remedy. The following are some anemia characteristics to consider:

- Is menstruation normal?
- How does the complexion appear?
- Does constipation, poor digestion, or any other symptom accompany the common anemia symptoms?

The typical remedies for anemia are calcarea phosphoricum, china officinalis, ferrum metallicum, and natrum muriaticum. The following biochemic tissue (mineral) salts may also be used: calcarea phosphoricum and ferrum phosphoricum.

For anemia characterized by heavy blood loss during menstruation and exhaustion, among other details, here's a sample homeopathic remedy: Take one dose of china officinalis, 30c, every 12 hours. (The *30c* refers to the potency of the remedy.)

Anxiety is the body and mind's response to a dangerous or distressing situation. Everyone experiences some degree of anxiety at some time. However, anxiety can occur persistently, often triggered by vague notions of a threat, and interfere with normal activities. When this happens, it's called an anxiety disorder.

CONVENTIONAL APPROACH

Allopathic medicine aims to relieve the symptoms of persistent anxiety with drug therapy and to treat any underlying disorders or conflicts with psychotherapy.

DRUG TREATMENT

Some of the more commonly used medicines include

- benzodiazepine drugs (a type of tranquilizer), such as diazepam and oxazepam, which limit brain activity, temporarily creating a state of relaxation (Because they are potentially habit-forming, they should be used only for short periods of time. Side effects can include daytime drowsiness, reduced concentration, and confusion.)
- buspirone, which may relieve symptoms after several weeks of use (Side effects can include dizziness, drowsiness, nausea, headache, and nervousness.)
- beta blockers, including propranolol, which can temporarily ease some of the physical symptoms of anxiety
- antidepressants, which can also relieve symptoms
- barbiturate drugs, which are used only rarely for their sedating effect (These drugs carry the risk of addiction and should, therefore, be used sparingly and only on a temporary basis.)

PSYCHOLOGICAL TREATMENT

People with anxiety may be helped by talking with trained therapists about their symptoms, feelings, behavior, history, and concerns. The treatment approach can be very simple (consisting of support and advice) or elaborate (involving an extensive psychoanalysis of the patient). One-on-one and group therapy are both options.

ALTERNATIVE APPROACHES
MEDITATION

Meditation can help people with anxiety by making them calmer and less vulnerable to stress and tension. People performing meditation exercises take an active role in their treatment, teaching themselves how to quiet or clear the mind.

Various clinical studies have shown that during meditation the body is altered in ways that are beneficial for people with anxiety: For example, the rate of metabolism drops and blood pressure decreases.

Studies have also revealed anxiety-reducing results with Transcendental Meditation (TM), a type of meditation used in Ayurvedic medicine. Meditation can be performed several times a

SYMPTOMS

- ☑ Pronounced or exaggerated heartbeat
- ☑ Shortness of breath and sighing
- ☑ Muscle tension, including head, neck, and backaches
- ☑ Restlessness during waking and sleeping hours
- ☑ Irritability
- ☑ Difficulty concentrating
- ☑ Upset stomach and diarrhea

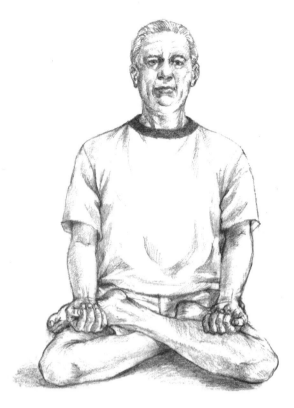

week (even daily) or just before an anxiety-provoking situation, such as giving a speech.

Here's a sample meditation that can be practiced every morning:

- Sit on the floor with your legs crossed, keeping your spine straight. Use a cushion if needed. Try to eliminate as many noises and distractions as possible, including unplugging the telephone.
- Select one word or sound that is pleasant or meaningful to you (sometimes called a *mantra*). Mentally repeat your selection, over and over again.
- Try to do this for about 20 minutes. If your mind wanders off to another thought, gently return it to the process of repeating your word or sound.

HOMEOPATHY

Homeopathic medicine is particularly promising for psychological conditions such as anxiety. Treatment stimulates the ability of the mind and body to return to a healthy state. Homeopathy uses highly diluted doses of natural substances, which would bring on anxiety symptoms if given in full strength to a healthy person. The substances are from plant, mineral, and animal sources.

The classical homeopath individualizes a remedy for each patient, depending on the particular symptoms and the general state of physical and emotional health. Here are some characteristics of anxiety to consider and report to a practitioner:

- Does a specific activity (anything from taking a test in school to meeting new people) bring on an anxiety attack?
- How do you react to other people during an attack? Insecure or overly confident?
- Which physical symptoms are present along with the feelings? Pronounced heartbeats, dry mouth, digestive upsets, others?

WHO USES ALTERNATIVE MEDICINE?

According to the landmark 1993 Harvard Medical School survey on alternative medicine, more than 25 percent of people with anxiety use unconventional therapies to find relief. They most commonly relied on relaxation techniques and guided imagery.

- What makes the anxiety better or worse?
- Are there certain times of the day or night when the symptoms are worse or better?

Common remedies for anxiety include argentum nitricum, gelsemium sempervirens (for test anxiety), lycopodium (for performance anxiety), aconite, arsenicum, kaliphos, and phosphorus.

For anxiety that makes the person nervous and fidgety and is accompanied by diarrhea or gas, among other details (consult a practitioner), here's a sample homeopathic remedy: Take one dose of argentum nitricum, 6c, every six hours. (The *6c* refers to the potency of the remedy.) Stop treatment as soon as the symptoms end.

HERBAL MEDICINE

Several herbs have the ability to act on the nervous system, bringing on states of relaxation and tranquility. Others can relax tense muscles, ease stress-related headaches, soothe an upset stomach, or encourage sound sleeping.

Kava kava, a member of the pepper family, can induce calm feelings and ease muscle tension. It's available in tincture and capsule form.

Skullcap, an herb that was used extensively in Native American medicine, may ease emotional tension and headaches as well as improve sleep. It is commonly used in capsule form, as a tea (made with the fresh herb), or as a tincture.

Valerian root has a calming, sleep-inducing effect for most people. (A few

experience the opposite effect.) The herb should be taken in low doses before bedtime. It can be taken as a tea made with fresh or dried root, but the taste and smell are rather unpleasant; extract and capsule form may be easier to tolerate.

Some other herbs that can be helpful include
- chamomile
- lemon balm
- passionflower
- St.-John's-wort
- vervain

These herbs generally perform their functions without major side effects and the threat of withdrawal symptoms that pharmaceuticals carry. However, herbs should be used only to provide short-term or occasional anxiety relief. Successful anxiety treatment requires learning to cope in the long term by reducing stress and other anxiety triggers.

An herbalist may prescribe the following kava kava treatment: Take 100 to 200 mg of a 30 percent standardized extract daily until anxiety subsides. You may have to take the herb for a day or so to produce any effects.

HYPNOTHERAPY

Hypnotherapy holds that people with anxiety can learn to release tension and effectively respond to stressful situations if their minds are prepared to do so. During a hypnotic trance, the subconscious mind is given gentle, positive suggestions, which are selected according to what situations and circumstances trigger an anxiety attack.

Examples of these suggestions may include

- "I feel better about myself each day, and other people notice this."
- "Meeting with my boss is not a bad thing; communication makes my job more enjoyable and generally easier to do."

OTHER THERAPIES

AROMATHERAPY—Essential oils from benzoin, lavender, and marjoram may be helpful.

BIOFEEDBACK TRAINING—Several types of biofeedback, including electrodermal activity and finger pulse, can teach a person to prevent anxiety and panic attacks. The training is typically coupled with relaxation techniques.

BODYWORK—Massage, dance therapy, and other forms of bodywork can reduce stress and improve the sense of well-being.

GUIDED IMAGERY AND CREATIVE VISUALIZATION—Mental exercises can bring a relaxed state similar to that of hypnotherapy.

NUTRITIONAL THERAPY—Treatment may include dietary changes (such as eliminating caffeine and food additives) and nutritional supplements (such as calcium and magnesium).

YOGA—Postures and breathing exercises may improve energy levels, boost blood circulation, and ease tension.

QIGONG—Exercise and mental techniques, part of traditional Chinese medicine, can improve breathing and reduce stress.

The treatments can be guided by a hypnotist or done by the person with anxiety (called self-hypnosis).

Here's a sample self-hypnosis session for someone experiencing anxiety attacks before speaking in public:

- Sit in a comfortable position.
- Close your eyes and breathe slowly and deeply, focusing on each inhalation and exhalation.
- Imagine you are boarding an elevator on the top of a skyscraper.
- The door closes and you slowly travel downward.
- Look up at the digital sign that displays each floor number as you go down.
- Focus on each number as it appears on the display. As the numbers count backward, you are going into a deeper and deeper state of relaxation.
- Imagine exiting the elevator and entering a comfortable room, decorated just the way you would decorate it. Walk around the room as much as you want.
- When you're ready, find an inviting chair and sit down.
- In your head, repeat to yourself: "I look good and feel confident as I stand at the podium. I am prepared to talk about something I know very well and enjoy talking about. I'm speaking to people who admire me and are genuinely interested in what I have to say."
- When you feel comfortable leaving your hypnotic state, count from ten to one, suggesting to yourself that you will emerge relaxed and confident.

ARTHRITIS IS A PAINFUL DISEASE OF THE JOINTS. OSTEOARTHRITIS (OA) AND RHEUMATOID ARTHRITIS (RA) ARE THE TWO MAJOR TYPES. IN OA—WHICH OFTEN AFFECTS THE HIPS, KNEES, FEET, AND SPINE—THE JOINT CARTILAGE DETERIORATES OVER TIME. IN RA, THE MEMBRANES LINING THE JOINTS BECOME INFLAMED, LIMITING THE JOINT'S RANGE OF MOTION. THE BODY'S IMMUNE SYSTEM ATTACKING ITS OWN TISSUES IS THE MOST LIKELY CAUSE OF RA.

CONVENTIONAL APPROACH

Because no cure is available, allopathic medicine's treatment for arthritis is aimed at relieving symptoms. The typical treatment program consists of drug therapy, exercise, and rest.

DRUG TREATMENT

Here are a few of the many medications used to treat the symptoms of arthritis:

- Aspirin (a nonsteroidal anti-inflammatory drug) in low doses can suppress pain, but high doses are needed to fight inflammation. The side effects of high-dose aspirin therapy include stomach bleeding, ulcers, and ringing in the ears.
- Other nonsteroidal anti-inflammatory drugs, such as ibuprofen and naproxen, can be effective but may cause side effects such as nausea, diarrhea, stomach ulcers, and intestinal bleeding.
- Corticosteroids can reduce inflammation and suppress the activity of the immune system. With long-term use, they can cause weight gain, diabetes, osteoporosis, and eye problems.
- Disease-modifying antirheumatic drugs (including oral and injectable gold) may be effective for people with RA. They can offer short-term relief but have significant side effects.
- Anticancer drugs, such as methotrexate, may be helpful for people with RA but may also dangerously suppress the immune system.

SURGICAL TREATMENT

Some severe cases of arthritis may require surgery to remove the lining around the joint and, with OA, any stray bone and cartilage fragments. Artificial joints may be implanted to replace those damaged beyond repair.

OTHER TREATMENT

Moderate daily exercise can keep joints flexible and protect them from further stress. Care should be taken not to exercise too long or hard and to get adequate amounts of rest. Applying cold (in the form of ice packs or wet towels) or heat (warm baths or heating pads) can ease pain. Maintaining a healthy body weight reduces extra burden on sore joints.

ALTERNATIVE APPROACHES

Many practitioners of alternative therapies disagree with the attitude of allopathic doctors toward arthritis. Instead of sidestepping the issue of cause, these alternative treatments recognize particular triggers that can be respon-

SYMPTOMS

☑ Swelling, tenderness, pain, and stiffness in one or more joints

☑ Limited movement

☑ Red, hot, or burning skin over the joints (RA only)

☑ Decreased appetite, weight loss, fever, and extreme fatigue (RA only)

In RA, the pain is often greatest after the joint has been kept still for a long time. In OA, the pain may increase after overuse. OA can affect just one joint, whereas RA usually affects multiple joints.

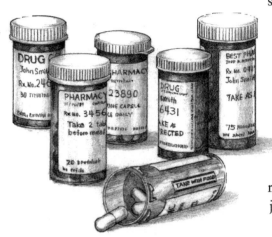

sible. In fact, some practitioners of alternative medicine believe that aspirin and other nonsteroidal anti-inflammatory drugs may actually encourage the progression of OA. These medicines have been suspected of interfering with the body's repair and maintenance of joint cartilage.

NUTRITIONAL THERAPY

According to nutritional therapy, diet plays a large role in both causing and treating arthritis. The disease is triggered in part by a complex mix of nutritional deficiencies, excesses, and sensitivities—a mix that is specific to each type of arthritis and each person. Therefore, a treatment program of dietary changes and supplements needs to be highly individualized. In many cases nutritional therapy can halt the progression of arthritis, and in a few cases, it can even reverse it.

Animal foods—Avoiding animal foods is one way of reducing some arthritis symptoms. This may be because arachidonic acid, a fatty acid found in these foods, can provoke joint inflammation. Aside from arachidonic acid, a diet high in animal protein delivers a lot of phosphorus but not a lot of calcium. This starts a chain reaction in the body, causing some calcium to leach out of the bones and a few calcium deposits to settle around the joints (a common characteristic of people with OA). To remedy this situation, calcium and magnesium supplements are often prescribed together with dietary changes.

A group of researchers with the University of Oslo in Norway showed that people with RA who followed a vegetarian diet for one year experienced a significant improvement in symptoms when compared with people in a control group who followed an ordinary diet. After a weeklong fast, the patients in the study group consumed a vegan diet (with no beef, poultry, seafood, dairy products, or eggs) and avoided all gluten (a wheat protein) for three and a half months. Then they switched to a lactovegetarian diet (with dairy

GET THAT BODY MOVING

Daily exercising is an important part of any arthritis treatment program and can—among other benefits—reduce pain, improve joint motion, and even ease depression. The workouts should include stretching, strengthening, and endurance (aerobic-conditioning) exercises and be accompanied by adequate rest periods. Exercises such as swimming that don't exert a lot of weight on the joints are typically recommended. However, weight-bearing exercises hold the promise of stimulating bone growth and strengthening connective tissue.

A team of researchers at the Charlotte Rehabilitation Hospital in North Carolina set out to see if weight-bearing exercises—in particular, Tai Chi Chuan, a traditional Chinese exercise—would be safe for people with rheumatoid arthritis. After ten weeks of Tai Chi instruction either once or twice a week, the study participants experienced no aggravation of joint symptoms.

products being the only animal foods allowed) for the rest of the year.

Food allergies—Food allergies or sensitivities have been implicated in many cases of arthritis, particularly RA. An elimination diet (in which certain foods are avoided for days or weeks and then reintroduced one by one) can be helpful in pinpointing what triggers or worsens a person's particular symptoms. Common culprits include

- wheat
- corn
- dairy products
- beef
- citrus fruits
- salt
- caffeine

In addition, some people with OA or RA may be sensitive to the "nightshade" foods, including tomatoes, white potatoes, eggplant, and all peppers except black pepper. Many have found relief by avoiding these foods.

Fish oils—Clinical studies have shown that fish oils can alleviate some RA symptoms. These oils, found in cold-water fish and in oil from the herb evening primrose, contain essential fatty acids that can work toward controlling inflammation in the body. Other essential fatty acid oils such as flax, borage, sesame, sunflower, and pumpkin are also gaining popularity.

Glucosamine sulfate—Glucosamine sulfate is one of the building blocks of cartilage. Studies have shown it to be useful in treating arthritis, especially OA. Not only does glucosamine sulfate help to rebuild the joint surface, but according to at least one study, it may be more effective at controlling pain than ibuprofen.

Weight control—Excess body weight means excess pressure on a lot of the body's joints. Therefore, people with arthritis, especially OA, should strive to maintain their ideal body weight. One way this can be achieved is by following a low-fat, whole-foods vegetarian diet. However, avoiding the essential fatty acids in an effort to cut fat may be detrimental in the long run (see Fish oils above).

After performing an exam and a detailed nutritional profile, a naturopathic physician may recommend several dietary measures. One part of the prescription might call for supplementing with 800 to 1,000 mg of calcium and 400 to 800 mg of magnesium per day. Sufficient calcium and magnesium may protect the integrity of bones and prevent bone spurs and other painful conditions associated with arthritis.

HERBAL MEDICINE

Herbs can do much more than ease pain for people with arthritis. They can fight inflammation, encourage the re-

---

WHO USES UNCONVENTIONAL THERAPIES?

The landmark 1993 Harvard Medical School survey on alternative medicine had this to say about people with arthritis: Eighteen percent reported using one or more unconventional therapies for their joint problems in a one-year period. They most often turned to chiropractic and relaxation techniques.

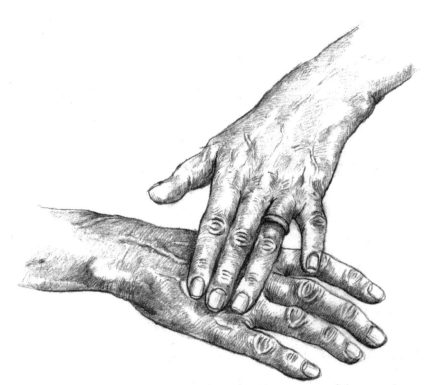

pair and maintenance of damaged cartilage and bones, and cleanse toxins from the joints.

Devil's claw root, gingerroot, meadowsweet leaves and flowertops, and white willow bark all act as anti-inflammatory agents that can relieve pain. (In fact, aspirin contains a chemical that's the synthesized version of a substance found in meadowsweet and willow.)

Comfrey, applied to the joints as a cream or infused oil, speeds healing of cartilage and bones, especially in cases of OA. Celery seeds can promote urination, thereby eliminating toxins from the body.

Other helpful herbs include boswellia (frankincense), capsicum (cayenne), feverfew, and licorice. It's important to note that the goal of herbal therapy is not to suppress pain totally, as this symptom signals people with arthritis to rest.

An herbalist may prescribe the following remedy to relieve joint pain:

- In a teapot or a saucepan, combine ¹/₂ teaspoon powdered devil's claw root with 1 cup of boiling water.
- Cover and steep for 10 minutes.
- Drink 1 cup daily.

DETOXIFICATION, FASTING, AND COLON THERAPY

Detoxification therapy can cleanse the body—in particular the joints—of any built-up toxins that might be causing the limited motion and pain of arthritis. Fasting for a week or more, taking only water and perhaps herbal teas, can be especially helpful. During a fast, all or most of the arthritic symptoms often disappear. Once the fast is over, the symptoms return for some people, but others experience a complete remission. If food allergies or sensitivities are suspected, a fast can flush out any allergenic substances and prepare the body for dietary alterations. A long-term fast such as this must be supervised by an experienced practitioner. A juice diet, such as drinking only carrot and celery juice for a week, can also be helpful but should be undertaken under strict supervision.

If you decide to undertake a long-term fast, you'll need to be regularly monitored for blood pressure, electrolyte levels, and several other bodily changes. Ask your health practitioner for advice.

MIND/BODY MEDICINE

Several factors besides the inflammatory response of tissues greatly influence the course of arthritis, including a person's attitude toward the disease, level of emotional stress, and ability to cope. The hopeful news is that the person with arthritis has control over these factors. Various mind/body techniques can lead to an easing of arthritic pain, improved range of motion, easier sleeping, and a strengthened immune system. These techniques include

- creative visualization
- guided imagery
- progressive relaxation
- support groups
- self-hypnosis
- meditation

The notion that the mind can relieve some symptoms of arthritis was popularized by the Arthritis Self-Help Course, an educational program developed at the Stanford University Arthritis Center. The course is typically taught by people with arthritis, not by doctors or nurses. Although the course follows the allopathic treatment approach, it also teaches mind/body techniques and basic how-to strategies (from opening jars to avoiding depression). Graduates of the course experience reduced joint swelling and greater mobility.

 Here's a simple relaxation technique that can reduce pain and may reduce inflammation:

- Wearing loose clothing, sit or lie down in a comfortable position.
- Begin breathing deeply and slowly.
- With each breath, invite a different part of your body to relax.
- Imagine each inhaled breath as light going to the joints of your body and each exhaled breath as the pain flowing out of your joints.
- Continue the slow, deep breathing for as long as you are comfortable.
- When you are ready, slowly return to your normal rate and rhythm of breathing and open your eyes slowly.

OTHER THERAPIES

AROMATHERAPY—Massages with essential oils of juniper, thyme, rosemary, or chamomile, may be helpful.

AYURVEDIC MEDICINE—Therapeutic diet, herbal therapy, oil massages, and breathing exercises are aimed at eliminating the causes of arthritis.

CHIROPRACTIC—Treatment can reduce pain and increase joint flexibility for people with osteoarthritis.

ENVIRONMENTAL MEDICINE—Certain foods, molds, chemicals, and other substances can all trigger arthritis. After extensive testing, treatment involves avoidance and desensitization.

HOMEOPATHY—Common remedies include bryonia alba, pulsatilla nigricans, and rhus toxicodendron.

HYDROTHERAPY—Cold or hot compresses, or alternating hot and cold compresses, can be used for pain relief and to stimulate blood circulation.

OSTEOPATHY—Manipulation can be particularly beneficial for people with osteoarthritis.

TRADITIONAL CHINESE MEDICINE—Arthritis may result from blocked energy, or qi; acupuncture can restore the energy flow. (The National Institutes of Health's Office of Alternative Medicine recently funded a study on acupuncture treatment for osteoarthritis.) Treatment may also include herbal therapy.

Asthma

Asthma is a disease that makes the airways to the lungs prone to bouts of narrowing, resulting in breathing difficulties. Things that trigger asthma attacks include respiratory infections, substances that cause allergies (such as pollen, dust mites, animal dander, certain foods), airborne irritants (cigarette smoke, air pollution, and perfumes), exercise, emotional stress, and certain weather conditions.

SYMPTOMS

- ☑ Dry coughing and wheezing
- ☑ Shortness of breath
- ☑ Chest tightness
- ☑ Rapid heartbeat and sweating (during severe attacks)

CONVENTIONAL APPROACH

With no cure for asthma, allopathic medicine focuses on keeping attacks under control. As with allergies, conventional medicine advises that asthma sufferers try to avoid the known triggers. The following drugs can be taken to prevent attacks or to ease those that have already started:

- Bronchodilators (such as albuterol, metaproterenol, or theophylline) work to expand the airways.
- Corticosteriods relieve inflammation in the airways, making the channels less vulnerable to triggers.
- Cromolyn may also prevent attacks for chronic sufferers. Compared with other asthma drugs, it has fewer side effects.

ALTERNATIVE APPROACHES

Asthma deaths are on the rise in America. Increases in air pollution can take partial blame, but practitioners of alternative medicine point to the rise to illustrate that conventional medicine is not doing the trick and that more treatment approaches should be considered.

MIND/BODY MEDICINE

For people with asthma, the mind can be a powerful tool in the healing process. It can communicate with the body, giving instructions and assisting in easier breathing, relaxing, handling stress, boosting the immune system, and managing the action of the lungs' airways—all factors that play a role in asthma.

Many therapies related to mind/body medicine hold the promise to reduce asthma symptoms and even eliminate future attacks. Those treatments include

- biofeedback to learn how to chase away tension and anxiety and loosen the muscles of the upper body
- breathing exercises to relax and emphasize breathing through the nose rather than through the mouth
- guided imagery and creative visualization to picture the airways widening, allowing air to flow easily in and out of the lungs, and to envision the weakening of allergens, so they can no longer trigger an attack
- hypnotherapy to regulate breathing
- meditation to clear the mind and to push out emotional upset that can contribute to an asthma attack
- yoga to regulate and slow breathing and calm the mind

Breathing exercises, such as those practiced in yoga, prepare you for the movements and poses to follow. Here's an example of a breathing lesson that can help asthma sufferers:

- Get in a comfortable position, perhaps sitting with legs crossed on a floor mat. Keep your spine straight.
- Breathe in slowly and deliberately, sticking out your stomach as air comes into your lungs. This should take about six seconds.
- Exhale, drawing your stomach back in. Again, take about six seconds.
- Repeat this ten times.

NUTRITIONAL THERAPY

Nutritional therapy can help people with asthma by removing all possible food allergens, fortifying against certain vitamin or mineral deficiencies, and fighting off colds or other infections. A vegan diet, which contains no animals products whatsoever (including milk and eggs), can prevent some asthma attacks. Swedish researchers followed a group of asthma sufferers who were dissatisfied with the success of conventional therapies and wanted to try a vegan diet of mainly raw foods. Nine patients dropped out after two months. But for the 24 who stayed with the diet for one year, 92 percent reported an improvement or complete elimination of symptoms.

Large doses of vitamin C can strengthen the immune system and may even prevent the airways of the lungs from narrowing in response to an asthma trigger. Vitamin C is also valuable for its antioxidant properties, as are vitamin E, beta-carotene, and the mineral selenium.

Also, the mineral magnesium may work to widen the airways. Bioflavonoids (hesparidin methyl chalcone and quercetin), vitamin B_6, vitamin B_{12} (es-pecially in children), and essential fatty acids can also be useful.

Increasing magnesium intake may be very helpful for some asthma sufferers. In the diet, the mineral is supplied by avocados, oatmeal, tofu, and other foods. It is difficult to get enough magnesium to be effective, though, so magnesium supplementation may be in order. A sample prescription would be 500 mg daily (a little less than twice the recommended dietary allowance for the mineral).

OTHER THERAPIES

ACUPUNCTURE—Treatments can correct any imbalances in vital life energy (perhaps along the lung, spleen, or kidney system meridians) that may be triggering the breathing problems.

CHIROPRACTIC—Asthma may be a symptom of a misalignment of the spinal vertebrae, which chiropractic adjustments can correct.

ENVIROMENTAL MEDICINE—Food allergies, molds, pollen, chemicals, and more can trigger asthma. Treatment may include desensitization, avoidance of triggers, and nutritional supplements (such as antioxidants).

HERBAL MEDICINE—Ginger, cayenne, Indian tobacco (*Lobelia inflata*), ma huang (*Ephedra sinica*), turmeric, skunk cabbage, and goldenseal all hold promise for asthma sufferers.

HOMEOPATHY—Specific remedies must be tailored to the individual, but common prescriptions include aconitum napellus, ipecacuanha, and natrum sulphuricum.

Back & Neck Pain

BACK AND NECK PAIN ARE TWO OF THE MOST COMMON AILMENTS. THE PAIN MAY OCCUR IN THE MUSCLES, SPINAL JOINTS, OR NEARBY NERVES. IT CAN RESULT FROM MUSCLE STRAIN, DAMAGED SPINAL DISKS (THE CUSHIONS BETWEEN THE VERTEBRAE), POOR POSTURE, BEING OVERWEIGHT, PREGNANCY, SOME FORMS OF ARTHRITIS, KIDNEY INFECTION, AND SEVERAL OTHER FACTORS.

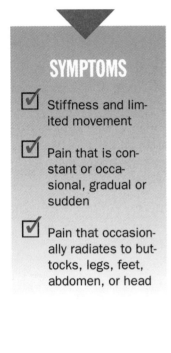

SYMPTOMS

☑ Stiffness and limited movement

☑ Pain that is constant or occasional, gradual or sudden

☑ Pain that occasionally radiates to buttocks, legs, feet, abdomen, or head

CONVENTIONAL APPROACH

Allopathic medicine commonly treats back and neck pain with a combination of rest, drugs, and surgery. If the pain is caused by a known disorder, such as osteoarthritis, then treatment is tailored to that ailment.

DRUG TREATMENT

Several medicines are recommended to relieve pain, stiffness, and other symptoms:

- Analgesics (painkillers), including aspirin and acetaminophen, reduce pain. Potential side effects range from stomach bleeding to liver damage. Other narcotic painkillers, such as codeine and meperidine, can be helpful but should be used only for short periods because of their habit-forming nature.
- Nonsteroidal anti-inflammatory drugs, such as ibuprofen and naproxen, can also ease pain but may cause nausea, diarrhea, and intestinal bleeding, among other side effects.
- Muscle-relaxant drugs, such as carisoprodol, diazepam, and methocarbamol, may cause weakness and drowsiness.
- Tricyclic antidepressants, in low doses, may encourage sound sleeping. Side effects may include dry mouth, blurred vision, and dizziness.

SURGICAL TREATMENT

A damaged disk that has ruptured and is putting pressure on the spinal nerves can be surgically repaired. Surgery is also used to widen the space between the vertebrae. Numerous critics, including some doctors, complain that many back surgeries are unnecessary and potentially harmful.

OTHER TREATMENT

Sleeping on a firm mattress, applying ice and then heat, and wearing a back or neck brace can relieve some of the pain and promote healing. A sudden onset of pain requires bed rest, but only for a short period. Resting should be followed by regular, gentle exercise.

ALTERNATIVE APPROACHES

More and more, allopathic doctors are beginning to recognize the benefits of several alternative therapies—in particular chiropractic, osteopathy, and acupuncture—in the treatment of back and neck pain.

CHIROPRACTIC

Chiropractic medicine, with its emphasis on the spine, is particularly effective in easing pain and improving function in the back and neck. The therapy works on the basis that misalignments in the vertebrae interfere with the nervous system, which prevent the body from operating at its peak. Adjustments and manipulations, performed with the chiropractor's hands, can return any misaligned vertebrae to their ideal positions. The body is then ready to take over the healing process.

A chiropractic examination includes palpations (examination with the hands) and sometimes X rays. A treatment for back pain may include "short-lever" thrusts to specific points on the spine, often performed by the chiropractor once a week or more until the pain is reduced. Instruction for the patient in exercising and posture is also included.

Many research trials have shown that manipulation is an effective treatment for several types of lower-back pain, especially in cases in which the pain comes on strongly and suddenly. In addition, a survey of patients with lower-back pain reported that those who went to chiropractors were more satisfied with their treatment than those who saw medical doctors.

Only a trained practitioner is qualified to perform chiropractic techniques. In addition to adjustments, some chiropractors may add dietary changes and other therapies to their treatments.

YOGA

Yoga teaches good posture and deep, relaxed breathing and strengthens and limbers the muscles. All of these benefits can ease back and neck pain and prevent injuries and strains from recurring. The mix of yoga exercises and movements de-

---

THE POPULAR ALTERNATIVES

According to the landmark 1993 Harvard Medical School survey on alternative medicine, more than one-third of the people with back problems turn to alternative therapies for treatment. They most often reported using chiropractic and massage.

---

pends on the cause of the pain and where it is located. The sessions usually last from 20 to 60 minutes and are performed anywhere from once a week to every day. Of course, it's preferable to prevent back and neck pain with yoga rather than to treat it.

Here's a sample yoga exercise—the "cat stretch"—that's often recommended for lower-back pain:

- Wear comfortable clothing.
- Get on your hands and knees. Placing your hands shoulder distance

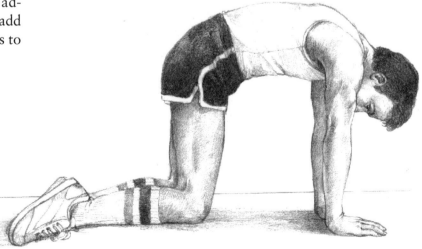

apart and your knees hip distance apart, look straight ahead. Your arms and back should be straight, as if you are a table.

- Inhale deeply.
- As you exhale, slowly and gently arch your back up, tighten your stomach, and hang your head down. Hold for several seconds.
- As you inhale, slowly and gently arch your back down and lift your head up. Hold this position for several seconds.
- Repeat four times.

BODYWORK

Several forms of bodywork can improve movement and posture, relieve pain, and aid in the healing process. Massage is perhaps the most recognized bodywork therapy for this type of pain. It relaxes muscles and increases blood circulation to the area (crucial to the healing process).

Several studies have shown that people with back pain receive positive results with forms of Swedish massage. In particular, deep-tissue massage can ease long-held muscle tension. As the name implies, it involves the application of firm pressure and slow strokes to muscle layers deep below the skin surface. One word of caution: The sudden and severe onset of pain will require time to heal before beginning deep-tissue massage treatments.

Other bodywork therapies can also be helpful in treating back and neck pain:

- Alexander technique offers simple, guided exercises that enhance posture, ease pain and tension, and allow better, more efficient use of the body.
- Feldenkrais method teaches new ways to move the body, helping to relax cramped or tense muscles.

In addition to specific exercises, the Alexander technique offers tips to perform everyday activities better. The following are some of those tips:

- Sit with your back firmly against the back of a chair. If the chair offers poor support, put a small pillow between your lower back and the chair.
- Also when sitting, pull the chair in close to the desk or table. Do not lean over the desk.
- Beware of low handrails. Do not hunch your shoulders to grip them. Instead, keep good posture and only run your fingers along the rail to guide you.

OSTEOPATHY

Osteopathic medicine holds much promise for people with back and neck pain. Similar to chiropractic, this therapy recognizes misalignments of the spine. Osteopathy takes a broad view of the body and sees misalignments as

---

KEEP ON MOVING

The common advice for people struck with a sudden case of back pain used to be to rest in bed and take it easy for several weeks. However, researchers now believe excessive rest can contribute to weak muscles and slow the healing process. Instead, they advise resuming gentle exercises, such as yoga, as soon as possible.

blocking healthy blood flow and nervous system functioning.

Treatment of back and neck pain can include manipulation of the back, arms, legs, and other joints, as well as massage and instructions on proper posture. The osteopath also looks to see if seemingly unrelated health problems, such as sinus problems, are contributing to the back or neck pain. Finally, the osteopath may prescribe drugs or surgery if necessary. Researchers have shown that osteopathic manipulation of the spine can restore function to backs that were immobilized by lower-back pain.

A licensed doctor of osteopathy is the only person qualified to use osteopathic manipulation. However, many specific therapies similar to osteopathic manipulation (chiropractic adjustment, naturopathic manipulation, bodywork techniques) can be prescribed for back and neck pain and are performed by various practitioners.

NEURAL THERAPY

Neural therapy may bring relief to people with long-term back and neck pain. The treatment involves injecting local anesthetics (including procaine, novocaine, or lidocaine) into specific sites on the body, such as particular nerves, acupuncture points, and even scar tissue. These injections are thought to unblock or stabilize the flow of electrical energy through the body.

Patients of neural therapy have reported pain reduction or even complete pain remission. Some detective work is required to find the appropriate injection site. For example, a scar on the leg may be causing an energy interference that produces pain in the lower back.

Various health care practitioners—including some naturopathic, osteopathic, and conventional doctors—are trained in neural therapy. Seek out a therapist with experience in this technique.

OTHER THERAPIES

AYURVEDIC MEDICINE—Treatment can include meditation, herbal therapy, and massages with warm oil.

BIOFEEDBACK TRAINING—Electromyographic biofeedback and relaxation exercises can lead to pain reduction.

GUIDED IMAGERY AND CREATIVE VISUALIZATION—Exercises may help people relieve pain and ease muscle tension.

HERBAL MEDICINE—White willow bark, cayenne, burdock, cramp bark, and chamomile can be used to relieve pain. Hypericum can be applied topically in lotion or oil form for sharp nerve pain.

HOMEOPATHY—Common remedies include arnica montana, calcarea fluorica, ruta graveolens, and rhus toxicodendron.

HYDROTHERAPY—Alternating hot and cold compresses (ending with cold) and exercises performed in a pool of water can be helpful.

TRADITIONAL CHINESE MEDICINE—Acupuncture is particularly recommended for treating back and neck pain. Herbal therapy, relaxation techniques, and Tai Chi exercises are also useful.

Bladder Infection

THE URINARY BLADDER CAN BECOME INFECTED WITH BACTERIA THAT NORMALLY INHABIT THE INTESTINAL TRACT. BLADDER INFECTION IS MUCH MORE COMMON IN WOMEN THAN IN MEN BECAUSE A WOMAN'S URETHRA—THE PASSAGE THAT LEADS FROM THE BLADDER TO THE OUTSIDE OF THE BODY—IS MUCH SHORTER THAN A MAN'S, THUS ALLOWING BACTERIA TO TRAVEL TO THE BLADDER MORE EASILY. BLADDER INFECTIONS CAN APPEAR AGAIN AND AGAIN, AND THE KIDNEYS AND OTHER PARTS OF THE URINARY TRACT MAY ALSO BECOME INFECTED.

SYMPTOMS

- ☑ Burning and stinging sensation when urinating
- ☑ Cloudy, bloody, or unusual-smelling urine
- ☑ Frequent urges to urinate that produce only small amounts of urine
- ☑ Waking up at night with the urge to urinate
- ☑ Pain in the lower abdomen or back
- ☑ Fever, nausea, and vomiting (usually signs that infection has moved to kidneys)

CONVENTIONAL APPROACH

TREATMENT

Allopathic medicine typically relies on drug therapy to treat bladder infections. One of several antibiotics is commonly prescribed to eliminate the infection. They can include

- trimethoprim (alone or in combination with sulfamethoxazole)
- amoxicillin
- nitrofurantoin
- cotrimoxazole

PREVENTION

Some women are prone to repeated bladder infections. To prevent them, low doses of antibiotics may be prescribed for half a year or longer, or they can be taken each time after sexual intercourse. Doctors sometimes advise women to follow several self-help measures, which can include

- drinking enough water so the urine is pale in color
- never resisting the urge to urinate
- wiping with toilet tissue from the front to back
- emptying the bladder immediately before and after sex

ALTERNATIVE APPROACHES

Practitioners of several alternative therapies frown on conventional medicine's dependence on antibiotics—drugs that can disrupt the body's normal balance of bacteria and may trigger yeast infections and other conditions. However, the alternative and conventional approaches do share one aspect of bladder infection treatment: Self-help measures such as drinking a lot of water and cranberry juice and maintaining good toilet hygiene are important.

HERBAL MEDICINE

Herbs can be used to fight infection, soothe the inflamed urinary tract, and encourage urination (which flushes bacteria out of the system). Uva ursi (also known as bearberry and upland cranberry) can be effective in clearing infections from the urinary tract and triggering urination. Its leaves are often taken as a tincture or tea. Because it can be toxic, only small doses of this herb should be used. Follow the directions from your doctor or on the product's label.

Echinacea (or purple coneflower) and goldenseal are commonly prescribed to boost the immune system and as a natural antibiotic. They can be taken in tincture or capsule form. (For suggestions on how to use purple coneflower, see Appendix 3.)

Marshmallow root and couch grass can relieve the inflamed lining of the urinary tract. For example, marshmallow root teas can be used. Other herbs that are helpful in treating bladder infection include
- alfalfa
- buchu
- celery
- juniper berries
- yarrow
- parsley

A sample herbal remedy might be to take one teaspoon of uva ursi tincture three times a day. The tincture can be added to a cup of warm water before drinking.

NUTRITIONAL THERAPY

Nutritional therapy offers several ways to treat and prevent bladder infections. Cranberries are often prescribed to increase the acid content of urine, making it unfriendly to bacteria. It's also thought that certain substances in cranberries may prevent bacteria from attaching themselves to the walls of the urinary tract. Research has confirmed that cranberry juice can effectively treat bladder infections. The juice should not contain added sugar, though, which may weaken the immune system. The fruit also can be taken in capsule form; this method can be desirable as it avoids the excess sugar in most cranberry juice formulas, but the patient must remember to maintain her fluid—especially water—intake.

Vitamin C (ascorbic acid) supplements may be used for the same antibacterial functions as cranberries. Other supplements that can aid in the treatment of recurrent infections include
- bioflavonoids
- vitamin A
- vitamin E
- zinc

If antibiotics are included in the treatment program, then the body's "good" bacteria should be reestablished with *Lactobacillus acidophilus* supplements or yogurt with live cultures.

Finally, good eating habits can contribute to a healthy immune system and lessen susceptibility to bladder infection. Many practitioners of nutritional therapy recommend eating a diet high in fresh vegetables, whole grains, and organic foods and low in sugars, refined carbohydrates, saturated oils, and animal products. Any food allergies should be ruled out with the help of an elimination diet (see Allergies, page 22).

A naturopathic physician may recommend drinking one quart of unsweetened cranberry juice

---

SEX MAY BE TO BLAME

Bacteria that have migrated from the intestinal tract to the urinary tract are often to blame for bladder infecitons. Sexual intercourse is one way to help the bacteria travel. (This may explain why nuns are reported to have very low rates of bladder infections.) Urinating before and after intercourse may help to flush the offending bacteria out of the urinary tract before it can get a foothold and multiply.

daily as soon as the symptoms of bladder infection begin.

HOMEOPATHY

Homeopathic medicine works to treat bladder infections by giving highly diluted doses of a natural substance that would produce the same infection if given in full strength to a healthy person. The substances are taken from plant, mineral, or animal sources. To find a remedy appropriate for the patient's symptoms, a homeopath questions the patient on details of the infection and assesses the general state of physical and emotional health. Using these clues, the remedy is then individualized to the patient. Some characteristics to consider:

- Did the symptoms come on slowly or quickly?
- Has the need to urinate changed? How has it changed?
- Is the urine unusual-looking?
- What is the nature of the pain?

Common remedies for bladder infection include

- berberis
- cantharis
- pulsatilla
- sarsaparilla

For a bladder infection characterized by a burning sensation when urinating and a general feeling of restlessness, among other details, here's a remedy a homeopath may prescribe: Take one dose of cantharis, 12c, every six hours for mild infection or 30c every two to three hours for more severe, acute infection. (The *12c* and *30c* refer to the potency of the remedy.)

AROMATHERAPY

Aromatherapy can relieve the pain of bladder infections. The essential oils of the following herbs are commonly used:

- sandalwood
- cedarwood
- pine
- tea tree
- juniper

These oils are often administered with body compresses and massages and in warm sitz baths and regular baths. It is important that these therapies not be used in conjunction with homeopathic treatments.

Here's a sample aromatherapy treatment: Mix ten drops of essential sandalwood oil with one ounce of massage oil (such as almond oil). Rub the mixture over the bladder area, three times a day.

OTHER THERAPIES

CHIROPRACTIC—Some cases of bladder infection may benefit from a rebalancing of the lower spine.

DETOXIFICATION, FASTING, AND COLON THERAPY—Short fasts can purify the urinary tract.

HYPNOTHERAPY—Warm or hot sitz baths and compresses can relieve the pain of bladder infection. These and other forms of hydrotherapy can increase blood circulation and encourage the healing process.

TRADITIONAL CHINESE MEDICINE—Bladder infection is often attributed to an excess of damp heat in the bladder. Treatment can include acupuncture, acupressure, and herbal therapy.

BURSITIS IS AN INFLAMMATION OF ONE OF THE BODY'S BURSAE (THE FLUID-FILLED SACS THAT CUSHION THE JOINTS). THIS PAINFUL CONDITION CAN BE CAUSED BY A MILD INJURY, REPEATED USE (SUCH AS PROLONGED KNEELING ON A HARD SURFACE), ARTHRITIS, OR INFECTION. COMMONLY AFFECTED JOINTS ARE THE SHOULDER, ELBOW, KNEE, AND HIP.

CONVENTIONAL APPROACH

For most cases of bursitis, allopathic medicine recommends resting the joint, cold and heat treatments, and drug therapy. Initially, ice packs can be applied to the joint to reduce pain and inflammation. Once the pain has eased (usually in two to five days), heating pads may be used. As healing begins, exercise should be slowly increased.

Drug therapy starts with high doses of nonsteroidal anti-inflammatory agents, such as ibuprofen, indomethacin, and naproxen, to kill the pain and reduce inflammation. Possible side effects include nausea, indigestion, diarrhea, and stomach ulcer. Narcotic analgesics (painkillers) may also be added to the treatment. If this fails to offer relief, the bursa may be drained and corticosteroid drugs may be injected into it. The joint is sometimes splinted after this procedure. High doses of corticosteroids can weaken the immune system. If an infection is present, antibiotics are first recommended.

In severe cases of bursitis, the lining of the fluid-filled bursa can be surgically removed.

ALTERNATIVE APPROACHES
CHIROPRACTIC

Chiropractic medicine holds promise for most people with musculoskeletal disorders such as bursitis. Performing adjustments or manipulations with the hands, the chiropractor directs treatment not just toward the injured joint but toward the whole body, unblocking any nerve interference that may be caused by a misaligned vertebra. For example, some forms of bursitis may result from a misplacement of a cervical (neck) vertebra.

The treatment goals are to reduce inflammation in the joint, restore proper posture and movement, and bring the body back to its healthy state, preventing the bursitis from occurring again.

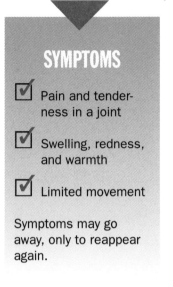 Only a trained practitioner is qualified to perform spinal manipulation. Chiropractors specialize in treating the spine and other joints. Osteopaths and naturopathic physicians may also employ these techniques, while physical therapists and massage therapists often incorporate elements such as trigger point therapy into their work. The treatment may also include an exercise and diet program.

ACUPUNCTURE

Acupuncture can relieve the pain of bursitis and restore function to the joint. But perhaps more important, this therapy can address the underlying im-

SYMPTOMS

☑ Pain and tenderness in a joint

☑ Swelling, redness, and warmth

☑ Limited movement

Symptoms may go away, only to reappear again.

balance in energy, or qi, that predisposed the person to bursitis in the first place.

In assessing a patient with bursitis, the acupuncturist looks beyond the symptoms to understand the health of the entire person. A complete physical is done (noting, among other things, the pulse and color of the tongue), and a history is taken. As needed, tiny needles are inserted in certain points on the body to replenish or disperse energy, bringing it back to its ideal level. These points can also be stimulated with needles and electrical current, as well as with pressure, heat, and cold.

OTHER THERAPIES

HERBAL MEDICINE—Arnica oil, comfrey, turmeric, and willow may be helpful.

HOMEOPATHY—Common remedies include bryonia alba and rhus toxicodendron.

HYDROTHERAPY—Relief may come from several days of ice pack applications followed by alternating hot and cold compresses, as well as castor oil packs applied to the joint (see Appendix 3).

NUTRITIONAL THERAPY—A poor, vitamin-deficient diet may predispose someone to bursitis. Among other things, increase intake of vitamins C and A and avoid caffeine.

OSTEOPATHY—Treatment involves aligning the spine, mobilizing the joints, and correcting posture to help blood flow freely in the body.

YOGA—This therapy can improve breathing, body posture, and muscle strength.

Chinese herbs are often added to an acupuncture treatment.

An acupuncturist, traditional Chinese physician, or naturopathic physician can perform acupuncture. For your first visit, be prepared to discuss in detail your bursitis symptoms, as well as your general health, diet, and lifestyle.

BODYWORK

Several forms of bodywork can be helpful for people with bursitis. None of these therapies claim to cure the condition. Rather, they can ease pain and bring the body back to a healthier, prime state, allowing it to heal itself. For example, massage therapy can reduce the pain of bursitis and increase blood supply to the tissues. A Swedish massage treatment for bursitis may use rhythmic, flowing strokes that are directed toward the heart.

Several bodywork techniques hold promise for bursitis sufferers:

- Applied kinesiology focuses on muscles to correct imbalances in the body's energy system (also involving diet and exercise regimens).
- Feldenkrais method uses specific movements to retrain the body to function at peak efficiency.
- Reflexology applies pressure to certain reflex points on the feet and hands to help the body heal itself.
- Rolfing involves the manipulation of the muscles and connective tissue to realign the body within the field of gravity.

A trained practitioner is needed to perform any of these bodywork therapies.

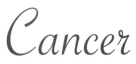

CANCER IS AN UMBRELLA TERM FOR MORE THAN 100 DIFFERENT DISEASES THAT SHARE A COMMON TRAIT: ABNORMAL CELLS THAT GROW UNCONTROLLABLY. THESE MUTATED CELLS CAN SHOW UP ON ALMOST ANY PART OF THE BODY, TYPICALLY DAMAGE NEIGHBORING BODY TISSUE, AND MAY SPREAD THROUGHOUT THE BODY.

CONVENTIONAL APPROACH

Allopathic medicine's treatment program and cure rate for cancer vary greatly, depending on the type of cancer and whether or not it has spread. Some treatments are aimed at curing the patient; other treatments take a less optimistic approach and are designed to improve the symptoms or quality of life.

Options for treatment include surgery, radiation, and drug therapy. They may be used alone (such as having only radiation for cervical cancer or only drug therapy for leukemia) or in combination.

SURGICAL TREATMENT

A cancerous tumor and surrounding tissue (such as muscle and lymph nodes) can be surgically removed, as long as the cancer has spread little or not at all. In some cases, part of the tumor may be cut out in preparation for other treatments.

RADIOTHERAPY

Ionizing radiation (high-energy X rays) can be aimed at the tumor in hopes of killing all of the cancer cells or shrinking the tumor (making it easier to remove surgically). Common side effects include hair loss, anemia, and fatigue. Radiation also carries the risk of triggering second tumors and other health problems.

DRUG TREATMENT

Chemotherapy works to destroy or inactivate cancerous cells, but it also harms some healthy cells in the process. It can involve any of a number of combinations of drugs given orally or by injection. It carries a number of potential side effects, including hair loss, nausea, anemia, water retention, fatigue, and bone marrow damage, which can weaken the immune system. Another drug treatment, hormone therapy, is sometimes used for prostate or breast cancers.

ALTERNATIVE APPROACHES

Perhaps more than any other ailment, cancer begs for alternatives to the conventional approach. America's cancer death rate continues to rise, and cancer is expected to nudge out heart disease and become the number one killer of American adults by the turn of the century.

For many people with cancer, selecting a treatment approach—whether to include elements of conventional medicine, alternative medicine, or both—is excruciatingly difficult. These people may decide to follow a conventional treatment program, using alternative therapies to ease the side effects of radiation or drug therapy, strengthen the immune system, and improve their well-being and outlook. Still other people prefer to rely only on alternative

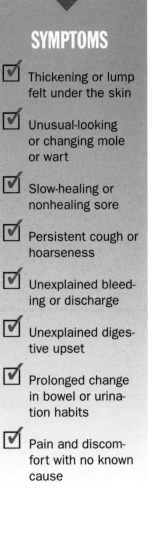

SYMPTOMS

- ☑ Thickening or lump felt under the skin
- ☑ Unusual-looking or changing mole or wart
- ☑ Slow-healing or nonhealing sore
- ☑ Persistent cough or hoarseness
- ☑ Unexplained bleeding or discharge
- ☑ Unexplained digestive upset
- ☑ Prolonged change in bowel or urination habits
- ☑ Pain and discomfort with no known cause

treatments, many of which focus on restoring general health.

NUTRITIONAL THERAPY

Nutritional therapists hold that a certain diet and certain supplements are an important part of the cancer treatment process. The goals include

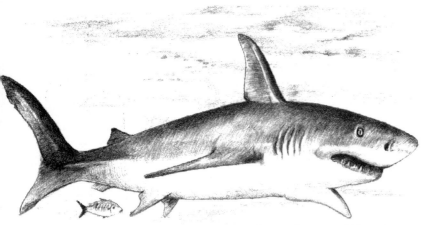

encouraging the proliferation of healthy cells, enhancing the immune system, and inhibiting cancerous tumors from growing. In general, the diet of someone with cancer should be

- rich in organic whole grains, vegetables, and fruits
- high in fiber
- low in refined sugars and low in sodium
- low in fat (deriving about 15 percent of daily calories from fat)

A vegetarian diet, with no meat, poultry, and fish, is recommended on the basis that it doesn't supply excess iron, a mineral that many types of tumors require to grow. The fat, chemicals, and other hormones found in red meat and chicken and the mercury and other pollutants found in fish caught in polluted water are also of great concern.

Shark Cartilage—Shark cartilage holds promise for people with cancer. Here's why: Cartilage—whether it comes from sharks or humans—has no need for an attached network of blood vessels to supply nutrients and oxygen and carry away wastes. Because of this, cartilage carries a substance that prevents blood vessels from forming. A cancerous tumor, on the other hand, does need a blood supply to thrive. Taking cartilage supplements can prevent the tumor from getting what it needs. Under this treatment, people with advanced cancer have reported their tumors stabilizing in size or shrinking.

Vitamin C—High doses of vitamin C are often prescribed to cancer patients. Researchers, including the famous vitamin C guru and Nobel laureate Linus Pauling, have found that people with cancer can experience shrinkage in tumor size after vitamin C treatments. It may also reduce some of the side effects of chemotherapy and radiation treatment.

Vitamin C is an antioxidant, which renders free radical compounds powerless. Occurring naturally in the body,

---

WHO USES ALTERNATIVE MEDICINE?

According to a 1988 nationwide survey commissioned by the American Cancer Society, 9 percent of people with cancer have used one or more alternative therapies for their disease. They most often turned to guided imagery, hypnotherapy, psychic healing, and special diets, and nearly 60 percent considered these therapies somewhat or very effective.

free radicals have the ability to damage tissue and speed the aging process. Antioxidants are often recommended to prevent some forms of cancer. Other nutrients that are antioxidants include

- beta-carotene
- vitamin A
- vitamin E
- selenium

Vitamin C functions to fight cancer in two other important ways as well: 1) It enhances the body's production of the connective tissue collagen, which can help to wall off the tumor; and 2) it enhances immune function, allowing the body to destroy cancer cells.

Other Emerging Supplements—Coenzyme Q_{10} has been shown to be very effective in the treatment of breast cancer at doses of 390 mg daily. Melatonin in fairly high doses (10 to 50 mg at bedtime) has been shown to improve the quality of life of patients with advanced solid tumors. And pH-modified citrus pectin was recently reported to aid in the prevention of metastatic (spreading) tumors of several types, including cancers of the breast, prostate, and skin. Because most cancer patients die as the result of a metastatic tumor and not the primary tumor, this is a potentially significant treatment option.

Prevention—Of course, it's better to prevent cancer than treat it after it has developed, and diet is estimated to be a contributing factor in 35 percent of cancer deaths. A first preventive step is avoiding the possible triggers of various types of cancer, which include

- high-fat diet
- lack of fiber
- deficiency in vitamin A
- food additives

THE NEXT BREAKTHROUGH?

Antineoplastons are one of the most promising alternative cancer therapies, yet their recognition has been suppressed by established conventional medicine. These naturally occurring peptides (compounds made up of amino acids) have been given to people with advanced cancer, causing many of them to experience remission. The developer of this therapy, Stanislaw Burzynski, M.D., Ph.D., of Houston, Texas, has been under fire by the American Cancer Society, Food and Drug Administration, and other government agencies for more than 10 years in an effort to halt his medical practice and research.

A practitioner of nutritional therapy may prescribe 10 grams of vitamin C per day. This is a high dose that will require monitoring by the practitioner. Higher doses—30 grams or more—are sometimes given intravenously to cancer patients.

MIND/BODY MEDICINE

Mind/body medicine recognizes that the mind plays a vital role in healing and recovery. In cancer treatment, various mind/body therapies can be used to control pain, relieve stress and anxiety, ease depression, and fortify the immune system.

If nothing else, these therapies seek to make people with cancer feel good about themselves and their lives.

Guided imagery, for example, encourages patients to picture their bodies' reaction to cancer in either medically accurate or highly personalized creative terms. Repeated use of these exercises is thought to contribute to a stronger immune system.

Other helpful mind/body therapies for cancer treatment include
- prayer and mental healing
- spirituality
- psychic healing
- biofeedback training
- meditation
- hypnotherapy

Guided imagery exercises should be performed two to three times a day, for about 20 minutes each time, during the cancer treatment program. Before starting each exercise, progressive muscle relaxation can be done as a way of "warming up." It involves letting go of tension in small, isolated steps:
- Sit in a comfortable chair or lie on a firm surface. Wear loose clothing.
- Close your eyes and begin breathing slowly and deeply.
- When relaxed, begin to visualize the white blood cells of your body as a large, highly organized troop of protective white knights.
- Imagine them finding and fighting off the small and weak cancerous cells.
- Feel this energy and activity happening inside your body.

OTHER THERAPIES

AYURVEDIC MEDICINE—Treatment may include herbal therapy, dietary changes, and meditation.

ENVIRONMENTAL MEDICINE—Cancer may be triggered by pollutants (such as asbestos), electromagnetic radiation, nutrient deficiencies, and other factors. Treatment can include, following a detoxification program, removing dental amalgam fillings.

HERBAL MEDICINE—Iscador (extracted from mistletoe), Venus flytrap, garlic, and astragalus can be effective. Two herb formulas, Hoxsey tonic and Essiac tea, have well-known anticancer properties.

TRADITIONAL CHINESE MEDICINE—Acupuncture, moxabustion, herbal therapy, qigong, and other therapies can be used to treat cancer. Beware that acupuncture may encourage certain types of cancer to spread.

OXYGEN THERAPY

Oxygen therapy employs two oxygen compounds, ozone and hydrogen peroxide, to wipe out cancer cells, which cannot withstand high oxygen concentrations. For example, research shows that ozone therapy can reduce the size of cancerous tumors.

Hydrogen peroxide is typically delivered to a patient via an intravenous drip, which lasts about one hour. Ozone treatment, on the other hand, involves drawing less than one pint of blood from the patient, mixing it with different amounts of ozone and oxygen, and then reintroducing it back into the blood vessels. Ozone can also be delivered through the rectum.

Oxygen therapy has more acceptance in Europe than in the United States. Nonetheless, several states permit medical doctors to use it in their practices.

Carpal Tunnel Syndrome

CARPAL TUNNEL SYNDROME IS AN INFLAMMATION OF THE NERVE THAT RUNS FROM THE FOREARM TO THE FINGERS, AS A RESULT OF THE NERVE BEING SQUEEZED IN THE TUNNEL OF WRIST BONES (CARPALS) AND LIGAMENTS (THE TISSUES THAT CONNECT BONES). IT CAN BE CAUSED BY REPETITIVE WRIST MOTION (SUCH AS TYPING), SUDDEN WEIGHT GAIN, OR FLUID ACCUMULATION.

CONVENTIONAL APPROACH

The first step in allopathic medicine's treatment program is resting the wrist and protecting it in a splint. If the pain continues, drug therapy and surgery are available.

Several medications are available to ease symptoms and encourage healing:

- Nonsteroidal anti-inflammatory drugs, such as aspirin, ibuprofen, and naproxen, are effective in fighting pain and inflammation.
- Corticosteroids can be injected under the ligament in the wrist to bring temporary relief.
- Diuretic drugs are used if any fluid is accumulating in nearby tissues.

Some severe cases may require surgery to cut the wrist ligament in the hopes of easing pressure on the nerve. Many people who undergo surgery see a return of symptoms within two years.

ALTERNATIVE APPROACHES
HOMEOPATHY

Homeopathic medicine works to treat carpal tunnel syndrome by giving highly diluted, nontoxic doses of a natural substance that would produce the same aching symptoms if given in full strength to a healthy person. The substances are taken from plant, mineral, or animal sources. To tailor a remedy for carpal tunnel syndrome, a classical homeopath questions the patient on the symptoms and assesses the general state of physical and emotional health. Using these clues, the remedy is then individualized to the patient. The following are some carpal tunnel syndrome characteristics to consider:

- When is the pain at its worst? Before or after movement?
- Does cold or heat ease the pain?
- Where on the body do the symptoms occur? On fingers, wrists, hands, arms, shoulders?

Some typical remedies for carpal tunnel syndrome are causticum, colchicum autumnale, hypericum perfoliatum, ruta graveolens, and rhus toxicodendron.

For a case of carpal tunnel syndrome characterized by a wrist that feels bruised, sore, and stiff, among other details, here's a sample homeopathic remedy: Take one oral dose of ruta graveolens, 6c, every six hours. (The 6c refers to the potency of the remedy.) Stop treatment as soon as the symptoms end.

HERBAL MEDICINE

Several herbs can provide relief by reducing inflammation. The flowering tops of St.-John's-wort, when applied to the skin as a cream, can ease inflammation of muscles and connective tissues. Meadowsweet leaves and

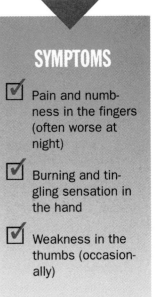

☑ Pain and numbness in the fingers (often worse at night)

☑ Burning and tingling sensation in the hand

☑ Weakness in the thumbs (occasionally)

Symptoms sometimes move up the arm and shoulder and may affect one or both hands.

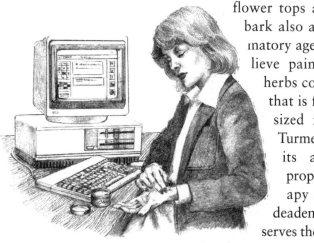

flower tops and white willow bark also act as anti-inflammatory agents, which can relieve pain. (Both of these herbs contain a substance that is found in a synthesized form in aspirin.) Turmeric is also used for its anti-inflammatory properties. Herbal therapy seeks to ease, not deaden, the pain, as pain serves the important role of signaling you to rest your wrist.

OTHER THERAPIES

ACUPRESSURE—Pressure applied to specific points, often on the wrist on the meridians of the large and small intestines, can relieve pain.

BODYWORK—Gentle wrist exercises and neck stretches can ease the pain of carpal tunnel syndrome and help release the pinched nerve.

CHIROPRACTIC—Spinal manipulation can relieve the compressed wrist nerves.

HYDROTHERAPY—Cold compresses or alternating hot and cold compresses can provide relief.

HYPNOTHERAPY—Trances employ the mind and body to reverse carpal tunnel syndrome.

NEURAL THERAPY—Injections of anesthetics, at certain points of the body, may treat the pain of chronic carpal tunnel syndrome.

OSTEOPATHY—Manual procedures can restore function to the wrist.

Here's a sample herbal remedy for carpal tunnel syndrome: Apply St.-John's-wort cream to the wrists once a day, as needed.

NUTRITIONAL THERAPY

Nutritional therapy can be used to fortify the body, treating and preventing wrist problems. Several studies have shown that many people with carpal tunnel syndrome are deficient in vitamin B_6 and that daily supplementation can ease the painful, tingling, and numbing symptoms. The vitamin treatment—sometimes combined with a high-potency B-complex supplement—can take about two months before it begins to work.

It is believed that certain seemingly unrelated dietary factors contribute to this vitamin deficiency, including high-protein diets, eating foods that contain yellow (hydrazine) dyes, and the use of oral contraceptives. These contributing factors should be avoided. In general, a sound diet should emphasize whole grains, seeds, nuts, and vegetables. Avoid excess protein and limit intake of sugars and caffeine.

A form of nutritional therapy called enzyme therapy may also be useful. Supplementation with the pineapple-derived enzyme bromelain has proved helpful for some patients. The enzyme is taken in capsules between meals.

The recommended dietary allowance for vitamin B_6 is 2 mg. However, to treat carpal tunnel syndrome, a naturopathic physician may prescribe 100 mg per day. High doses of this vitamin may be toxic, so a physician's monitoring is required.

Chronic Fatigue Syndrome

CHRONIC FATIGUE SYNDROME IS AN ILLNESS THAT PRODUCES SEVERE AND OFTEN DISABLING FATIGUE AND EXHAUSTION, ACCOMPANIED BY PAIN IN VARIOUS PARTS OF THE BODY. IT CAN LAST FOR MONTHS OR YEARS. ITS CAUSE IS UNKNOWN; IT MAY BE CAUSED BY MANY FACTORS, INCLUDING A MALFUNCTIONING IMMUNE SYSTEM, CHRONIC INFECTION, ALLERGIES, AND OTHERS.

CONVENTIONAL APPROACH

The allopathic medical community does not agree on what chronic fatigue syndrome is or even that it's a real illness. Usually, therefore, conventional treatment is aimed at relieving the symptoms and ignores possible causes.

DRUG TREATMENT

Commonly used medications include
- analgesics (painkillers), including aspirin and acetaminophen, for headaches and various pains
- nonsteroidal anti-inflammatory drugs, such as ibuprofen and naproxen, that can also relieve pain
- antihistamines, which can improve breathing and may induce sleep
- benzodiazepines to encourage sleep
- antidepressants
- antivirals

ALTERNATIVE APPROACHES

Chronic fatigue syndrome may puzzle conventional doctors, but a patient has many options in alternative therapies. In fact, naturopathic physicians, with their broad range of therapeutic options, may be the best qualified practitioners for these patients.

NUTRITIONAL THERAPY

Nutritional therapy's approach to chronic fatigue syndrome is twofold. It works to strengthen the health, in particular the immune system, and eliminate any dietary items that might be causing or aggravating the condition.

The most basic prescription is to eat an unrefined whole-foods diet, high in complex carbohydrates and fiber and low in sugar, fats, and protein (especially from animal sources). Adding raw garlic to the diet is also suggested for its potential to fight viruses, bacteria, and fungi. Eliminating caffeine because of its negative effects on the adrenal gland is also important.

An investigation into any food allergies or sensitivities that may be aggravating the symptoms is also recommended. An elimination diet will identify any culprits. In an elimination diet, frequently eaten foods and common food allergens (such as milk) are avoided for approximately two weeks. Foods are then reintroduced one at a time, making note of any change in symptoms. Foods that bring on or worsen symptoms should be avoided.

The following specific supplements can support the activities of the immune system and adrenal glands and are, therefore, frequently prescribed to people with chronic fatigue syndrome:
- vitamin C
- beta-carotene
- pantothenic acid (vitamin B_5)
- zinc
- magnesium (especially mixed with malic acid)
- adrenal extract

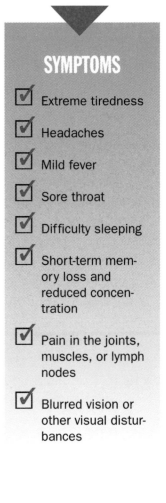

SYMPTOMS

- ☑ Extreme tiredness
- ☑ Headaches
- ☑ Mild fever
- ☑ Sore throat
- ☑ Difficulty sleeping
- ☑ Short-term memory loss and reduced concentration
- ☑ Pain in the joints, muscles, or lymph nodes
- ☑ Blurred vision or other visual disturbances

An overgrowth of the yeast *Candida albicans* has been linked to some cases. This yeast normally lives in the body, but certain factors (such as repeated treatment with antibiotics) cause it to multiply beyond healthy ranges. A diet free of sugars, including corn syrup, honey, dairy products (lactose), and fruit, is typically part of the program to treat yeast overgrowth. Products with baker's yeast, alcoholic beverages with brewer's yeast, and other aged or fermented foods are also to be avoided. Adding an antifungal substance such as garlic, caprylic acid, or grapefruit seed extract may also be useful.

Here's a sample nutritional prescription for chronic fatigue syndrome: Take a high-potency six-a-day multiple vitamin and mineral supplement and two adrenal extract tablets three times a day. Magnesium and malic acid (150 mg elemental magnesium) three times daily is also good, but check the amount of magnesium in the multimineral supplement.

ACUPUNCTURE

Acupuncture stimulates the body to heal and protect itself from disruptive forces—from viruses and poor diet to stress. Treatment for chronic fatigue syndrome typically focuses on points along the meridians (the energy channels) of the kidney, liver, lungs, and spleen, which control aspects of the immune system. Tiny needles are inserted in points on these meridians to replenish or disperse the flow of energy, or qi, bringing it to its ideal level.

In devising a personalized treatment, the acupuncturist looks beyond the symptoms to understand the health of the entire person. An acupuncturist will diagnose the problem with a physical and a medical history. Acupuncture treatment is often coupled with herbal therapy, dietary changes, and exercises.

An acupuncturist or naturopathic physician can perform acupuncture. For your first visit, be prepared to discuss in detail your symptoms and your general health, diet, and lifestyle.

OTHER THERAPIES

AYURVEDIC MEDICINE—Treatment includes dietary changes, herbal therapy, and stress-reduction techniques.

DETOXIFICATION, FASTING, AND COLON THERAPY—Fasts, special diets, and colonic irrigation can cleanse from the body toxins that are weakening it.

ENVIRONMENTAL MEDICINE—Certain chemicals, foods, emotional or physical stress, and infections can trigger chronic fatigue syndrome. Treatment involves desensitization and avoidance.

HERBAL MEDICINE—Echinacea, goldenseal, licorice, astragalus, panax ginseng, Siberian ginseng, and hypericum can be effective.

HOMEOPATHY—Specific remedies must be tailored to the individual.

OSTEOPATHY—Treatment involves physical manipulation, with drugs added if needed.

YOGA—Exercises and breathing techniques can give the body energy and reduce stress.

COLITIS IS AN INFLAMMATION OF THE MUCOUS MEMBRANE THAT LINES THE COLON (LARGE INTESTINE). THE INFLAMMATION CAN RESULT FROM A BACTERIAL OR VIRAL INFECTION OR THE USE OF ANTIBIOTIC DRUGS, AMONG OTHER CAUSES. ULCERATIVE COLITIS IS A MUCH MORE SERIOUS AND LONG-TERM INFLAMMATION AND ULCERATION OF THE COLON. IT HAS BEEN LINKED WITH AN INCREASED RISK OF COLON CANCER. ITS CAUSE IS UNKNOWN.

CONVENTIONAL APPROACH

COLITIS

Allopathic medicine usually suggests self-treatment measures and drug therapy for people with colitis. Bed rest is also beneficial. To deal with severe diarrhea, the patient should drink only water, tea (not black tea, which can be irritating), and clear broths and avoid all foods. However, this should not be done for more than five days without a doctor's supervision. If an infection is present, several antibiotic drugs may be effective.

ULCERATIVE COLITIS

Because no cure is available, treatment is aimed at relieving the symptoms. Common medications include
- corticosteroids
- sulfasalazine
- immunosuppressive drugs used when other drugs are not effective

When symptoms don't respond to courses of medication, all or part of the colon and rectum can be surgically removed.

ALTERNATIVE APPROACHES

Several alternative therapies offer ways other than drugs or surgery to treat an inflamed colon. *In cases of ulcerative colitis, the treatments should not be self-administered.*

HERBAL MEDICINE

Several herbs can offer relief from colitis as well as ulcerative colitis. Herbs called demulcents can soothe the mucous membranes that line the colon and trigger the production of more mucus to ease irritation and lessen symptoms. Slippery elm bark and marshmallow root are two commonly used demulcents.

Robert's Formula, a well-known naturopathic herbal remedy, is often prescribed to heal intestinal irritation and inflammation. It contains slippery elm, marshmallow root, comfrey, echinacea (purple coneflower), goldenseal, and other herbs, as well as cabbage powder.

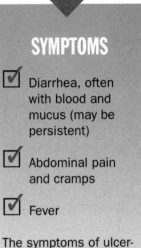 A naturopathic physician may recommend taking two doses of Robert's Formula three times a day, with meals. (See Appendix 3 for a sample recipe.)

NUTRITIONAL THERAPY

Nutritional therapists contend that altering the diet may eliminate ulcerative colitis or reduce its harmful effects. Food allergies (or sensitivities) are thought to contribute to the onset of colon inflammation. Wheat, corn, and dairy products are common allergens. Following an elimination diet will re-

SYMPTOMS

- ☑ Diarrhea, often with blood and mucus (may be persistent)
- ☑ Abdominal pain and cramps
- ☑ Fever

The symptoms of ulcerative colitis may go away, only to reappear later. Most cases of ulcerative colitis initially appear in people 20 to 30 years of age.

veal if any foods make the symptoms worse.

Once the colon is inflamed, it no longer performs at peak. This can lead to an upset in the normal bacterial makeup of the intestines and to nutritional deficiencies. A therapy called probiotics aims to reestablish the ideal levels of the natural intestinal bacteria. Bacteria such as *Lactobacillus acidophilus* can be taken in powder, capsule, or liquid form (however, this bacteria should be avoided if the patient is lactose intolerant).

OTHER THERAPIES

AROMATHERAPY—Massages with essential oils (such as patchouli and peppermint) can offer relief from colitis.

AYURVEDIC MEDICINE—Using herbal therapy, meditation, and dietary changes, Ayurvedic practitioners can treat both colitis and ulcerative colitis.

CHIROPRACTIC—A chiropractor can readjust the spine, the misalignment of which can affect the functioning of the digestive tract.

DETOXIFICATION, FASTING, AND COLON THERAPY—Water or juice fasts can give the colon's inflamed lining time to heal. Fasting is also used to cleanse the body before food allergy tests begin.

HOMEOPATHY—Homeopathy is a very important therapy for colitis, but a complete evaluation by a professional is necessary.

TRADITIONAL CHINESE MEDICINE—Treatment may include acupuncture, moxibustion, herbal therapy (including herbal enemas), and yoga (including breathing exercises).

Another serious concern in both types of colitis is nutritional deficiencies. Nutritional deficiencies may result for several reasons:
- People with the disorder may eat less than needed as a way of avoiding diarrhea and abdominal pain.
- Chronic diarrhea can lead to the loss of nutrients.
- Some of the drugs used in conventional treatment (such as corticosteroids) may interrupt nutrient metabolism.
- Mucosal irregularities can result in poor nutrient absorption.

These patients, therefore, can benefit from taking supplements orally or by injection (sometimes as much as five times the recommended dietary allowance) and eating smaller, more frequent meals.

An elimination diet can help the health practitioner and patient link any foods with an aggravation of symptoms. Here's how it might work:
- For two to three weeks, the patient's commonly eaten foods are eliminated from the diet. Instead, the diet should consist of foods—such as rice, lamb, iceberg lettuce, cranberries, cherries, apples, olive oil, apricots, peaches, and spinach—that are not usually associated with allergies.
- If symptoms have subsided or not appeared by the end of this period, then the food challenges can begin. If the symptoms are still present, then more foods should be eliminated from the diet.
- Reintroduce the commonly eaten foods one at a time, every two days, noting if any symptoms appear.

ANY OF ABOUT 200 VIRUSES CAN CAUSE THE COMMON COLD AND BRING ON THE ALL-TOO-FAMILIAR SYMPTOMS THAT CAN RANGE FROM AN ANNOYING SCRATCHY THROAT TO A THROBBING HEAD COLD THAT BRINGS YOU TO A HALT. COLD VIRUSES SPREAD RELATIVELY EASILY FROM PERSON TO PERSON AND HIT MOST PEOPLE IN THE WINTER.

CONVENTIONAL APPROACH

Allopathic medicine hasn't found a cure for the common cold, but research continues. In the meantime, when a cold hits, most people who follow conventional medicine take treatment into their own hands. They turn to the massive array of over-the-counter cold remedies, which may offer temporary or partial relief from cold symptoms. These treatments often contain a combination of ingredients:

- Pain relievers, such as aspirin and acetaminophen, can be used for headaches and body aches and to reduce fever. Side effects range from stomach irritation to nausea. (Children under 18 years old with fevers should not be given aspirin, which may lead to the potentially fatal disorder called Reye syndrome.)

- Caffeine is sometimes included to boost the pain reliever's effectiveness, although caffeine's ability to do this is doubtful.

- Antihistamines, such as chlorpheniramine and diphenhydramine, may stop a runny nose and suppress coughing. Their most notable side effect is drowsiness; others include dry mouth and blurred vision.

- Decongestants, such as pseudoephedrine and phenylephrine, can relieve a stuffed-up nose. Tremors and heart palpitations may result. When taking the drug in the form of nose drops or sprays, the symptoms can return in a more severe form when the dose wears off.

Doctors sometimes prescribe antibiotics to their patients with common colds, although this treatment is only good for bacterial infections and does nothing to kill a cold virus.

ALTERNATIVE APPROACHES

Many alternative therapists believe the symptoms of the common cold should not be suppressed. They are the body's way of fighting a cold virus and, therefore, should be encouraged to do their work. Alternative treatments hold promise to shorten the duration of a cold and maybe even prevent one.

NUTRITIONAL THERAPY

According to nutritional therapy, eating certain foods and taking supplements can mean the difference between catching a lot of colds and few colds, as well as between colds that drag on and colds that disappear quickly.

A sound diet does go a long way toward fostering a strong immune system that can stand up to cold viruses. This sound diet means cutting down on sugars, fats, and alcohol and loading up on fresh vegetables, whole grains, easy-to-digest proteins, and essential fatty acids. Milk and dairy products should also be eliminated from the diet, either

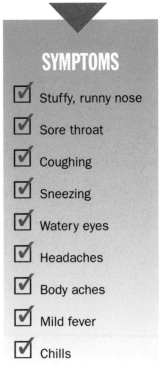

SYMPTOMS

- ☑ Stuffy, runny nose
- ☑ Sore throat
- ☑ Coughing
- ☑ Sneezing
- ☑ Watery eyes
- ☑ Headaches
- ☑ Body aches
- ☑ Mild fever
- ☑ Chills

during a cold or year-round. They can trigger the body's production of mucus, compounding the problems of a cold.

After a cold has started, large doses of vitamin C can ease the symptoms and may even shorten the sickness. Numerous studies have proved this effect, which is usually attributed to the vitamin's antioxidant properties. Whether vitamin C can actually prevent colds is still being debated.

Zinc may also speed up the recovery from a cold, perhaps by blocking viruses from multiplying. Several studies have illustrated this effect: A group of Texas researchers, for example, compared the effectiveness of zinc gluconate lozenges to a placebo. After seven days of treatment, 86 percent of the patients who took the zinc got rid of their cold symptoms. Less than half of the patients who took the placebo were symptom free.

A possible prescription for vitamin C might be to take 4,000 to 5,000 mg per day until the cold symptoms go away. The doses should be spaced out during the day—in four or five doses—or the excess vitamin will simply be eliminated in the urine. Some practitioners recommend up to 1,000 mg per hour if your bowels can handle that much. Eating oranges is helpful, but stay away from juices that contain a lot of sugar.

HERBAL MEDICINE

In the effort to stave off the common cold, herbs can be used to strengthen the body's immune system. When a cold virus has already taken hold, herbs can ease—not mask—a battery of symptoms: sore throat, stuffy nose, overproduction of mucus, fever, and other symptoms.

Echinacea (or purple coneflower) may perform two valuable functions for people with colds: weakening cold viruses and stimulating the body's defenses to work better. Taking this herb—usually in the form of a tincture—can shorten the duration of a cold. Goldenseal is often combined with echinacea in herbal cold treatments. It's also an immune-booster, and the herb may lessen mucus in the nose and throat as well. (For suggestions on how to use purple coneflower, see Appendix 3.)

Other immune-fortifying herbs include garlic, ginger, and astragalus. The list of herbs that can make cold symptoms bearable is quite long. Most of the following can be made into teas that can soothe symptoms:
- chamomile
- elder flowers
- hyssop
- peppermint
- rose hips
- yarrow

 At the first sign of a cold, an herbalist may prescribe 15 to

---

VITAMIN C TO THE RESCUE

Since Nobel-winning chemist Linus Pauling wrote the landmark book *Vitamin C and the Common Cold* in 1970, the benefits of this nutritional treatment have been examined in about 20 experiments. Most have confirmed the vitamin's ability to shorten colds or ease their symptoms.

20 drops of echinacea tincture four times a day. The drops can be diluted in a cup of warm water. Stop the treatment as soon as the cold symptoms disappear.

TRADITIONAL CHINESE MEDICINE

Traditional Chinese medicine attributes the common cold to causes that originate outside of the body—the so-called external factors such as wind and cold. Poor diets and too much stress are just two of the things that can knock out the body's resistance and make it vulnerable to these external factors. The factors involved then determine the specific cold symptoms a person will have. The therapies of traditional Chinese medicine work to restore the flow of the body's energy, or qi, and return yin and yang to harmony.

Herbal therapy in the traditional Chinese treatment of colds involves a mix of herbs such as ma huang (Chinese ephedra), lian qiao (forsythia), and jin yin (honeysuckle). These are usually given in the form of a decoction—a concentrated extract. The herbs used depend on the factors causing the illness. For example, warming herbs are prescribed if the illness is caused by cold.

Traditional Chinese medicine sometimes employs acupuncture to replenish or disperse energy. Colds due to both wind and cold, for example, may respond to acupuncture at the points Dazhui (Du14), Fengchi (GB13), and Quchi (LI11).

Acupressure—similar to acupuncture, except finger and hand pressure is used instead of needles—may also be useful.

Here's a sample acupressure treatment for colds that have symptoms of fever and headaches:

- Wear loose clothing and sit in a comfortable position.
- To find pressure point LI11, bend the right elbow. With your left thumb, apply firm pressure to the top of the elbow crease. (Use your other fingers on your left hand to cradle the elbow.)

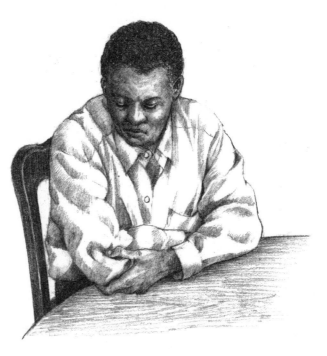

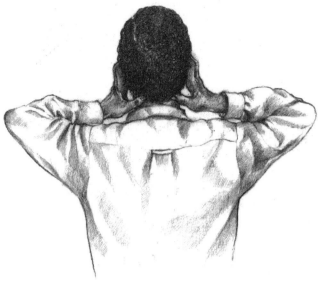

- Hold for one to two minutes.
- Repeat on the left elbow.
- Next, to find pressure point GB20, put both hands behind the head. Place your thumbs at the base of the skull on either side of the spine.

OTHER THERAPIES

AYURVEDIC MEDICINE—Treatment usually involves a special diet (including lots of whole grains but no dairy products, for example) and herbs (such as cinnamon, ginger, or licorice).

DETOXIFICATION, FASTING, AND COLON THERAPY—Water and herbal tea fasts and juice diets, lasting only a couple of days, can be helpful.

HOMEOPATHY—Specific remedies must be tailored to the individual, but common prescriptions include aconitum napellus, belladonna, euphrasia, and natrum muriaticum.

HYDROTHERAPY—Treatment may involve nasal flushing, steaming hot baths, and alternating hot and cold compresses, applied to the neck.

- Tilt your head back slightly.
- Apply pressure with the thumbs for about one minute.

AROMATHERAPY

Aromatherapy holds that the essential oils of certain plants can gently relieve cold symptoms and may even help fight viruses. Commonly used oils include

- eucalyptus to clear breathing and ease a cough and fever
- lavender to alleviate congestion, enhance sleep, and stimulate the immune system
- hyssop to aid free breathing and induce sweating
- peppermint to ease congestion, correct any digestive disturbances, and cleanse and cool the body
- yarrow to reduce fever, promote sweating, and clear breathing passageways

Depending on the essential oil, it can be used alone or in combination with others. They are often mixed with steaming water and inhaled or combined with a massage oil and worked into the chest.

The following aromatherapy treatment can help bring up phlegm from the airways, making breathing easier:

- Boil about eight cups of water.
- Remove the pan from the stove top, and add three to four drops of essential eucalyptus oil.
- Hold your head over the pan, and then create a tent over your head with a towel, trapping in the steam. (Let the water cool off if it's too hot.)
- Inhale the vapors for no more than ten minutes.

Constipation

CONSTIPATION IS THE INFREQUENT AND DIFFICULT MOVEMENT OF THE BOWELS. ITS CAUSES ARE NUMEROUS, INCLUDING A DIET LOW IN FIBER, IRREGULAR TOILET HABITS, IRRITABLE BOWEL SYNDROME, DIABETES, HYPOTHYROIDISM, CHRONIC TENSION, AND EVEN DEPRESSION.

CONVENTIONAL APPROACH

Allopathic medicine offers several self-treatment approaches to constipation, including

- adding fiber to the diet, from sources such as fruits, vegetables, bran, or fiber supplements
- drinking at least eight glasses of water daily
- adopting regular toilet habits and never ignoring the urge to have a bowel movement
- exercising
- using enemas

In addition, several forms of laxative medications are available but should only be used on a short-term basis.

ALTERNATIVE APPROACHES

The ideal frequency of bowel movements is much debated by conventional and alternative medicine. On the whole, alternative therapists recommend at least one per day.

NUTRITIONAL THERAPY

A nutritional therapist's view of constipation is quite straightforward: What goes in the mouth affects how waste products will or—in the case of constipation—will not exit the body. And constipation is more than uncomfortable: It causes toxins to linger in the bowels, a problem that has been linked to a number of ailments.

The diet must be high in fiber to encourage regular bowel movements, and water and other fluids need to accompany the fiber so the stool has the proper consistency. Fiber can be added with whole foods or powder (such as flaxseed powder). A nutrient deficiency (perhaps magnesium or vitamin C) may also cause constipation, in which case supplements can help.

Prunes and prune juice have a laxative effect, but they can also have an addictive effect; that is, the bowel becomes dependent on them.

For regular bowel movements, try to eat at least 30 grams of insoluble fiber per day. Read food labels. Good sources are

- bran
- fresh fruits and vegetables
- brown rice

BIOFEEDBACK TRAINING

Biofeedback training can give the person with constipation greater control over the digestive system. With the help of monitors that "feed back" certain biological levels, the therapy instructs people to alter involuntary functions of the body.

In one type of training, electrodes are attached to the skin around the anus to give the patient readings on the tightness or looseness of local muscles. The biofeedback technician teaches the patient to relax the muscles around the anus while pushing stool through the bowels. The therapy usually includes

SYMPTOMS

- ☑ Hard, dry stools
- ☑ Fewer bowel movements than normal (Depending on the person, the normal number of movements can be as many as three a day or as little as three a week.)
- ☑ Pain in the lower abdomen or when passing stool (occasionally)
- ☑ Rectal fissures
- ☑ Hemorrhoid development

relaxation techniques, such as progressive muscle relaxation, that can be done at home to reinforce the effects of the training.

At least two studies have shown the effectiveness of biofeedback training for children whose constipation is attributed to the improper tightening of anal muscles.

Progressive muscle relaxation aided by biofeedback monitoring involves letting go of tension in the body in little, isolated steps. Here's a sample exercise for progressive relaxation:
- Wearing loose clothing, lie down on a padded surface or sit in a comfortable chair.
- Close your eyes and tighten the muscles in your feet. Then release these muscles.
- Next, direct your attention to your calves, tensing and then easing these muscles in the same fashion.

OTHER THERAPIES

CHIROPRACTIC—Some cases of constipation can be relieved by realigning the spine.

DETOXIFICATION, FASTING, AND COLON THERAPY—Certain forms of enemas and colonic irrigation can be effective for constipation.

HOMEOPATHY—Common remedies range from nux vomica to alumina.

YOGA—Several breathing exercises and poses can clear the body's energy flow, encouraging movement of the bowels.

- Continue up the body, including your arms and ending with your scalp.

HERBAL MEDICINE
Many herbs can effectively relieve the occasional bout with constipation. In fact, several laxatives used in conventional medicine contain ingredients derived from herbs, such as cascara and senna.

The aged bark of cascara encourages the movement of stool by irritating the bowels. Often taken in tincture or pill form, it's considered a strong laxative and may cause cramping. Other, milder laxative herbs include dandelion root and burdock root and leaves. Yellow dock can also be used to soften stools. These are commonly taken as tinctures.

Psyllium seed husks can be used to make a homemade bulking agent (similar to the commercially prepared psyllium products). Psyllium adds form and softness to the stool. It is important to drink enough water with these products: at least eight ounces with the dose and eight ounces after.

Although herbalists consider herbs to have fewer side effects than drugs, the plants still should only be used infrequently. If the bowels are repeatedly blocked, the cause should be corrected.

The list of other herbs with promising laxative qualities includes
- aloe
- dong quai
- licorice

A sample herbal prescription might be to mix one dropperful of cascara tincture with a cup of warm water. Drink the mixture just before bedtime.

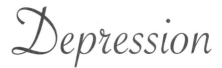

Depression

CLINICAL DEPRESSION IS AN ILLNESS THAT CAUSES A PERSON'S MOOD AND BE-HAVIOR TO CHANGE FOR LONG PERIODS OF TIME. IT'S MAINLY CHARACTERIZED BY FEELINGS OF SADNESS, IRRITABILITY, OR INDIFFERENCE. DEPRESSION MAY RE-SULT FROM A CHEMICAL IMBALANCE IN THE BRAIN, AND EPISODES CAN BE TRIG-GERED BY A TRAUMATIC EVENT, PROLONGED STRESS, AND OTHER FACTORS.

CONVENTIONAL APPROACH

To treat clinical depression, allo-pathic medicine relies on drug therapy, psychotherapy, or both. According to National Institute of Mental Health es-timates, this treatment program is ef-fective for about 80 percent of people with depression. The problem is the majority of people with depression never seek treatment.

DRUG TREATMENT

Antidepressants are the drugs of choice and are used to correct chemi-cal imbalances in the brain. Often they need to be taken for six to eight weeks before their effects begin, and treat-ment usually lasts 6 to 12 months or more. The three types of antidepres-sants are
- tricyclics, such as desipramine and imipramine
- monoamine oxidase (MAO) in-hibitors, including phenelzine and tranylcypromine
- serotonin reuptake inhibitors, such as fluoxetine (Prozac) and sertraline

Depending on the drug, the side ef-fects can include blurred vision, drowsiness, insomnia, impotence, ab-normal heartbeat, and increased blood pressure, among others. To treat manic depression (a type of depression with severe mood swings), several other drugs may be used, including lithium and anticonvulsants.

PSYCHOLOGICAL TREATMENT

Talking with trained therapists about one's symptoms, behavior, his-tory, and future may help some peo-ple with depression. Areas of concern may include negative thinking and un-happy personal relationships. Treat-ment can be simple (consisting of support and advice) or extensive (in-volving in-depth analysis).

OTHER TREATMENT

Severe cases of depression can be treated with electroconvulsive therapy, which sends an electric current through the head.

ALTERNATIVE APPROACHES

The following alternative medicine treatments for depression should be ac-companied by regular exercise, relax-ation measures, and participation in support groups.

NUTRITIONAL THERAPY

Nutritional therapy offers a lot of promise for treating clinical depression that is triggered by chemical imbal-ances in the brain or nutritional defi-ciencies. Whereas allopathic medicine uses drugs to correct the brain's chem-ical upsets, nutritional therapy employs certain nutritional supplements to do the same thing.

Here's how the theory goes: The body requires certain building-block

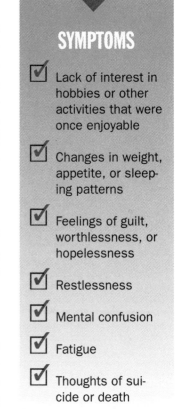

SYMPTOMS

☑ Lack of interest in hobbies or other activities that were once enjoyable

☑ Changes in weight, appetite, or sleep-ing patterns

☑ Feelings of guilt, worthlessness, or hopelessness

☑ Restlessness

☑ Mental confusion

☑ Fatigue

☑ Thoughts of sui-cide or death

chemicals before it can make important biochemicals. For example, the amino acid tryptophan is needed for the synthesis of serotonin, a mood-regulating chemical in the brain, and the amino acid tyrosine is needed for the brain chemical norepinephrine. So, adding these amino acids should help reestablish a healthy balance of brain chemicals.

Many nutritional practitioners report positive results with this approach. In addition, researchers have found that some people with depression are deficient in one or more nutrients, several of which play a role in the function of certain brain chemicals. These nutrients include

- ascorbic acid (vitamin C)
- cyanocobalamin (vitamin B_{12})
- folate (vitamin B_9)
- niacin (vitamin B_3)
- pyridoxine (vitamin B_6)
- riboflavin (vitamin B_2)
- L-tyrosine
- DL-phenylalanine

Depending on the deficiencies, supplementation is recommended. A nutritional treatment program for depression may also include an investigation into food allergies and low blood sugar, among other possible causes.

A high-potency B-complex supplement combined with one of two amino acids—L-tyrosine (1,500 mg twice daily) or DL-phenylalanine (1,000 mg twice daily)—can be an effective treatment. Take the amino acid doses in the morning and afternoon, as they can cause sleeplessness.

HERBAL MEDICINE

Several herbs can restore function to the nervous system, ease muscle tension, and promote sleep, among other mood-altering actions. Patience is required, however, as they usually work slowly. St.-John's-wort has long been used to treat emotional upsets. This herb's flowering tops are commonly taken in the form of a tea or tincture. According to a recent clinical study, St.-John's-wort eased the symptoms of mild to moderate depression for two-thirds of the people tested. Other helpful herbs include

- borage
- lady's slipper
- oatstraw
- skullcap
- valerian
- vervain
- ginkgo

For someone with mild to moderate depression, an herbalist may prescribe taking 300 mg of St.-John's-wort three times a day. Look for standardized extract in capsules (standardized to at least 3 percent hypericin).

TAKING CHARGE OF DEPRESSION

Twenty percent of people with depression turn to alternative therapies for treatment, according to a 1993 survey by Harvard Medical School researchers. It seems these people prefer to play an active role in their treatment: The most frequently used therapies were relaxation techniques and self-help groups.

HOMEOPATHY

Homeopathic treatment for depression stimulates the mind and body to return to a healthy, fully functioning state. For example, a homeopathic remedy may help someone open up to express oneself better and talk about troubles and concerns, thereby furthering the recovery process. This therapy uses highly diluted doses of natural substances, which would cause the symptoms of depression if given in full strength to a healthy person. The substances are from plant, mineral, and animal sources.

A remedy is tailored specifically to individual patients and depends on their particular emotional and physical symptoms, as well as their general state of health. Common remedies for depression include china officinalis, ignatia amara, natrum muriaticum, pulsatilla nigricans, aurum, and sepia.

For acute depression or grief associated with the loss of a loved one or the end of a relationship, take ignatia, 30c, twice daily at least 20 minutes apart from meals. (The *30c* refers to the potency of the remedy.) Take the remedy for a week or less if symptoms improve sooner.

WAVE THERAPY

Light therapy is particularly effective for people with seasonal affective disorder—a depression that's triggered by a lack of light and usually occurs during months when there are fewer hours of daylight. A typical treatment calls for sitting in front of a full-spectrum fluorescent light (one that's approximately 12 times brighter than ordinary indoor light) for about two hours per day. This therapy is widely used by both conventional and alternative medicine.

Here's some helpful light therapy tips for people with seasonal affective disorder:
- Exercise outdoors each day around noontime.
- Trim trees and bushes that prevent sunlight from coming through windows.
- Plan a winter vacation in a sunny, southern location if possible.

OTHER THERAPIES

ACUPUNCTURE—Treatment aims to rebalance the flow of vital energy, or qi, and focuses on points along certain meridians, such as the heart meridian.

AROMATHERAPY—Essential oils from benzoin, bergamot, jasmine, and neroli may be helpful. They can be added to baths, mixed with steaming water and inhaled, or massaged into the body.

BODYWORK—Massage can ease depression, as shown in recent clinical studies.

ENVIRONMENTAL MEDICINE—Certain foods, chemicals, and other environmental factors are thought to trigger depression in susceptible people. Treatment includes avoidance and dietary changes.

GUIDED IMAGERY AND CREATIVE VISUALIZATION—Mental exercises can encourage relaxation and improve mental outlook.

YOGA—Postures and breathing exercises instill energy and confidence and reduce stress.

Dermatitis

Dermatitis is an inflammation of the skin that can have many causes, including allergy or infection. Many types of dermatitis are more commonly known as eczema. Some classifications include atopic dermatitis (related to an allergy), contact dermatitis (related to an allergy or irritant), and seborrheic (related to irregularities of the the sebaceous, or oil, glands).

SYMPTOMS

- ☑ Skin is red or brownish, blistering, oozing, crusting, or scaly.

- ☑ Itching varies from mild to intense.

- ☑ It commonly occurs on scalp, face, neck, upper chest, elbow bends, wrists, backs of knees, or ankles.

- ☑ With infants, it appears on face, scalp, or diaper area.

CONVENTIONAL APPROACH

Allopathic medicine works to relieve the pain of dermatitis rashes and, in some patients, attempts to shorten and ease the course of the disease. Medications and some lifestyle adjustments are the main weapons in conventional medicine's arsenal.

Dermatologists may instruct patients on ways to eliminate irritants, such as scratchy clothing and certain lotions, and how to bathe properly. A physician may also advise stress-reduction techniques to eliminate or alleviate anxiety-induced flare-ups.

Treatments can include

- medications applied to the skin, including corticosteroid ointments or tar creams, which stop the redness, itching, and inflammation but can bring side effects such as thinning of the skin
- oral drugs including antihistamines (to control allergy-induced itching), antibiotics (to fight infection), and corticosteroids (to reduce inflammation), with side effects ranging from simple drowsiness to chronic high blood pressure
- ultraviolet light therapy in severe cases, but the risks and benefits must be weighed carefully

After treatment, dermatitis may return, and then another course of treatment is necessary. Although some dermatitis conditions are thought to be related to allergies, the sufferers often do not test positive for the offending allergens.

ALTERNATIVE APPROACHES
TRADITIONAL CHINESE MEDICINE

With dermatitis, traditional Chinese medicine aims to correct imbalances in the total body, not just in the skin. The menu of treatments can include herbal medicine, acupuncture, and dietary recommendations.

A traditional Chinese physician tailors the therapy to the needs of each dermatitis sufferer. For example, two people with the same condition won't necessarily take the same herbs or follow the same exercise regimen.

Researchers in London showed that traditional Chinese herbal therapy benefits both adults and children with atopic dermatitis. In one trial, adults were given either a daily mixture of ten herbs (which had been simmered in water) or a placebo. Contrary to the medicine's philosophy, which usually prescribes medicine on an individual basis, these researchers gave the identical herbal formula to all study patients. Nonetheless, after two months, those taking the herbs experienced significantly less redness, scaling, and other symptoms than the subjects taking the placebo.

A dermatitis treatment might call for a daily herbal tea, made by boiling and then simmering dried herbs for an hour and a half. The tea could include the following traditional Chinese herbs (a chien is a traditional unit of measure for herbs that equals about 3.75 grams or about ⅛ ounce):

- 1.5 chien *Clematis armandii*
- 1.5–2 chien *Dictamnus dasycarpus* (bai xian pi)
- 1–1.5 chien *Glycyrrhiza glabra* (licorice)
- 2 chien *Ledebouriella seseloides* (fang feng)
- 2 chien *Lophatherum gracile* (dan zhu ye)
- 2–3 chien *Paeonia lactiflora* (red peony)
- 2–3 chien *Rehmannia glutinosa* (di huang)
- 1.5–2 chien *Schiaonepeta tenuifolia*
- 2–3 chien *Tribulus terrestris* (ci ji li)

Because traditional Chinese medicine's remedies are individualized, it is necessary to contact a qualified practitioner to obtain an accurate diagnosis and a specific prescription for your condition.

NUTRITIONAL THERAPY

According to nutritional therapy, certain foods can be one of the triggers of dermatitis, especially in children. Removing the perpetrators from the diet can give the body more tolerance for other triggers, such as stress, dust mites, or animal dander. Dairy products, eggs, and wheat are common culprits.

Dermatitis patients may not necessarily test allergic to the foods whose elimination helps their skin condition. For this reason, some practitioners prefer to use the terms "food intolerance" or "food sensitivities" instead of "food allergies."

Dermatitis sufferers may also benefit from adding essential fatty acids, which promote healthy skin. In one study, a group of Italian researchers treated two- to four-year-old children suffering from atopic eczema with daily doses of evening primrose oil (rich in essential fatty acids). After four weeks, the children's symptoms dramatically improved. These young pa-

OTHER THERAPIES

ACUPUNCTURE—Treatments can correct any imbalances in vital life energy (perhaps along the lung, large intestine, or liver system meridians) that may be triggering skin inflammation.

DETOXIFICATION, FASTING, AND COLON THERAPY—The skin reveals any upsets or impurities inside the body, so detoxification therapy is helpful.

HOMEOPATHY—Specific remedies must be tailored to the individual, but common prescriptions include graphites, rhus toxicodendron, and sulphur.

HYPNOTHERAPY—Hypnotic trances can give the subconscious mind suggestions regarding stress reduction and the healing of the inflammation.

MEDITATION—Regular meditation is useful for stress reduction and deep breathing, both important to a well-rounded dermatitis treatment program.

tients continued the treatment for 20 weeks with the same results and experienced no adverse side effects. Other studies have also confirmed these positive findings.

Supplementation with vitamin A, vitamin E, and zinc can also be useful in some cases of atopic dermatitis.

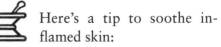 To see if any foods are related to your skin reaction, a nutritional practitioner may suggest an elimination diet. Cut the following items from your diet for two to three weeks:

- milk
- cheese
- eggs
- pork
- fish
- shellfish
- nuts
- all fruit (including tomatoes)
- wheat
- yeast

Keep note of the changes in your skin condition. If there's been an improvement after two to three weeks, the practitioner may suggest a food challenge: Reintroduce the foods one at time, starting with the one you used to eat most often. If none of your symptoms return in a day or two, keep that food in your diet. Naturally, if the redness and inflammation resurface, eliminate the culprit from your diet for good. Continue to reintroduce other foods every two to three days and keep track of the results.

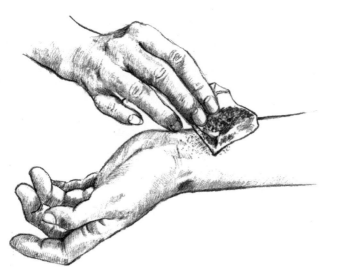

HERBAL MEDICINE

Herbal medicine practitioners think that some parts of the body—such as the liver or the nervous system—may need strengthening and tuning to head off a case of dermatitis. Several herbs can assist in cleansing the body and getting rid of toxins. Burdock, for example, is a liver tonic; when the liver is working well to filter toxins from the blood, the skin is generally healthier. Similarly, red clover is a very effective blood purifier.

Other herbs can directly ease the pain of itchy, inflamed skin. For example, preparations made from licorice root, calendula (marigold) flower heads, and especially ginkgo all have potent anti-inflammatory effects when used topically.

Here's a tip to soothe inflamed skin:

- Dip a chamomile tea bag in comfortably warm water.
- Hold on the lesion for a couple of minutes.
- Reheat and repeat if desired.

In cases where the dermatitis covers a large area, chamomile extract in a cream form may be easier than using the tea bags.

$\mathcal{D}$iabetes

DIABETES MELLITUS IS A DISORDER THAT PREVENTS THE BODY FROM EFFECTIVELY CONVERTING CARBOHYDRATES (SUGARS AND STARCHES) INTO ENERGY. INSULIN-DEPENDENT (TYPE I) DIABETES OCCURS WHEN THE PANCREAS GLAND STOPS PRODUCING INSULIN (A HORMONE THAT HELPS IN THE CONVERSION PROCESS), WHEREAS NON–INSULIN-DEPENDENT (TYPE II) DIABETES HAPPENS WHEN THE BODY DOESN'T PROPERLY USE THE INSULIN IT HAS.

CONVENTIONAL APPROACH

There is no one cure for diabetes, so allopathic medicine focuses on managing the disease. Depending on the type of diabetes, an effective treatment program can include any combination of drug therapy (including insulin injections), dietary changes, weight control, and exercise. The goal is to keep glucose (blood sugar) within healthy limits and to stave off any complications (such as kidney damage, visual problems, and heart disease).

People with type I diabetes require daily injections of insulin, while people with type II need injections only if their diabetes can't be controlled with lifestyle changes or oral hypoglycemic drugs. Insulin overdoses can lead to hypoglycemia, which carries the risk of insulin shock, which can cause disorientation, mood swings, profuse perspiration, convulsions, loss of consciousness, and even death.

People with type II diabetes may need hypoglycemic drugs if they can't maintain their blood glucose levels with dietary alterations, weight loss, and exercise. These oral medicines trigger the pancreas to make more insulin.

The dietary guidelines for diabetes usually emphasize eating more complex carbohydrates, moderating protein, and limiting fats. Meals should be small and eaten throughout the day, with snacks added. If weight loss is needed (as it often is with type II diabetes), calorie intake is restricted. Finally, regular exercise is recommended to keep blood glucose levels in check.

ALTERNATIVE APPROACHES

The following alternative therapies all recommend that diabetes treatment be accompanied by an exercise regimen (including walking, jogging, or swimming) and a weight-loss program.

NUTRITIONAL THERAPY

A correct diet offers people with type I diabetes the chance to stay healthy with less insulin and offers people with type II the possibility to manage the disorder without any drugs. Furthermore, a proper diet may even prevent diabetes.

Many practitioners of nutritional therapy believe that a typically Western, high-fat diet limits the way cells can use naturally occurring insulin and injected insulin. But fat isn't the only concern: High amounts of protein tax the kidneys, which may already be stressed because in diabetes excess blood sugar is excreted through these organs. Therefore, dietary recommendations call for lowering fat significantly and reducing protein.

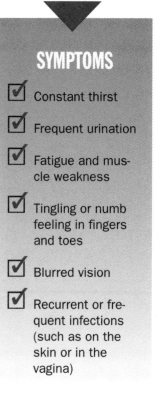

SYMPTOMS

- ☑ Constant thirst
- ☑ Frequent urination
- ☑ Fatigue and muscle weakness
- ☑ Tingling or numb feeling in fingers and toes
- ☑ Blurred vision
- ☑ Recurrent or frequent infections (such as on the skin or in the vagina)

In the place of fat and protein, unrefined carbohydrates should be significantly increased. Often as much as 75 percent of the daily calorie intake should come from carbohydrates—an amount much larger than conventional medicine recommends.

Carbohydrates provide fewer calories per gram than fats do. Because weight loss is often critical for people with diabetes (especially type II diabetes), eating a lower-calorie, yet filling, diet is important. In addition, carbohydrates supply a lot of fiber, which can positively affect the levels of blood sugar. Good carbohydrates to focus on include

- fresh vegetables
- fresh fruits (in moderation because of their high sugar content)
- whole-wheat bread, oatmeal, and other whole grains
- legumes (dry peas and beans)

Other research seems to advocate a diet with lower levels of carbohydrates and higher levels of protein and fat, but evidence is not yet conclusive. Moderation on all levels may be the best approach.

Surveys report that vegetarians, who eat no meat, poultry, or fish, have lower rates of type II diabetes than nonvegetarians. One reason for this may be that vegetarians' bodies are typically leaner than their meat-eating counterparts. Studies of the Pritikin diet—which is high in complex carbohydrates and fiber, is low in cholesterol and fat, and avoids meat—have shown that people can control their type II diabetes without drugs.

Nutrients such as the mineral chromium and niacin (in small doses) may boost the power of insulin and can be taken in supplement form. Other helpful supplements include

- vitamin B_6
- vitamin C
- vitamin E
- manganese
- magnesium
- vanadium (in the form of vanadyl sulfate)

Bioflavonoids, such as naringen (from the inside of grapefruit skins), hesperidin, and quercetin, can help alleviate some of the degenerative effects of high blood sugar. They block the buildup of sorbitol, a substance that may be responsible for the kidney, eye, and nerve damage caused by diabetes.

In addition to changes in the diet, a naturopathic physician may recommend the following supplements to someone with type II diabetes:

- 400 µg chromium picolinate daily
- 400 mg magnesium daily
- 1 gram vitamin C daily
- 400 IU vitamin E daily

A WORD OF CAUTION

People with diabetes, especially those with the insulin-dependent (type I) disorder, should not abandon their conventional treatment to experiment with alternative therapies on their own. Always consult a qualified practitioner of alternative medicine. For example, there have been reports of people with type I diabetes who traded their insulin treatments for faith healing, resulting in some damage to their kidneys or eyes.

HERBAL MEDICINE

In the treatment of diabetes, herbs are mainly used for their ability to control elevated levels of glucose (sugar) in the blood. Several herbs can have beneficial effects:

- Bilberry leaves can be made into a tea or, more often, taken in capsule form as a standardized extract (standardized to contain 25 percent anthocyanosides). This herb often requires several months of treatment before its effect begins.
- Fenugreek seeds are used in powdered form or as a tea.
- Bitter melon is available in extract form (made from the unripe fruit) or as juice (from the fresh fruit).
- Garlic and onion can easily be added to meals. These may also ward off heart disease, a possible complication of diabetes.

Any of these herbs could decrease insulin (or hypoglycemic drug) requirements. Therefore, a person with diabetes should be under the strict supervision of a health care professional and carefully monitor blood glucose levels whenever starting a new treatment regimen.

An herbalist may prescribe *Gymnema sylvestre* (800 mg three times per day) and fenugreek in the form of a tea (a couple cups daily).

TRADITIONAL CHINESE MEDICINE

Traditional Chinese medicine often treats diabetes with a combination of herbal therapy, acupuncture, calorie-restricted diets, and exercise (including qigong). Some traditional Chinese physicians have identified close to 20 different diabetes syndromes, which vary according to the degree of imbalance in vital life energy, or qi, as well as yin and yang.

The treatment goal is to return the flow of vital life energy to its ideal state. The physicians often prescribe multi-herb diabetes treatments, which are boiled with water and then taken as tea. Several of the herbs, such as panax ginseng, are selected for their mild ability to lower blood sugar levels.

Several types of practitioners are qualified to offer acupuncture and Chinese herbal treatment, including acupuncturists and some naturopathic physicians and medical doctors.

OTHER THERAPIES

BIOFEEDBACK TRAINING—Electromyographic biofeedback and relaxation techniques can teach people with diabetes to reduce stress, which is important because stress hormones can increase the levels of blood sugar.

HOMEOPATHY—Treatment can lower the need for insulin injections and other drug therapy.

HYDROTHERAPY—Alternating hot and cold compresses and showers, as well as castor oil packs over the abdomen (see Appendix 3), may be helpful.

HYPNOTHERAPY—Hypnotic trances can be used to lower stress and offer the subconscious mind suggestions that the body needs less insulin.

YOGA—Studies have shown that regular sessions of poses and breathing exercises can improve blood sugar levels.

Diarrhea

DIARRHEA IS THE PASSING OF LARGE VOLUMES OF UNFORMED, OFTEN LIQUID STOOL. IT HAPPENS WHEN THE INTESTINES HAVEN'T ABSORBED ENOUGH LIQUID FROM THE FECES OR HAVE ADDED MORE FLUID. IT CAN BE A SYMPTOM OF EATING CONTAMINATED FOOD OR AN INTESTINAL DISORDER, AMONG OTHER THINGS.

SYMPTOMS

Diarrhea is itself a symptom. It is usually limited in duration and not that serious, but it should be monitored by a professional if it

☑ lasts for weeks

☑ is accompanied by dehydration (especially in children)

☑ is accompanied by blood in the stool

CONVENTIONAL APPROACHES

Many allopathic doctors recognize that diarrhea that lasts less than a day or two and only occurs occasionally in a healthy adult is best left alone. However, some physicians still prescribe drugs that stop diarrhea in these cases. Antidiarrheal medications include
- narcotics (loperamide, codeine phosphate, and diphenoxylate combined with atropine), which may slow the movement of feces
- bulk-forming agents (kaolin, methylcellulose, and psyllium), which can remove some liquid from the feces

Both of these categories of medication can lead to constipation.

ALTERNATIVE APPROACHES
HERBAL MEDICINE

Several herbs can offer relief from diarrhea and may also prevent future bouts. The alkaloid substance berberine, found in some herbs, may weaken the microorganisms that often cause short-term diarrhea. Goldenseal and barberry are used for this purpose; they can be taken as a tea or a tincture. People traveling to countries where the food or water may be contaminated can use these herbs in capsule form.

Robert's Formula, a naturopathic herbal remedy, is often prescribed to offer relief from diarrhea that's caused by intestinal irritation such as irritable bowel syndrome or colitis. It contains goldenseal, as well as slippery elm, marshmallow root, echinacea (purple coneflower), and other herbs. (For suggestions on how to use purple coneflower, see Appendix 3.)

Other herbs, such as chamomile, peppermint, or fennel, can be taken as teas to soothe the digestive tract.

A naturopathic physician may prescribe taking three doses of Robert's Formula a day for certain cases of diarrhea caused by inflammation or ulceration such as irritable bowel syndrome or colitis. (See Appendix 3 for the recipe for Robert's Formula.)

HOMEOPATHY

Homeopathic medicine works to treat diarrhea by giving highly diluted doses of a natural substance that would produce diarrhea if given in full strength to a healthy person. The remedy stimulates the body to overpower whatever is causing the diarrhea.

A homeopath questions the patient on details of the diarrhea and assesses the general state of physical and emotional health. Using these clues, the remedy is then individualized to the patient.

The following are some diarrhea characteristics a homeopathic physician might consider:
- How does the stool look and smell?
- Does vomiting, stomach pain, or fever accompany the diarrhea?

- Is the diarrhea better or worse at certain times of the day?

Homeopathic remedies require an evaluation by a professional practitioner. The following are common homeopathic remedies for diarrhea:

- Arsenicum album for diarrhea from bad food (especially fruit) or water; that is characterized by chilly, burning pains, restlessness, weakness, and anxiety; and that is worse between 1:00 and 3:00 A.M.
- Chamomilla for diarrhea accompanied by extreme irritability, peevishness, cramping, and sensitivity to pain; resulting in greenish stools; and occurring in children or colicky infants.
- Podophyllum for copious, painless, often mustard yellow diarrhea in infants and children usually during the summer months.
- Sulphur for diarrhea that drives the patient from bed in the early morning (5:00 or 6:00 A.M.); causes burning pains and a red irritated anus; makes the patient hot and prone to perspire; and has the odor of rotten eggs.

NUTRITIONAL THERAPY

Nutritional therapy recognizes that diarrhea may be caused by eating too much of a particular food or by eating something the person cannot tolerate. In addition, certain supplements can help the body recover from diarrhea. Indulging in too many servings of fresh fruit, for example, leads to loose bowel movements. A food allergy or intolerance to lactose (found in milk and most cheeses) may be to blame for diarrhea that returns again and again.

People with chronic diarrhea may want to keep a food diary, which can point to a particular item that triggers an attack. Doses of the normal intestinal organism *Lactobacillus acidophilus* may be recommended to restore any "good" intestinal bacteria that was lost during a bout with diarrhea; this is especially important if antibiotics were prescribed recently. Vitamin and mineral supplements (including potassium) may also be needed. Electrolyte formulas are available over the counter, but homemade broths such as miso soup or carrot broth with salt can also be effective.

A sample prescription for *Lactobacillus acidophilus* might be to take half a teaspoon of the powder three times a day. It's best to take the dose between meals on an empty stomach.

OTHER THERAPIES

ACUPUNCTURE—Certain techniques can redirect the energy flow that relates to the spleen, stomach, and intestine. Burning moxa in the navel area can be very helpful.

AROMATHERAPY—Diarrhea can be treated by massaging diluted essential oils (such as 1 part peppermint oil diluted with 20 parts almond oil) into the skin.

MEDITATION—Relaxation techniques can reduce stress, which may trigger diarrhea.

YOGA—Yoga can also be used to ease stress.

Diverticular Disease

DIVERTICULAR DISEASE MOST OFTEN AFFECTS THE COLON. ITS TWO STAGES ARE 1) DIVERTICULOSIS, THE ABNORMAL PRESENCE OF TINY POCKETS (CALLED DIVERTICULA) THAT BULGE OUT FROM THE WALL OF THE COLON, AND 2) DIVERTICULITIS, IN WHICH BODY WASTES OR BACTERIA BECOME TRAPPED IN THE POCKETS, LEAVING THEM INFLAMED AND SOMETIMES PIERCED WITH HOLES. MANY PEOPLE WHO HAVE THE FIRST STAGE OF THE DISEASE NEVER PROGRESS TO THE SECOND.

SYMPTOMS

FOR DIVERTICULOSIS:

☑ Abdominal cramps or pain

☑ Bloated feeling

☑ Alternating bouts of diarrhea and constipation

☑ Bleeding from the rectum (rare)

Symptoms occur in only about 20 percent of people with diverticulosis.

FOR DIVERTICULITIS:

☑ Severe pain and firmness in the abdomen, usually in the lower left portion

☑ Fever

CONVENTIONAL APPROACH

Allopathic medicine offers several ways to manage diverticular disease. The common treatment program consists of drug therapy and dietary changes. For some cases of diverticulitis, surgery is also prescribed.

Several drugs are used to relieve the symptoms of diverticular disease:

- Antispasmodic drugs, such as belladonna alkaloids, can eliminate abdominal cramps.
- Sedatives, including phenobarbital, are often combined with antispasmodic medications.
- Antibiotics, such as cephalexin, can be helpful if infection results from wastes or bacteria trapped in the intestinal pockets.

Diverticular disease often results from eating a diet low in fiber and high in refined foods. Therefore, doctors often prescribe slowly incorporating more fiber-rich foods and fiber supplements into the diet.

For some cases of diverticulitis, doctors recommend surgical removal of part of the colon.

ALTERNATIVE APPROACHES
HOMEOPATHY

Homeopathic medicine can offer relief from the symptoms of diverticulosis by providing highly diluted doses of a natural substance that would produce the same symptoms if given in full strength to a healthy person. Before selecting a remedy, a homeopath questions the patient on details of the diverticulosis and assesses the general state of physical and emotional health. The following characteristics of the symptoms are carefully studied:

- Do you have pain or cramps in the abdomen?
- Does warmth or coldness ease the symptoms?
- Are bowel movements irregular? In what way?

Although homeopathic treatments need to be individualized and prescribed by a professional, common remedies may include

- belladonna
- bryonia alba
- colocynthis
- magnesia phosphorica

For a bout with diverticulitis that includes abdominal cramps, among other symptoms, and is made better by warmth, here's a sample homeopathic remedy: Take one dose of colocynthis, 6c, every six hours. (The *6c* refers to the potency of the remedy.) Stop treatment as soon as the symptoms go away. Homeopathic treatments, however, require a professional evaluation; remedies are highly individualized.

NUTRITIONAL THERAPY

According to nutritional therapy, a high-fiber diet that's low in fat and sugar can prevent the symptoms of diverticulosis and the development of diverticulitis. Many practitioners recommend a vegetarian diet as an effective way of meeting these suggestions. Fiber, of course, can make stool softer and easier to pass through the bowels. Lowering the intake of fat and sugars may also allow food to move through the digestive tract quicker and with fewer complications. Foods with a lot of fiber include brown rice, whole grains, fruits, vegetables, and legumes.

Certain items that can become trapped in the intestinal pockets should be avoided, including nuts, berries with seeds, and popcorn. For the fiber to have a positive effect on bowel movements, you should increase your daily intake of water by more than five glasses. Some researchers say that vegetarians have a lower rate of diverticular disease; studies have shown that Seventh-Day Adventist vegetarians (who eat no beef, fowl, or seafood) have a diet that is higher in fiber and lower in fat than the diet of the general population and lower rates of diverticular disease and colon cancer.

For someone with diverticulosis, a naturopathic physician may recommend adopting a vegetarian diet. The following are a few food selection tips:

- Eat a wide variety of whole grains, beans, and vegetables, all of which provide protein.

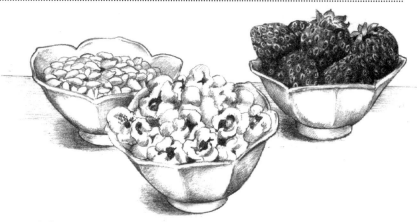

- Avoid food items such as seeds and popcorn that are small enough to become trapped in intestinal pockets.
- Protein combining (eating beans together with rice, for example) is not necessary to get needed protein.
- Do not overload your meals with eggs and dairy products; this will result in a diet high in fat and cholesterol.
- Cook vegetables first if raw ones cause irritation.

OTHER THERAPIES

ACUPUNCTURE—Pressure on specific points may be used to relieve pain and rebalance qi.

DETOXIFICATION, FASTING, AND COLON THERAPY—Fasting can be beneficial when the colon is irritated or inflamed. Colonic therapy is not recommended, however.

HERBAL MEDICINE—Commonly used herbs include slippery elm and chamomile. Robert's Formula, a naturopathic herbal remedy (see Appendix 3), is also often prescribed.

HYDROTHERAPY—Treatment may include warm sitz baths, cold compresses on the abdomen, and castor oil packs (see Appendix 3).

Ear Infection

A PAINFUL INFLAMMATION OF THE EAR CAN BE CAUSED BY BACTERIA OR FUNGI IN THE EAR OR BY AN INFECTION OF THE NOSE AND THROAT (SUCH AS A COLD). EAR INFECTION IS CLASSIFIED ACCORDING TO WHERE IT STRIKES: EAR CANAL INFECTION (KNOWN AS OTITIS EXTERNA, OR SWIMMER'S EAR) AFFECTS THE PASSAGEWAY FROM OUTSIDE THE HEAD TO THE EARDRUM. MIDDLE EAR INFECTION (OTITIS MEDIA) OCCURS AROUND THE EARDRUM. EARACHES ARE MOST COMMON IN CHILDREN.

SYMPTOMS

- ☑ Earache
- ☑ Discharge from the ear canal
- ☑ Red and swollen skin on the ear canal
- ☑ Itchiness (ear canal infection only)
- ☑ Feeling of fullness in the ear
- ☑ Ringing or some hearing loss (middle ear infection only)
- ☑ Fever (middle ear infection only)

CONVENTIONAL APPROACH

DRUG TREATMENT

Conventional medicine usually relies on one or more drugs to treat cases of ear infection:

- Painkillers—aspirin, acetaminophen, and nonsteroidal anti-inflammatory drugs (including ibuprofen and naproxen)—can offer relief.
- Decongestants, in the form of over-the-counter tablets, nose drops, or nose spray can be helpful.
- Antibiotics (such as amoxicillin) can eliminate an infection caused by bacteria.

In stubborn cases of middle ear infection, surgery is used. The eardrum is punctured, and any blocked fluid is sucked out.

ALTERNATIVE APPROACHES

Many alternative therapies consider the conventional approach to ear infections too aggressive.

NUTRITIONAL THERAPIES

According to nutritional therapy, certain foods can make the body prone to ear infections. And still other foods can ready the immune system to fight off infections. Food allergies may be responsible for repeated ear infections, especially in young children. Testing can be done to pinpoint allergens (foods that trigger an allergic reaction), or all common food allergens can be eliminated from the diet under the supervision of a trained professional. Supplementation of vitamin C, vitamin A, and zinc may also be helpful in warding off infections. Beta-carotene, bioflavonoids, and foods that tonify the kidneys are often helpful, as well.

For middle ear infection in a child, a holistic practitioner may recommend removing common allergens from the diet, including

- dairy products, including milk and cheese
- eggs
- wheat
- corn
- peanuts

Eliminating heavy proteins and sugars is also recommended.

HOMEOPATHY

Homeopathy has claimed a lot of success in treating ear infections in children. To stimulate the body to fight the infection, the therapy uses highly diluted, nontoxic doses of a natural substance that would produce the symptoms of an ear infection if given in full strength to a healthy person. A homeopathic remedy for ear infection depends on the person's specific symptoms. The homeopathic practitioner considers characteristics such as the following:

- What is the quality of the pain? Sharp, throbbing, dull?
- Are there any associated symptoms? Discharge from the ear, throat, nose?
- What makes the symptoms better or worse? Swallowing, applying heat, applying cold?
  Possible remedies include
- belladonna
- chamomilla
- lycopodium
- pulsatilla

A sample homeopathic remedy is one dose of belladonna, 30c, every half hour. (The *30c* refers to the potency of the remedy.) Stop treatment as soon as the ear pain has improved.

HERBAL MEDICINE

Herbs can offer relief to people with ear infections and may fend off future earaches. Mullein flowers can be used for their ability to soothe inflamed tissue. Infused oil from this herb is commonly prescribed as eardrops, but only if the eardrum is intact. Crushed garlic is thought to kill bacterial infections, and the immune boosters echinacea (purple coneflower) and goldenseal may also be helpful. (For suggestions on how to use purple coneflower, see Appendix 3.)

A possible herbal treatment for middle ear infection could be four drops (two drops for younger children) of warmed garlic oil in the ear, using a cotton ball to prevent leakage, as needed. The eardrum should first be examined to make sure it's not punctured.

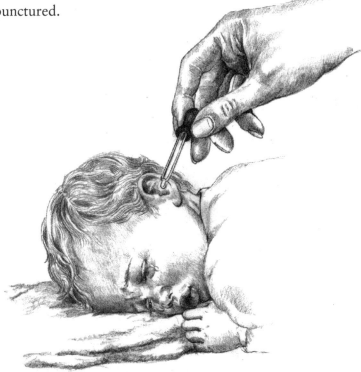

OTHER THERAPIES

CHIROPRACTIC—Manipulations or adjustments, such as on the neck or base of the skull, offer a lot of promise to adults and children with ear infection.

CRANIOSACRAL THERAPY—Blockages in the fluid surrounding the skull and spinal column may trigger the infections. Manipulation to clear these blockages is helpful.

ENVIRONMENTAL MEDICINE—Pollutants, animal dander, food allergies, mold, and more can contribute to an ear infection. Treatment may include avoidance of triggers, desensitization, and a rotation diet.

HYDROTHERAPY—Treatment can involve gargling with warm salt water and hot compresses.

Fever

THE BODY'S NORMAL TEMPERATURE IS AROUND 98.6°F (AS MEASURED IN THE MOUTH). TO QUALIFY AS A FEVER, THE TEMPERATURE USUALLY HAS TO TOP 100°F. A FEVER IS A SYMPTOM OF AN INFECTION, SUCH AS THE FLU, THE MEASLES, OR TONSILLITIS, OR ANOTHER AILMENT RANGING FROM DEHYDRATION TO HEART ATTACK.

SYMPTOMS

Fever is itself a symptom, but it may also be associated with the following:

☑ Headache

☑ Thirst

☑ Redness in face

☑ Bouts of severe coldness and shivering alternating with profuse sweating (occasionally)

☑ Mental confusion (rarely)

CONVENTIONAL APPROACH

Allopathic medicine offers a choice of drugs that can lower body temperature and make the patient more comfortable:

- Over-the-counter painkillers (including aspirin and acetaminophen) can be effective in reducing fever. Children under 18 years old with fevers should never be given aspirin, which could bring on the potentially fatal disorder called Reye syndrome.
- Medications to treat the cause of the fever, such as antibiotics in the case of a bacterial infection.

Fevers that run for more than three or four days or go above 104°F require the attention of a doctor. Fevers in infants and the elderly should also receive careful observation.

ALTERNATIVE APPROACHES

Many alternative therapies disagree with some allopathic doctor's belief that a fever should be suppressed. Instead, these therapies hold that a fever is the body's way of fending off an infection, a process that should be allowed to run its course. In fact, a fever may actually shorten the length of an illness. (Not lowering fevers is usually considered safe for temperatures under 103°F in adults; the cutoff point for infants is about 104°F.) Certain treatments can be employed to beef up the immune system, giving it more strength against the invaders.

HOMEOPATHY

Homeopathic medicine works to treat a fever by giving highly diluted doses of a natural substance that would produce a fever in a healthy person. The remedies stimulate the body to work at the cause of the fever. A homeopath studies the person's specific symptoms, as well as the general state of health, to devise a fever remedy. There are dozens of fever characteristics that are considered in finding a treatment. Consider the following:

- Does a dry heat accompany the fever?
- Is one cheek redder or warmer than the other?
- Is it accompanied by a backache?
- Does urinating make it better?

Common homeopathic remedies for fevers include

- belladonna
- nux vomica
- pulsatilla
- ferrum phosphoricum

All of these remedies are from plant sources, but a group of French researchers tested an all-purpose animal-based homeopathic remedy for fever (defined as more than 100°F, measured rectally) and other flu symptoms. About twice as many patients on the homeopathic treatment found recovery within 48 hours as those patients with no treatment.

A sample homeopathic prescription might be to take one dose of belladonna (with a potency of 12c) two times a day, stopping as soon as the fever subsides.

HERBAL MEDICINE

Herbs can be used to encourage the action and completion of a fever and to strengthen the immune system. Yarrow, black elder, linden flowers, cayenne, and boneset may induce sweating, among other functions. Many of these herbs are often taken as teas, either individually or combined. Echinacea (purple coneflower) is considered a classic for enhancing the immune system. (For suggestions on how to use purple coneflower, see Appendix 3.) The leaves of feverfew can also be helpful, especially in cases of fever accompanied by a headache, but avoid this remedy during pregnancy. Garlic, ginger, and phytolacca (strong) have also proved useful.

An herbalist might prescribe a tea of black elder: Pour 2 cups of hot water over 30 grams of dried flowers. Let the tea steep for 15 minutes. Strain it and drink it throughout the day.

HYDROTHERAPY

Treatment with hot or cold water, or a treatment alternating the two temperatures, can stimulate healing in the body. Heat, for example, stimulates the immune system. Cooler water can reduce fever, which is necessary for es-pecially high temperatures. Some of the techniques include

- bathing in warm water to promote sweating
- sponging off the body with water to slightly reduce a fever (Depending on the person's temperature and comfort level, hot, warm, or cold wet cloths can be used.)
- drinking fluids to make up for what is lost from perspiration and encourage the body to continue sweating
- taking a hot foot bath while placing a cold cloth on the head and wrapping the body in a blanket (especially good for fevers with headache)

A soothing hydrotherapy tip for someone with a fever: Take a warm (not hot) bath, especially if the fever is accompanied by shivering.

OTHER THERAPIES

AROMATHERAPY—The essential oils of bergamot, chamomile, or eucalyptus can be diluted and applied as a compress or inhaled.

AYURVEDIC MEDICINE—Treatment may involve a special, short-term diet and herbal therapy.

DETOXIFICATION, FASTING, AND COLON THERAPY—During the fever, water or herbal tea fasts or juice diets are beneficial.

TRADITIONAL CHINESE MEDICINE—Treatment can include acupressure, acupuncture, and herbal therapy.

Fibrocystic Breast Disease

IN FIBROCYSTIC BREAST DISEASE, BREASTS BECOME SWOLLEN OR DEVELOP LUMPS WHEN THE MENSTRUAL CYCLE BRINGS ABOUT HORMONAL CHANGES. THE LUMPS, WHICH OCCUR ALONE OR IN A GROUP, ARE NOT DANGEROUS; THEY CAN BE FLUID-FILLED TISSUE SACS (CYSTS) OR THICKENED MILK GLANDS. ALTHOUGH THE CONDITION IS CALLED A DISEASE, IT CAN ALMOST BE CONSIDERED NORMAL, AFFECTING UP TO 70 PERCENT OF WOMEN IN THEIR REPRODUCTIVE YEARS.

SYMPTOMS

☑ Breast pain and tenderness

☑ One lump or overall lumpiness in the breast

☑ Discharge from the nipple (rare)

Symptoms usually appear or worsen a week or so before the period begins.

CONVENTIONAL APPROACH

About three-quarters of breast lumps are not cancerous. Once breast cancer has been ruled out, allopathic medicine offers a treatment program for fibrocystic breast disease that is only aimed at relieving the intolerable symptoms.

Doctors may prescribe one of the following drugs:

- Diuretics remove water from the body by encouraging urination.
- Danazol, a synthetic male hormone, can greatly reduce breast pain. It should only be used by women with severe symptoms and for short periods of time.
- Tamoxifen, an anticancer drug, can also ease breast pain. Again, it should only be taken by those with severe symptoms.

If drugs fail to ease the symptoms, two surgical procedures are available. Lumps filled with fluid can be punctured with a needle and drained (called aspiration). Fibrous lumps can be removed.

ALTERNATIVE APPROACHES

Because excess estrogen in the body is believed to contribute to fibrocystic breasts, several alternative therapies focus on normalizing the levels of this hormone.

NUTRITIONAL THERAPY

With diet and supplements, nutritional therapy works to prevent breast swelling and lumps. A high-fat diet can encourage the body to produce too much estrogen. Hence, in cases of fibrocystic breast disease, eating only low-fat foods is recommended. Ideally, all animal products (including chicken, fish, milk, and cheese) should be eliminated from the diet. However, if animal foods are consumed, only use them if they're free of synthetic hormones. Increasing your intake of vegetables and whole grains can help the body get rid of excess estrogen.

Several researchers have linked the chemical methylxanthine with provoking the lumpiness and inflamed cysts of fibrocystic breasts. Avoiding foods with this chemical may reduce symptoms, but it may take a complete menstrual cycle before any change is noticed. Foods that contain methylxanthine include

- coffee (both caffeinated and decaffeinated)
- tea
- cola
- root beer
- chocolate

Vitamin E can serve several functions for women with fibrocystic breasts: It can ease inflammation, neutralize free radicals, and stabilize hormone levels. It's often taken in supplement form. The B vitamins may also be helpful.

A naturopathic physician may prescribe 400 to 800 IU of vitamin E each day. Usually, the doses begin at lower levels and build up to 800 IU. (High doses of vitamin E are not recommended for women with high blood pressure.)

HERBAL MEDICINE

Herbs can stabilize the levels of hormones in the body and encourage the peak functioning of the liver (which breaks down estrogens). Dong quai, a Chinese herb also called angelica, contains plant estrogens that lower the level of estrogen in a woman's body. It is commonly taken in capsule form. Dong quai is also high in vitamin E.

Chasteberry (also known as chaste-tree or vitex) directs its actions toward the brain's pituitary gland to trigger the production of hormones that cause the production of progesterone in the ovaries. Typically, the seeds are used in tincture or powdered (capsule) form.

Several other herbs can stimulate liver function, including

- burdock
- yellow dock
- dandelion root

Here's a sample herbal decoction to help eliminate breast lumps. Drink three cups of it per day.

- Mix together the following herbs in a large bowl: one part gingerroot, one part licorice root, one part chasteberry seeds, one part yellow dock root, two parts burdock root, three parts dandelion root, and four parts pau d'arco bark.
- In a saucepan, combine one quart of cold water and six tablespoons of the herb mixture. Bring it to a boil for 5 to 10 minutes. Reduce heat and cover. Simmer for 20 minutes.
- Remove pan from heat and let steep for 20 minutes.
- Strain and serve.

HYDROTHERAPY

Several forms of hydrotherapy, applied to the breasts, can stimulate blood circulation, helping to deliver nutrients and other beneficial substances to the cells and to clean away waste products. These treatments can also ease pain. Castor oil, made from the leaves of the castor-oil plant, is commonly applied to the breasts as a warm pack (as you would an ice pack). The cold-pressed oil contains a substance that stimulates cells important to the immune system. Alternating hot and cold compresses may also help.

A naturopathic physician may recommend placing castor oil packs (see Appendix 3) on the breasts once a day when symptoms are severe.

OTHER THERAPIES

AROMATHERAPY—Essential oils that target the actions of the liver can be very effective. They include carrot seed, celery seed, and rosemary.

BODYWORK—Gentle massage of the breasts and surrounding areas can stimulate blood circulation and promote healing.

Gastroenteritis

GASTROENTERITIS IS AN INFLAMMATION OF THE MUCOUS MEMBRANES THAT LINE THE STOMACH AND INTESTINES. IT'S A BROAD CATEGORY OF ILLNESS THAT CAN BE CAUSED BY BACTERIAL, VIRAL, OR PARASITIC INFECTIONS; FOOD INTOLERANCES; ANTIBIOTIC DRUGS; OR ANY OF SEVERAL OTHER FACTORS.

SYMPTOMS

☑ Nausea and vomiting

☑ Diarrhea, perhaps with blood and mucus

☑ Loss of appetite

☑ Pain and rumbling sounds in the abdomen

☑ Fatigue and muscle aches (occasionally)

These symptoms often strike with sudden intensity.

CONVENTIONAL APPROACH

Allopathic medicine's treatment program largely depends on the cause of the gastroenteritis, but it most often involves rest and medication. If the illness is mild, most people in good health can recover in two days.

The following types of drugs can relieve the symptoms of gastroenteritis:

- Antiemetic drugs reduce vomiting.
- Narcotics can limit diarrhea.
- Antibiotics may be helpful for bacterial infections.

ALTERNATIVE APPROACHES

Many alternative therapists recommend against suppressing the symptoms of gastroenteritis, believing instead that the body should be supported as it eliminates the cause of the illness.

HOMEOPATHY

Homeopathic medicine works to treat gastroenteritis by giving highly diluted doses of a natural substance that would produce the symptoms of gastroenteritis if given in full strength to a healthy person. The remedy stimulates the body to heal itself.

A homeopath will question you on details of the gastroenteritis. Using these clues, the remedy is then individualized to the patient. Some gastroenteritis characteristics to consider:

- Is vomiting present? How does it look and smell?
- Do you feel restless or prefer no movement?
- Does your body ache? Where?
- Are the symptoms made better by warmth or cold?

Common homeopathic remedies for gastroenteritis include minute quantities of arsenicum, ipecacuanha, and podophyllum. Arsenicum may be prescribed for gastroenteritis with

- vomiting and diarrhea
- bad water or food as the suspected cause
- restlessness or anxiety
- thirst for small sips of liquid, especially warm liquid
- burning pains

Podophyllum may be prescribed for gastroenteritis

- with painless, yellowish diarrhea
- with diarrhea that is more intense than vomiting
- in a child

Ipecacuanha may be prescribed for gastroenteritis with

- vomiting and gagging more intense than diarrhea
- vomiting that doesn't relieve nausea
- no thirst

For gastroenteritis characterized immediately above, here's a sample homeopathic remedy: Take one dose of ipecacuanha, 12c, every two hours. (The *12c* refers to the potency of the remedy.) Stop treatment as soon as the symptoms go away.

NUTRITIONAL THERAPY

Nutritional therapy works to replace the fluids and nutrients that are lost from vomiting and diarrhea. It may also help prevent future bouts with some types of gastroenteritis.

Some bacteria occur naturally in the intestines and promote good health. These are called *probiotics.* The bacteria *Lactobacillus,* taken in supplement or food form, can build up the intestines' store of "good bacteria" and lessen the body's susceptibility to invading bacteria, such as *Escherichia coli* (which can cause traveler's diarrhea). So, for example, some practitioners of nutritional therapy recommend taking *Lactobacillus acidophilus* before going on an overseas trip.

Gastroenteritis may also be prevented by never eating protein-rich foods (such as meat, eggs, and cream) that have been undercooked or stored without refrigeration.

Dehydration can result when large amounts of water and electrolytes (including sodium, potassium, and glucose) are passed out of the body. Preventing it calls for drinking a lot of water mixed with small quantities of table salt and sugar. Fruit juices spiked with salt and sugar and nonfat vegetable broths can effectively replace lost fluids and electrolytes. Mineral supplements can also be helpful.

Until the symptoms have passed, spicy foods, oils, caffeine, animal fats including milk, and anything else that may irritate the stomach and intestines should be avoided. A diet of clear liquids and broths is best at first. When symptoms improve, graduate to a BRAT (bananas, rice, apples, and toast) diet.

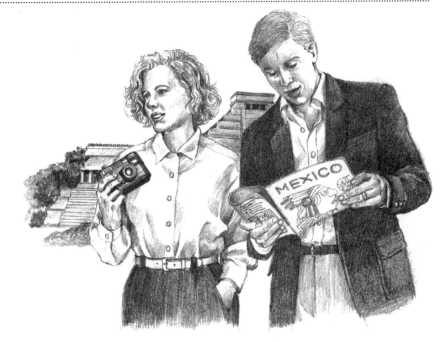

The following can help replace fluids and electrolytes: Grate a carrot and cook in two cups of water; remove the carrot, salt the broth, and drink. Cases of severe dehydration require medical attention.

OTHER THERAPIES

AYURVEDIC MEDICINE—Herbal therapy, meditation, and special dietary instruction are used to treat gastroenteritis.

HERBAL MEDICINE—A common treatment calls for fresh garlic and thyme tea.

TRADITIONAL CHINESE MEDICINE—A practitioner may use acupuncture, acupressure, herbal therapy, and qigong to rebalance qi and invigorate blood circulation.

MEDITATION—Reducing stress with meditation can prevent the production of gastric acid that further irritates an inflamed stomach.

Headaches

The pain of a headache can be steady or throbbing and range from simply uncomfortable to debilitating. The most common types are tension headaches and migraines. Stress, irregular sleep, hormonal shifts, depression, eyestrain, and certain foods, among other things, can trigger a headache.

SYMPTOMS

FOR TENSION HEADACHES:

- ☑ Dull constant ache
- ☑ Pain that begins at the forehead or back of head and then spreads to both sides

FOR MIGRAINES:

- ☑ Pounding ache, usually on one side of the head
- ☑ Nausea, vomiting, and sensitivity to light and sound (occasionally)

Slurred speech, appearance of flashing lights, and other warning signs (known collectively as an aura) can precede attacks

CONVENTIONAL APPROACH

Allopathic medicine usually combines medications, exercise, and stress reduction to prevent and to relieve headaches. Some conventional doctors have also recognized the benefits of a few alternative approaches, such as biofeedback training, meditation, and yoga. Nevertheless, painkillers and other medications are the heavy artillery in conventional medicine's war on headaches.

For tension and migraine headaches that occur once a week or less, over-the-counter pain relievers can be effective. They include

- aspirin
- acetaminophen
- a combination of caffeine with aspirin and/or acetaminophen
- nonsteroidal anti-inflammatory drugs, such as ibuprofen and naproxen sodium

If these medications fail to produce results, prescription painkillers may work. All of these measures carry warnings of side effects (from stomach ulcers to chest tightness) and dangerous interactions with other drugs.

Overuse of both prescription and over-the-counter pain remedies can lead to drug rebound headaches. When this happens, a once-effective drug no longer produces results, and when the dose wears off, another, worse headache appears.

In some cases, antidepressant medications are used to treat tension and migraine headaches. Drugs that regulate an aspect of brain activity or blood-vessel action may stop an oncoming migraine attack or prevent future ones. However, these medications, ranging from ergotamine to beta blockers, can bring severe side effects.

ALTERNATIVE APPROACHES

Alternative medicine emphasizes eliminating those things that cause or make the body vulnerable to recurrent headaches, recognizing that the pain is an important way for our bodies to alert us to trouble.

NATUROPATHIC MEDICINE

A naturopathic physician is interested in helping the body heal itself. To discover what could be causing the painful attacks, a naturopath would conduct a physical examination coupled with a dietary and nutritional evaluation and allergy tests. A naturopath would also look at possible hormone-related causes as well as bowel toxemia (the presence of toxins in the digestive tract).

In this investigation of suspects, diet receives careful scrutiny. Certain foods have been shown to bring on tension or migraine headaches in susceptible people. The list of common culprits includes

- aged cheese (especially yellow cheese)
- nuts
- citrus fruits
- chocolate
- hot dogs
- red wine
- coffee (and other caffeine sources such as soda)

Some of these foods contain substances that influence blood vessels in the head, which may explain their connection to headaches. With other foods, it's unclear why they are linked to headaches. Allergic reactions to food may be contributing to the pain. Sugar may contribute to headaches by causing wild fluctuations of blood sugar levels.

After an assessment, the naturopath would suggest a specific diet for the patient.

Supplements also may be prescribed if any important nutrients are missing from the diet, such as magnesium or niacin (both of which have an effect on the proper functioning of blood vessels) and quercetin (which can help block inflammation, among other functions). A naturopathic physician from Seattle reported that some of his patients have found immediate relief from headaches by taking magnesium supplements.

Finally, the naturopath would specify a program tailored to each headache patient that may include nutritional supplements, stress-reduction techniques, exercise, herbal medicine, acupuncture, naturopathic manipulation, and homeopathy.

For your first visit to a naturopathic physician, be prepared for a thorough discussion of your headaches as well as your general health, lifestyle, and diet.

To help your doctor and you pinpoint what triggers your headaches, it's a good idea to keep a diary of habits and symptoms for at least one month. Be sure to note the following:

- When did each headache occur? How long was the attack? Was it mild or severe?
- What did you eat minutes, hours, or a day before the headache?
- Did you work late that day? Oversleep? Did you feel stressed or overtired?
- Did anything remarkable or unusual occur before your attack?
- Women should also note their place in the menstrual cycle during the headache.

BIOFEEDBACK TRAINING

Biofeedback training can instruct headache sufferers on how to control certain involuntary functions of the body, such as heart rate or body temperature, which can, in turn, ward off headaches.

First, it is important to understand what happens in the head when a headache strikes. In the case of migraines, the blood vessels in the head narrow and then expand, causing pain. With tension headaches, the blood vessels constrict, but first the muscles in the head, neck, and shoulders become tense. Biofeedback training can help to stabilize or alter these blood vessel or muscle functions.

For example, a migraine sufferer could learn to raise the temperature of a part of the body, say the hands. This change in temperature would redirect the flow of blood from the painful vessels in the head to the hands. This is how it would work:

- A practitioner might use electrodes attached to the head and fingers hooked up to a biofeedback monitor, which reveals the current temperature of the hands and any tension in the head.
- The patient concentrates on the idea of submersing the hands in a tub of hot water.
- Meanwhile, the practitioner gives instructions on how to relax.
- The monitor shows the progress of the hand's actual temperature and the tension in the head.
- After several training sessions, the hands do change temperature. Eventually the patient can raise the temperature of the hands without the aid of the monitor.

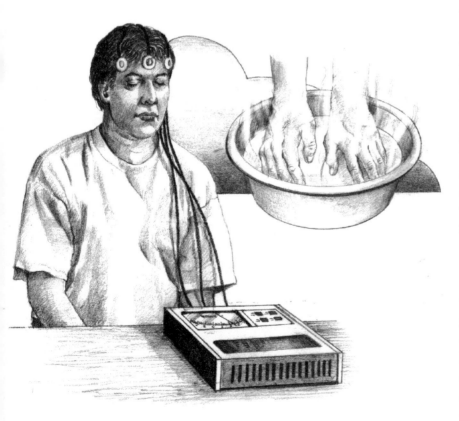

Biofeedback training requires an experienced practitioner. The lessons usually include relaxation techniques, such as progressive relaxation, that can be done at home while the training is ongoing. Progressive relaxation involves letting go of the stress in the body in little, isolated steps:

- Lie down or sit in a comfortable chair. Wear loose clothing.
- Close your eyes and imagine tightening the muscles in your feet. Then release these muscles.
- Next, direct your attention to your calves, tensing and then easing these muscles in the same fashion.
- Continue up the body, including your arms, until you end with your scalp.

ACUPUNCTURE

By inserting needles at specific points, acupuncture promises to restore the flow through the body's energy channels. The body is then able to heal itself. So, for example, when stress comes along, the body can weather it, and a tension headache doesn't result.

Sufferers of both tension and migraine headaches have found relief with acupuncture. In fact, researchers in New Zealand have shown that after as few as 12 treatment sessions, patients experience fewer and less-severe migraine attacks.

Several types of practitioners are qualified to offer acupuncture, including acupuncturists and some naturopathic physicians and medical doctors; different states have different licensing requirements. Be sure to inquire about the practitioner's training and experience. The needle therapy is often coupled with Chinese herbs,

WESTERN EXPLANATIONS

Western scientists have become increasingly intrigued by this use of acupuncture. One theory suggests that acupuncture releases endorphins, the brain's natural painkillers. Another states acupuncture may stabilize levels of serotonin, a chemical messenger in the brain.

changes in diet and lifestyle, vitamin supplements, and other measures.

HERBAL MEDICINE

Various herbs have proved beneficial in either preventing or relieving headaches. Whether taken as a single herb or combination, they can be used for their calming, regulating, and restoring properties.

Tension-headache sufferers, for example, can benefit from herbs that soothe the body and mind. Teas made from chamomile or passionflower help relax stiff muscles in the head and neck, reducing pressure on the blood vessels.

For centuries, the perennial herb feverfew has been used to treat migraines. Feverfew can reduce the number and intensity of attacks or even prevent them. The herb contains compounds that may perform several headache-blocking functions, such as improving the tone of blood vessels. It can be taken in fresh, capsule, tincture, or tablet form. (If you go for the straight-from-the-garden version, be aware of its bitter taste and its potential to cause mouth ulcers.)

Several scientific studies conducted in the past two decades have confirmed feverfew's effectiveness and lack of serious side effects. Researchers have shown that migraine sufferers who took daily doses of feverfew leaves experienced fewer and milder attacks when compared with those who did without the herb. The patients reported no serious side effects from the herb.

To safeguard against migraines, a sample prescription would call for about 50 mg of dried and powdered feverfew in capsules taken daily. During an attack, between 1 to 2 grams a day is necessary. It's always a good idea to consult an herbalist or naturopathic physician before beginning an herbal regimen.

OTHER THERAPIES

ACUPRESSURE—Treating the following acupressure points may bring headache relief: LI4 (located on the web between the thumb and index finger) and GB20 (on the back of head at the base of the skull).

CHIROPRACTIC—Adjustments or manipulations, especially of the neck vertebrae, can be useful in treating both tension and migraine headaches.

HOMEOPATHY—Specific remedies must be tailored to the individual, but common prescriptions include gelsemium sempervirens, iris versicolor, and pulsatilla.

MEDITATION—Mind-calming and mind-clearing sessions are especially beneficial in treating tension headaches.

YOGA—Regular practice can relieve tension and improve breathing and posture.

Heart Disease

CORONARY HEART DISEASE IS A CONDITION IN WHICH THE CORONARY ARTERIES (THE VESSELS THAT BRING BLOOD TO THE HEART MUSCLE) BECOME CLOGGED WITH DEPOSITS OF FAT, CHOLESTEROL, AND OTHER SUBSTANCES (COLLECTIVELY KNOWN AS PLAQUE), DEPRIVING THE HEART MUSCLE OF ENOUGH BLOOD. WHEN THE HEART IS IN THIS WEAKENED AND MALFUNCTIONING STATE, CHEST PAIN AND A HEART ATTACK MAY RESULT.

SYMPTOMS

Early heart disease has no symptoms. A blood cholesterol test can reveal one of the risks for the disease. Chest pain (angina pectoris)—a squeezing sensation felt in the center of the chest caused by exertion or strain and eased by resting—can be a precursor.

The warning signs of a heart attack include

- ☑ severe pain in the chest radiating to the neck, abdomen, or left arm

- ☑ weakness

- ☑ dizziness

- ☑ sweating

- ☑ nausea

- ☑ shortness of breath

CONVENTIONAL APPROACH

Allopathic medicine treats early heart disease, including instances of chest pain (called angina pectoris), with a program of drug therapy and lifestyle changes (such as exercise and suggestions for dietary modifications). More aggressive and expensive treatments, surgery and angioplasty, are growing in popularity and are used to treat both chest pain and damage from a heart attack.

DRUG TREATMENT

Medicines are prescribed to relieve chest pain, lower blood pressure or blood cholesterol levels, regulate abnormal heartbeat, or treat heart attacks. Their potential side effects range from throbbing headaches, dry mouth, and breathing difficulties to liver damage. Some examples of these medications are

- beta blockers, including atenolol and metoprolol, which stop some messages of the nervous system, keeping the heart from overworking
- calcium channel blockers, such as nifedipine and verapamil, which lower heart rate and hinder muscles from tightening around blood vessels
- lipid-lowering drugs, such as lovastatin, which reduce cholesterol levels in the blood

- nitrate drugs, including isosorbide dinitrate and nitroglycerin, which boost blood flow to the heart
- thrombolytic drugs, such as tissue plasminogen activator and streptokinase, which are given just after a heart attack to dissolve blood clots

SURGICAL TREATMENT

Coronary artery bypass surgery is recommended if drugs fail to bring results. It involves removing a section of blood vessel (such as from one of the legs) and transplanting it to the heart muscle to create a new pathway for the blood flow, bypassing a blocked coronary artery. A less-invasive surgical procedure, angioplasty, can stretch open a clogged coronary artery by inserting a thin, balloonlike device into the vessel and then inflating it. However, neither procedure corrects underlying factors, such as high blood cholesterol levels, or prevents more clogged arteries.

OTHER TREATMENT

Dietary recommendations call for restricting the amount of saturated fats and cholesterol. Doing this prevents or lowers high blood cholesterol levels, reducing the chances of having a heart attack. With guidance from a physician, a patient should adopt a regular exercise program. If applicable, patients should also quit smoking and lose excess body weight.

ALTERNATIVE APPROACHES

Many alternative therapies fault allopathic medicine for not placing enough attention on the possible triggers of heart disease. These therapies offer treatments that eliminate or lessen the need for drugs and surgery. Dean Ornish, M.D., a professor and researcher in San Francisco, has pioneered ways of reversing heart disease. His approach combines a number of alternative therapies, including vegetarianism (eating no meat, poultry, or fish), meditation, and yoga.

MEDITATION

Following the premise that stress can boost blood pressure and blood cholesterol levels, a relaxation-inducing therapy such as meditation is an important part of a heart disease treatment program. Meditation, however, does more than lower dangerously high levels of blood cholesterol and blood pressure in the body. This practice with ancient roots can quiet and clear the mind, improving a person's sense of peacefulness and control.

Research has shown that daily meditation can lower the blood pressure of those with hypertension. Studies of people with heart disease have proved that a treatment program that includes daily meditation (for 20 minutes or more) can increase blood flow to the heart and—perhaps equally important—boost feelings of well-being.

 Here's a sample meditation that can be done once a day:

SOBERING FACTS

Heart disease claims the title of the leading cause of death for adults in the United States. According to the American Heart Association, about every 20 seconds someone suffers a heart attack, and about every minute someone dies from one.

- Sit on the floor with your legs crossed, keeping your spine straight. Use a cushion if needed. Rest your arms loose and your hands close to your kneecaps, palms facing up. Try to eliminate as many noises and distractions as possible, including unplugging the telephone.
- Select one word or sound that is pleasant or meaningful to you. Mentally repeat your selection, over and over again.
- Try to do this for about 20 minutes. If your mind wanders off to another thought, gently return it to the process of repeating your word or sound.

HERBAL MEDICINE

Herbs can be used to relieve chest pain and possibly prevent heart attacks with little or no side effects. Hawthorn berries, for example, can reduce or eliminate chest pain by widening coronary arteries (which boosts blood circulation to the heart) and regulating abnormal heartbeats. Several European studies have confirmed these actions. The berries are available in several forms: as a tincture, extract, or capsule or in dried form (to make teas with or add to foods).

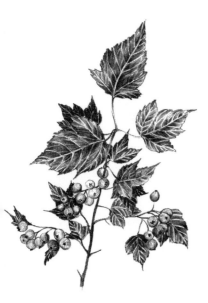

Hawthorn berry

Other helpful herbs include
- garlic to lower cholesterol, reduce blood clotting in blood vessels, and widen blood vessels
- ginger to reduce cholesterol and limit blood clotting
- ginkgo to facilitate blood flow and lower blood pressure

An herbalist may prescribe taking three droppers of hawthorn berry tincture or ¼ teaspoon of solid extract, three times a day.

NUTRITIONAL THERAPY

The right diet combined with nutritional supplements can be part of the recipe to prevent or reverse heart disease. Nutritional therapists assert that conventional medicine's dietary suggestions for heart disease do not go far enough. Instead of striving for a diet that derives up to 30 percent of daily calories from fat (as the American Heart Association recommends), nutritional therapy often calls for about half that.

For example, Dean Ornish's heart disease-reversing program includes a vegetarian diet that receives 10 percent or less of its calories from fat, severely reducing dietary cholesterol (the body also produces cholesterol) and saturated fat. Ornish's clinical studies of people with heart disease have shown that a complete treatment program that includes this very-low-fat vegetarian diet can lower blood pressure and blood cholesterol level and boost blood flow to the heart.

A significant majority of patients in these studies have experienced an "unclogging" of many blocked arteries after following Ornish's program, while patients in the control groups (receiving conventional therapies) have not. This recommendation of a vegetarian diet makes sense in light of population surveys that reveal fewer vegetarians die from heart disease than nonvegetarians. In addition, vegetarians typically have lower levels of total blood cholesterol and low-density lipoprotein cholesterol (known as bad cholesterol). As important as removing dietary cholesterol and saturated fat is eating plenty of foods that are unrefined, organic, high in fiber, and fresh. For one, these measures reduce the amount of the harmful oxidized cholesterol in the body.

Some practitioners of nutritional therapy, however, maintain that effective treatment and prevention of heart disease goes beyond restricting cholesterol and fat. Certain nutritional deficiencies may put people at risk for heart disease by
- contributing to weak blood vessel walls
- promoting vessel-blocking plaque buildup

THE POWER OF EXERCISE

Regular exercise, particularly aerobic exercise, is an essential part of heart disease prevention and treatment. The minimum should be 30 minutes of exercise three times a week. Positive results have been shown in clinical studies with yoga and daily walking, for example. If you have been inactive or have heart problems, consult your physician before embarking on an exercise program.

- encouraging blood to clot
- increasing blood cholesterol

Adding these important nutrients to the diet (by eating unrefined foods and taking supplements) is recommended:

- L-carnitine
- chromium
- coenzyme Q_{10} (ubiquinone)
- magnesium
- selenium
- vitamin B_6 (pyridoxine)
- vitamin C

Essential fatty acids can also be helpful. They can lower blood cholesterol and triglyceride levels, and flaxseed oil or fish oil capsules decrease the blood's clotting ability, thereby reducing the danger of blockages.

Dietary cholesterol is found only in animal foods, including meat, poultry, fish, egg yolks, and whole-milk dairy products. The ideal heart-treatment program allows just some egg whites and nonfat dairy products. Saturated fat is found in animal foods and a few vegetable foods (such as palm and coconut oils).

CHELATION THERAPY

According to chelation therapy, removing calcium from the bloodstream and out through the kidneys can help clear any plaque that has built up on blood vessel walls. That's because calcium contributes to the glue that holds plaque together. Once the calcium is gone, the plaque (containing deposits of fat, cholesterol, and other substances) breaks down on its own and also leaves the body.

The process of removing calcium and other minerals starts with intravenous injections of ethylenediaminetetraacetic acid (EDTA), an amino acid that binds to metallic ions in the body and renders them chemically inactive. These joined-together substances are then excreted by the kidneys in the urine.

Various clinical studies of chelation therapy have yielded promising results. In one trial, the majority of people with heart disease who were each given 20 chelation treatments experienced an improvement in chest pain. The reported side effects included nausea and dry mouth. The treatments are often combined with a supplemental regimen of vitamins, minerals, and trace elements (to replace any lost during the chelation process) as well as long-term dietary changes.

Only a licensed physician is qualified to perform chelation therapy. Look for someone who has been well-trained in this area.

OTHER THERAPIES

AYURVEDIC MEDICINE—Effective treatment may include dietary alterations, herbal therapy, and meditation.

GUIDED IMAGERY AND CREATIVE VISUALIZATION—People with heart disease can focus on images of clear arteries and a healthy heart.

TRADITIONAL CHINESE MEDICINE—Treatment involves acupuncture, acupressure, dietary changes, herbal therapy, and qigong.

YOGA—Poses and breathing exercises are an important part of a treatment program, as research has shown.

Heartburn

Heartburn is the burning sensation that results when acidic juices travel from the stomach up the esophagus. The technical term is acid reflux. It's usually caused by overindulging in food or alcohol, or by stress, but physical conditions such as hiatal hernia can also produce the symptom.

SYMPTOMS

☑ Pain in the stomach, center of the chest, and/or throat

☑ Belching small amounts of an acidic fluid

☑ Pain that increases when leaning forward or lying down

CONVENTIONAL APPROACH

Allopathic medicine suggests prevention to people with heartburn. Avoid the foods that trigger the discomfort (often fatty meats, chocolate, coffee, and hot peppers), and don't consume too much, too fast, too close to bedtime. Overweight people should lose some weight and avoid tight waistlines and belts. Propping up the head of the bed (to make it harder for stomach juices to move upward) can also help.

Drugs may be taken to prevent or stop heartburn:

- Antacids, available over the counter in liquid or tablet form, work to neutralize stomach acid.
- Histamine$_2$-receptor antagonists (including ranitidine hydrochloride), some available over the counter, may prevent heartburn.

ALTERNATIVE APPROACHES
HERBAL MEDICINE

Herbs can improve digestion and soothe the stomach. One commonly used herb is ginger. Fresh gingerroot is used to absorb the acid in stomach juices and can calm upset stomachs.

Although it sounds paradoxical, one of the most common causes of heartburn is not enough stomach acid. With less acid to aid in the breakdown process, food stays undigested in the stomach longer, thus increasing the chances of reflux. The group of herbs known as bitters signal the stomach to crank out more digestive juices. The herbs' bitter taste on the tongue is probably responsible for sending these messages to the brain and stomach. Bitters include gentian root, dandelion root, wormwood, and goldenseal root.

Carminatives, another group of herbs, can relieve stomach discomforts as well as gas. They include fennel seeds, lemon balm leaves, and peppermint leaves and stems.

The leaves and stems of meadowsweet can also pamper an irritated digestive tract. Meadowsweet protects and soothes mucous membranes and reduces excess acidity. The tincture form can be more palatable than teas, and for those who find alcohol irritating, the tincture can be put in hot water to evaporate the alcohol.

An herbalist may prescribe drinking a tea of gentian root about half an hour before a meal to prevent heartburn. Prepare the tea by simmering about a teaspoon of the chopped, dried root in a cup of water for 20 minutes. If the taste of the gentian root tea is too bitter, capsules are also effective.

BIOFEEDBACK TRAINING

Biofeedback training has shown promise in several digestive disorders, including heartburn. It can teach people with heartburn to control the action of their digestive systems as well as to reduce stress, thereby preventing the pain. Here's how it might work:

- The patient's abdomen, head, or other body part is hooked up to a biofeedback machine with sensors that measure unconscious bodily functions and give back readings (either visual signs or audible tones). This information lets the patient know which functions need to be controlled or relaxed.
- The biofeedback technician teaches techniques such as creative visualization, giving the patient ways to alter the bodily functions.
- After weeks of practice, the machines are no longer needed, and the patient can reinforce the lessons with techniques at home.

A biofeedback technician can perform biofeedback training after your health care practitioner has ruled out other, more serious digestive problems. A therapeutic course can last as long as four months.

TRADITIONAL CHINESE MEDICINE

According to traditional Chinese medicine, heartburn reveals an imbalance in the body's energy, or qi, and a disruption of the harmony between the body's opposing forces (yin and yang). For example, the painful, burning sensation may signal that the energy is blocked and that the stomach system has too much yang. The following therapies can offer relief:

- Acupuncture and acupressure—using needles or pressure points to clear the energy channels or strengthen or calm the energy.
- Traditional Chinese herbs—in the form of a preparation of a dozen or so herbs tailored to the patient's condition.
- Qigong—exercises can address heartburn by reducing stress and correcting the imbalances in an individual's qi that can contribute to heartburn.

Of course, traditional Chinese physicians stress prevention. They would devise an individualized program of diet, exercise, lifestyle adjustments, and relaxation techniques so each person with heartburn could do away with the condition for good.

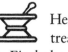

Here's a sample acupressure treatment for heartburn:

- Find the S41 point on the exact front and center of either ankle joint.
- You can "disperse" this point by pressing the thumb up and down on the spot for about two minutes.
- Repeat on the other ankle.

OTHER THERAPIES

BODYWORK—Various therapies can strengthen abdominal muscles, teach proper breathing, and ease tension.

DETOXIFICATION, FASTING, AND COLON THERAPY—Treatment may involve dietary alterations, fasts, and colonic irrigation.

MEDITATION—Regular meditation can reduce stress and anxiety, which may be contributing to heartburn.

NUTRITIONAL THERAPY—Recommendations include eating smaller meals, avoiding rich or spicy foods, and taking digestive enzymes.

Hemorrhoids

HEMORRHOIDS ARE ENLARGED BLOOD VESSELS UNDER THE LINING OF THE RECTUM AND ANUS. THEY ARE SIMILAR TO VARICOSE VEINS IN THAT THEY ARE BLOOD VESSELS THAT ALLOW BLOOD TO POOL, SWELLING THE TISSUES. HEMORRHOIDS CAN RESULT FROM EXTENDED PERIODS OF INACTIVITY, STRAINING TO HAVE BOWEL MOVEMENTS, CHRONIC DIARRHEA, OBESITY, OR PREGNANCY.

SYMPTOMS

☑ Bleeding from the anus (traces of bright red blood often appear on the toilet paper)

☑ Pain and itching around the anus

☑ Painful bowel movements

☑ Discharge of mucus and itchiness around the anus, usually a sign of a hemorrhoid that extends outside the anus

If bleeding is one of the symptoms, other, more serious conditions should be ruled out by a doctor before self-treatment begins.

CONVENTIONAL APPROACH

Straining to have a bowel movement can usually be avoided by adding more fiber and water to the diet. Stool softeners (such as methylcellulose and psyllium) can also be helpful. Also, exercising and keeping regular toilet habits can be effective.

Drugs can ease the pain of hemorrhoids. Most often they act as painkillers and sometimes contain corticosteroids to reduce inflammation.

Conventional medicine offers several procedures to eliminate hemorrhoids. Smaller, bleeding hemorrhoids can be injected with a chemical that shrinks them, and they then fall off. In a procedure called hemorrhoid banding, small rubber bands are placed around the base of hemorrhoids, causing them to shrink and fall off. Surgery to remove hemorrhoids is also available, but the procedure and recovery can be painful and may result in incontinence.

ALTERNATIVE APPROACHES

The treatment of hemorrhoids is one area in which alternative therapy is gaining acceptance with conventional physicians. Several therapies offer natural pain relief from hemorrhoids and aid in preventing them from returning.

NUTRITIONAL THERAPY

Nutritional therapy can reduce the pain of hemorrhoids and prevent future ones. One way to prevent the straining that can lead to hemorrhoids is to ensure softer stools—include unrefined fiber and lots of water and decaffeinated liquids. (Coffee and other drinks with caffeine act as laxatives and can train the colon to be lazy, only producing bowel movements with the help of artificial stimulation.)

Certain nutritional supplements such as vitamin C and the bioflavonoids can strengthen the tone of blood vessel walls and prevent hemorrhoids in other ways.

Excess body weight can also make someone susceptible to hemorrhoids, so weight loss is a good idea.

In addition to prevention, nutritional therapy can help ease the pain of hemorrhoids, as well. Certain foods, such as coffee, red pepper, mustard, and alcohol, can irritate hemorrhoids as they are passed out of the body. Avoid these.

Eating at least 30 grams of insoluble fiber and 10 grams of soluble fiber per day, together with drinking at least eight 8-ounce glasses of water, should eliminate problems with hard stool. Good sources of insoluble fiber include
- wheat bran
- fruits such as apples and pears
- vegetables such as carrots and spinach
- brown rice

Good sources of soluble fiber include

- oatmeal or oat bran
- barley
- lentils
- broccoli

HERBAL MEDICINE

Herbs can be used to shrink and strengthen the blood vessels around the anus, providing relief from the pain and bleeding of hemorrhoids. Witch hazel, a native American plant, acts as an astringent when applied to the hemorrhoids. It's often used in distilled or extract form. Another valuable astringent is stone root, often taken in capsule form.

Other herbs commonly used to treat hemorrhoids include

- bayberry bark
- butcher's broom
- calendula
- ginkgo
- pilewort
- plantain
- horse chestnut

Here's a sample herbal prescription for relief from hemorrhoids that are bleeding and itchy: Soak a cotton ball in distilled witch hazel and dab on the hemorrhoid and around the anus several times a day. (Be prepared: Witch hazel may sting during the application.)

HYDROTHERAPY

Hydrotherapists use applications of water to ease the pain of hemorrhoids and encourage the circulation of blood in the area around the anus. The types of hydrotherapy commonly used for hemorrhoids are

- alternating warm and cold sitz baths—soaking the area
- hot and cold compresses—alternating applications of comfortably hot and ice-cold washcloths
- cold compresses—applying ice-cold cloths only

Certain herbs, such as yarrow, can be added to the water in each of these treatments for an astringent effect.

Follow these steps for an alternating sitz bath:
- Fill the bathtub with four inches of comfortably warm water.
- Sit in the tub with your knees bent and near your chest.
- Sit for five minutes.
- Refill the tub with cold water.
- Sit in the cold water the same way for one minute.
- Repeat the procedure three times.

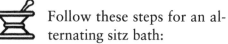

OTHER THERAPIES

AROMATHERAPY—Several essential oils, including cypress, geranium, and myrrh, can be used in sitz baths and as compresses.

AYURVEDIC MEDICINE—Treatment can involve dietary changes, stress reduction (including meditation), and herbal therapy (with astringent herbs).

DETOXIFICATION, FASTING, AND COLON THERAPY—Fasting can relieve constipation.

HOMEOPATHY—Common remedies include nux vomica, belladonna, hamamelis, and collinsonia.

YOGA—Yoga offers exercises to relieve constipation and improve circulation.

Herpes, Genital

Genital herpes is a disease that brings about a painful rash on the sex organs. It's caused by the herpes simplex virus type 2, which is usually contracted by having sexual contact with an infected person. According to conventional medicine, the virus never leaves the body but lies dormant for periods, probably in the nervous system. The rash and its accompanying symptoms can appear once or several times over a lifetime.

SYMPTOMS

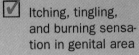 Itching, tingling, and burning sensation in genital area

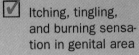 Small blisters on genitals and surrounding areas (The blisters pop to create painful open sores.)

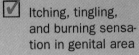 Accompanying headache, fatigue, fever, and swollen lymph nodes in the groin (occasionally)

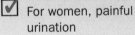 For women, painful urination

An attack of symptoms may be triggered by poor diet, emotional stress, overexposure to sun, and menstruation, among other factors.

CONVENTIONAL APPROACH

No cure is available for genital herpes. All allopathic medicine can offer is drug therapy and lifestyle changes that can ease the symptoms during a herpes attack and potentially reduce the number and frequency of future attacks.

Acyclovir, an antiviral drug available in capsule, ointment, and injection forms, slows the multiplication of the herpes simplex virus. If taken at the beginning of a symptoms attack, it can relieve the pain of open sores and allow them to heal faster.

This prescription medication can cause side effects such as headaches, dizziness, vomiting, and skin irritation. Daily doses of acyclovir capsules can cut the number and severity of future herpes attacks. But once the medication is discontinued, this preventive action ends.

Because outbreaks can be painful, painkillers can offer short-term relief, as can warm baths spiked with a small amount of sea salt. (Table salt also works, but sea salt is best.)

Because the open sores can carry the infectious agent, to prevent the spread of the virus, sexual contact should be avoided during a herpes attack and one to two weeks after the symptoms end. Also avoid kissing and sharing clothes and towels.

In women, genital herpes has been linked to cervical cancer. Therefore, annual or biennial Pap smears are recommended for women known to have the disease. Likewise, a pregnant woman who has an attack just when she's ready to deliver usually has a cesarean section to avoid infecting the baby.

ALTERNATIVE APPROACHES

Several alternative therapies offer ways to prevent herpes outbreaks from returning. These treatments should be coupled with

- good nutrition
- regular sleep
- exercise
- stress-reduction techniques

NUTRITIONAL THERAPY

Dietary changes and nutritional supplements can significantly lessen the severity and frequency of herpes outbreaks. One important step for people with genital herpes is to decrease the amount of the amino acid arginine in the body while increasing another amino acid, lysine.

Arginine assists the herpes simplex virus in multiplying, and lysine can help break down arginine and decrease its absorption in the body. One group of researchers gave lysine supplements to people infected with the herpes simplex virus who were showing the symptoms of a herpes attack. After a few days, the symptoms of more than 90 percent of the patients went away.

Lysine supplements are available, but whole foods that are high in lysine and low in arginine can be added to the diet as well. Foods high in lysine include

- beef
- brewer's yeast
- chicken
- dairy products (including milk and cheese)
- fish
- mung bean sprouts
- potatoes

Avoid those foods rich in arginine, including

- almonds
- carob
- chocolate
- cashews
- peanuts
- pecans
- sesame seeds

In general, a sound diet can bolster the immune system, perhaps delaying or blocking future herpes attacks. For example, the guidelines include eliminating most simple carbohydrates (sugars and sweets), avoiding alcohol, and skipping common food allergens such as wheat and dairy products. In their place, add a lot of fresh vegetables and fruits.

Other supplements that may be helpful include beta-carotene, vitamins C and E, zinc, and the B vitamins (especially vitamin B_6).

A naturopathic physician may recommend taking 300 to 500 mg of a lysine supplement a day to prevent future herpes attacks. Higher doses are used during an outbreak of symptoms.

HERBAL MEDICINE

Herbs can perform several functions for people with genital herpes, including overpowering the herpes simplex virus, boosting the body's own defenses by strengthening the immune system, and promoting the healing of sores with topical treatment.

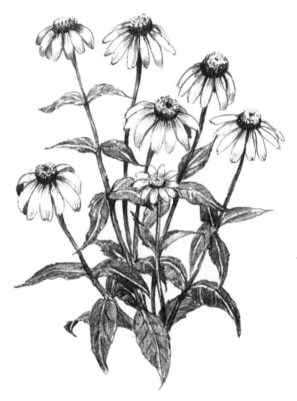

Echinacea (or purple coneflower) can strengthen the immune system.

An ingredient of licorice root, glycyrrhizic acid, may slow the multiplication and action of the herpes simplex virus. An ointment of licorice root, ap-

OTHER THERAPIES

HOMEOPATHY—Common remedies include dulcamara, natrum muriaticum, petroleum, rhus toxicodendron, and sepia. However, prescriptions must be tailored to the individual case and require consultation with a homeopath.

HYDROTHERAPY—Castor oil packs (see Appendix 3) applied to the abdomen, warm or sitz baths with salt added, and ice packs applied to the genital area can be helpful.

MIND/BODY MEDICINE—Because emotional tension may trigger an outbreak of symptoms, therapies that alleviate stress, such as meditation and guided imagery, are often recommended. Support groups may also be very useful.

TRADITIONAL CHINESE MEDICINE—Acupuncture and herbal therapy can be effective at minimizing outbreaks.

plied to the genital area, is commonly prescribed.

Echinacea (or purple coneflower) is one of the most widely used herbs in America. Its use in cases of herpes is warranted because of its well-established ability to strengthen the immune system. This herb is most often taken orally in either tincture or capsule form. (For suggestions on how to use purple coneflower, see Appendix 3.)

Raw garlic eaten on a regular basis can also help the body's defenses. Cal-endula (marigold) may fight the virus and encourage healing. Soaking in strong calendula tea is often prescribed.

Here's a sample herbal treatment: Apply glycyrrhizic acid gel (derived from licorice root) three times a day. (Patients who use high doses of licorice for more than one month need to be monitored for the potentially serious side effects of this treatment—namely, sodium retention and high blood pressure.)

OXYGEN THERAPY

Oxygen therapy may offer some promise for people with recurring and especially painful cases of genital herpes. Treatment with the oxygen compound ozone can be used to boost the immune system and fight off the herpes simplex virus.

In oxygen therapy, typically, less than one pint of blood is drawn from the patient, mixed with different amounts of ozone and oxygen, and then reintroduced into the veins. Therapy with hydrogen peroxide, another oxygen compound, may also be effective.

Oxygen therapy has more acceptance in Europe than in America. Nonetheless, several states permit medical doctors to use it in their practices. Check for the practitioner's experience with treating herpes.

High Blood Pressure

HIGH BLOOD PRESSURE, OR HYPERTENSION, INVOLVES A GREATER THAN NORMAL PRESSURE OF BLOOD COURSING THROUGH THE ARTERIES. THIS HIGH PRESSURE FORCES THE HEART TO WORK HARDER THAN NORMAL AND INCREASES THE RISK OF AN ANEURYSM (RUPTURE OF AN ARTERY), HEART ATTACK, STROKE, KIDNEY FAILURE, AND OTHER DISORDERS.

CONVENTIONAL APPROACH

Allopathic medicine's most effective program for lowering high blood pressure is a combination of drug therapy and lifestyle changes.

DRUG TREATMENT

The class of medicines called antihypertensive drugs employs several different methods to reduce blood pressure. Some are taken in combination, and they must be taken continuously to achieve the desired effect. These drugs include

- angiotensin converting enzyme (ACE) inhibitors, such as captopril and enalapril, which prevent or slow the constriction of blood vessels
- beta blockers, including atenolol and metoprolol, to stop some messages of the nervous system
- calcium channel blockers, such as nifedipine and verapamil, which hinder the constriction of blood vessels
- diuretics, including chlorthalidone and hydrochlorothiazide, to remove water and salt from the body via the urine, thus decreasing blood volume
- other vasodilator drugs, such as hydralazine and minoxidil, which trigger blood vessels to expand

LIFESTYLE CHANGES

Most people with hypertension can benefit from lowering sodium (salt) intake and reducing emotional stress. If applicable, patients should also quit smoking, drink less alcohol, and lose excess body weight.

ALTERNATIVE APPROACHES

Several alternative approaches emphasize the need to eliminate some of the triggers or causes of high blood pressure. The goal is for people with hypertension to cut down or eliminate their use of antihypertensive drugs.

NUTRITIONAL THERAPY

According to nutritional therapy, diet can make all the difference between high blood pressure and healthy blood pressure. Population surveys have shown that certain groups of people in some parts of the world have a high rate of hypertension, while others have a low rate. This difference is usually attributed to their food choices.

In general, the ideal diet to prevent or reduce blood pressure should emphasize fresh vegetables and fruits and whole grains and limit animal products, including milk and cheese. Fats and sugars should be avoided as much as possible. This sounds close to a vegetarian diet for good reason: Surveys of vegetarians, who eat no meat, poultry, or fish, show that they consistently have lower rates of hypertension than nonvegetarians.

The following are specific dietary guidelines:

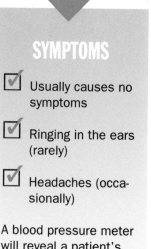

SYMPTOMS

- ☑ Usually causes no symptoms
- ☑ Ringing in the ears (rarely)
- ☑ Headaches (occasionally)

A blood pressure meter will reveal a patient's levels; anything more than 140/90 mm Hg is considered high.

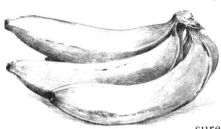

- Significantly reduce sodium (salt) in the diet.
  - Eat more foods rich in potassium, such as bananas, prunes, and tomatoes.
  - Increase intake of calcium and magnesium, but make sure the sources are low in fat and salt.
- Limit alcohol and caffeine intake.

People who are overweight are also at higher risk for high blood pressure. Maintaining ideal body weight is an important part of the treatment, and adhering to the above dietary guidelines should make this possible.

Several supplements are also commonly prescribed, including

- vitamin C
- vitamin E (although high doses may have the opposite effect)
- B complex vitamins
- potassium
- calcium
- magnesium
- zinc
- coenzyme Q_{10} (ubiquitone)
- fish oils (containing omega-3 fatty acids)

THE POWERS OF EXERCISE

The American Heart Association pinpoints a lack of exercise as one of the major factors contributing to hypertension and other cardiovascular problems. Regular exercise, especially aerobic exercise, serves many functions, including keeping the blood vessels elastic, removing excess salt from the body, and helping with weight loss.

Here are some tips to reduce sodium in your diet:

- Never use table salt.
- Try to replace as many processed foods with fresh foods as you can.
- Avoid hidden salt that can be found in processed foods (even sweet-tasting desserts).
- Go easy on the salad dressing.

MIND/BODY MEDICINE

For people whose hypertension is triggered or exacerbated by emotional stress and tension, mind/body medicine can be an effective treatment. Research has shown that several mind/body therapies have the power to decrease high blood pressure, sometimes by as much as 10 mm Hg.

Biofeedback training, which instructs people to alter certain involuntary functions of the body, is particularly recommended for people with hypertension. It involves using sensors to hook a patient up to a biofeedback monitor, which reveals the levels of heart rate, muscle tension, body temperature, or other functions. Using this information, the patient is taught to change one or more of these levels. Relaxation techniques and guided imagery exercises are usually part of the instruction.

One of two training types are typically used to treat hypertension: electromyograph biofeedback, which measures muscle tension (on the forehead, for example), and thermal biofeedback, which measures body temperature. A recent study at the Medical College of Ohio showed that patients who used diuretics and biofeedback were five times more likely to lower their high blood pressure than patients who only used drugs.

Other helpful mind/body therapies include

- Spirituality—Researchers have discovered links to fostering a religious commitment and reduced hypertension.
- Meditation—Researchers have also shown daily meditation to lower hypertension.
- Hypnotherapy—Hypnotic trances can relieve tension.
- Yoga—Poses and breathing exercises are effective stress busters.

Here's a sample relaxation breathing exercise that might be helpful in relieving stress:

- Sit or lie down in a comfortable position. Wear loose, nonrestrictive clothing.
- Close your eyes. Begin breathing slowly and deeply.
- When exhaling, imagine tension effortlessly flowing out of your body.
- As you inhale, picture yourself filling your body with fresh air and energy.
- Continue the slow, deep breathing for as long as you are comfortable.
- When you are ready, slowly return to your normal rate and rhythm of breathing.

HERBAL MEDICINE

Herbs hold a great deal of promise in preventing and treating high blood pressure and other heart conditions, and they have few or no side effects. Herbs have the ability to dilate vessels to increase circulation, regulate the heart rate, and encourage urination (to remove water), among other functions.

Commonly used herbs include

- cayenne to stimulate the flow of blood and reduce blood cholesterol levels
- garlic to widen blood vessels, lower blood cholesterol levels, and decrease blood clotting
- ginkgo to increase blood flow and dilate blood vessels
- hawthorn berries also to expand blood vessels

An herbalist may prescribe taking three droppers of hawthorn berry tincture, three times a day. Garlic—1 to 2 cloves daily—may also be added to the diet.

OTHER THERAPIES

ACUPUNCTURE—A series of treatments, often on the heart meridian, can lower blood pressure, with the results lasting for months or years.

BODYWORK—Massage is effective in relieving stress and tension.

DETOXIFICATION, FASTING, AND COLON THERAPY—Short, supervised fasts or juice diets and daily sauna treatments may be effective.

HOMEOPATHY—Specific remedies must be tailored to the individual.

OSTEOPATHY—Manipulations and other treatments can relieve muscle tension and improve posture and breathing.

QIGONG—This traditional Chinese technique also enhances breathing and posture; it also improves blood circulation and clears the mind.

Impotence

IMPOTENCE IS THE INABILITY OF A MAN'S PENIS TO BECOME ERECT OR STAY ERECT DURING SEXUAL INTERCOURSE. IN MANY CASES, A PSYCHOLOGICAL REASON—RANGING FROM STRESS AND FATIGUE TO DEPRESSION—IS TO BLAME FOR IMPOTENCE. OTHER CAUSES INCLUDE CERTAIN DRUGS, OLD AGE, A HORMONE IMBALANCE, SPINAL CORD INJURY, AND DIABETES MELLITUS, AMONG OTHERS.

SYMPTOMS

☑ Impotence is a symptom itself. It can develop suddenly or gradually. In some cases, erections during sleep and the ability to masturbate are still present.

CONVENTIONAL APPROACH

Allopathic medicine's treatment program for impotence depends on the cause. Counseling or sex therapy is often effective if psychological factors are at play. Otherwise, treatment options include drug therapy or surgery. (A do-it-yourself solution is a condomlike device that can produce a temporary erection.)

Medicines, such as papaverine, that widen the blood vessels can be injected into the penis to produce an erection. These can be used at home on a short- or long-term basis. Side effects can include nausea and drowsiness. Overdoses may lead to painfully prolonged erections, blood clotting, and gangrene (a death of body tissue). Several drugs can reverse a prolonged erection, if needed. If a certain medicine (such as an antipsychotic, antidepressant, or diuretic) is causing the impotence, then the dose may be lowered or another drug can replace the offending drug.

For impotence caused by malfunctioning blood vessels in the penis or lower body, surgery can often repair the vessels; the success of these procedures is highly variable. Penile implants are available for cases of impotence that don't respond to other therapies. A bendable silicone splint can be permanently inserted into the penis. Another option is implanting a pump-operated device that can be manually inflated and deflated.

ALTERNATIVE APPROACHES
HOMEOPATHY

Homeopathic medicine holds a lot of promise for men with impotence, particularly for those cases stemming from anxiety or other psychological reasons. This therapy uses highly diluted doses of natural substances that would produce the symptoms of impotence if given in full strength to a healthy person. The substances are from plant, mineral, or animal sources. A classical homeopath goes about tailoring a remedy for a patient by studying the symptoms as well as the general state of physical and emotional health. To pinpoint possible causes of the impotence, the following questions are useful:

- Has there been a recent illness?
- What is the patient's feeling about sex and his relationships?
- Has the penis been injured?

Patients receive the remedies tailored to their specific case. For example, the remedy argentum nitricum, made from silver nitrate, is often effective for men with impotence who easily become excited and anxious, which frequently leads to physical exhaustion. Fresh air or cold drinks make them feel better, and they typically have digestive problems. Other possible remedies for impotence include arnica montana, lycopodium, and sabal serrata.

Here's a sample homeopathic prescription for argentum nitricum: Take one dose of the remedy (with a potency of 6c) three times a day.

TRADITIONAL CHINESE MEDICINE

Traditional Chinese medical treatment seeks to bring the body's energizing life force, or qi, back into balance, thus eliminating the problems of impotence. One possible explanation of this condition is that it results from a deficiency in yang in the kidney system. (Together, yang and yin create harmony in the body.) Treatment typically involves a combination of acupuncture, moxibustion, herbal therapy, and dietary changes. Both the impotence and the patient's general health are addressed. Several clinical experiments and case studies have shown acupuncture to be a successful treatment of impotence for the majority of patients.

Regulations on who can practice acupuncture and other forms of traditional Chinese medicine vary from state to state. In addition to traditional Chinese physicians, some naturopathic physicians and medical doctors are trained in acupuncture.

HERBAL MEDICINE

Herbal medicine offers treatments that can influence hormones, act as sexual stimulants, and reduce anxiety and tension. Saw palmetto berries are often used to regulate the hormonal balance and may also act as an aphro-

disiac. The berries come from a small palm tree native to the southeastern coast of the United States and are often used as tinctures.

Damiana has long been used to stimulate sexual desire in men, as one of its botanical names, *Turnera aphrodisiaca*, testifies. It may also relieve anxiety.

Siberian ginseng (also known as eleuthero) can encourage relaxation. The root of this herb is available as a tincture or in capsule form.

Other helpful herbs include ginkgo and potency wood (also known as muira puama).

An herbalist may prescribe taking up to three capsules of damiana a day, before meals.

OTHER THERAPIES

CHIROPRACTIC—Manipulating the spine may restore function to the penis.

DETOXIFICATION, FASTING, AND COLON THERAPY—Fasts and other treatments can eliminate toxins from the body that may be contributing to impotence.

HYDROTHERAPY—Treatment may include alternating hot and cold sitz baths and short soaks in ice-cold water.

MIND/BODY MEDICINE—Biofeedback training, creative visualization, hypnotherapy, meditation, and other therapies employ the mind and body together to bring relaxation and encourage successful and enjoyable intercourse.

NUTRITIONAL THERAPY—Diet (such as limiting cholesterol) and supplements (such as zinc, vitamin B_6, and vitamin E) can be helpful for treating impotence.

Incontinence

INCONTINENCE IS THE INABILITY TO CONTROL URINATION OR BOWEL MOVEMENTS. THERE ARE SEVERAL TYPES OF URINARY INCONTINENCE, AND ITS CAUSES RANGE FROM INFECTIONS AND BLADDER STONES TO INJURY DUE TO CHILDBIRTH OR SURGERY. BOWEL INCONTINENCE CAN RESULT FROM A BLOCKAGE OF STOOL, SEVERE DIARRHEA, OR INJURY.

SYMPTOMS

 Involuntary passage of urine or small pieces of stool and watery stool

 Leaking urine after coughing, sneezing, lifting, or straining (called *stress incontinence*)

The incidence of urinary incontinence increases with age.

CONVENTIONAL APPROACH

Allopathic medicine's treatment program for incontinence can consist of drug therapy, surgery, and/or lifestyle changes.

DRUG TREATMENT

If a urinary tract infection or other ailment is to blame for the incontinence, then that ailment is treated with appropriate medication, such as antibiotics.

Anticholinergic drugs, such as propantheline and oxybutynin, may be effective in treating some types of urinary incontinence. They block some of the responses of nerves in the bladder. Potential side effects include dry mouth and eyes, mental confusion, and blurred vision.

Narcotics, such as loperamide, can be helpful for bowel incontinence. While they do slow the movement of stool through the intestine, they can also lead to constipation and are addictive.

SURGICAL TREATMENT

Several surgical techniques can be performed to repair damaged or weakened muscles and organs. For example, the urethra (the tube that empties the bladder) can be surgically tightened. In some cases, artificial muscles may be implanted.

OTHER TREATMENT

Depending on the type of urinary incontinence, doing specific exercises (called Kegel exercises) that work the muscles around the pelvis can be beneficial (this is most often helpful for women).

Bowel incontinence can be helped by adopting a high-fiber diet and regular toilet habits. Glycerin or laxative suppositories and enemas may also prove useful for some patients. If stool is severely blocked, a doctor may have to manually remove it. To prevent the soiling of clothes, diaperlike underpants are available.

ALTERNATIVE APPROACHES
BIOFEEDBACK TRAINING

Biofeedback training can help people with incontinence regain control over the muscles that regulate urination or bowel movements. The treatment uses monitors that "feed back" certain biological levels. Armed with this information, patients can learn to alter and control involuntary functions of the body.

Electromyographic biofeedback, which measures muscle tension, is often used to treat both urinary and bowel incontinence. For example, electrodes can be attached around the anus to measure electrical activity, which is translated into degrees of muscle pressure. The biofeedback trainer then instructs the patient on ways to tense up or relax these muscles around the anus, and the biofeedback monitor shows the progress.

For urinary incontinence, biofeedback also offers a way to check that patients are properly doing their exercises of the pelvis muscles. With women, a probe is inserted in the vagina to measure muscle contractions and relaxation.

About a dozen studies have shown that biofeedback training can improve bowel incontinence in more than 70 percent of patients tested. Other studies have reported 20 to 25 percent of patients being totally "cured" of urinary incontinence after undergoing a course of treatment with biofeedback training.

Biofeedback training can be used to reinforce the pelvic muscle exercises taught to women with certain types of urinary incontinence. The exercises, done four times a day, include the following steps:

- Tighten and then relax the muscles around the vagina and urethra as fast as you can. Do this about ten times. (To make sure you're using the right muscles, the next time you're sitting on the toilet, try to stop the flow of urine midstream. If you can stop the flow, then you're using those muscles.)
- Next, tighten the muscles, hold for four seconds, and then relax. Also do this about ten times.

HERBAL MEDICINE

Herbs can be especially effective in treating urinary incontinence. The group of plants called toning herbs can strengthen and restore the mucous membranes in the urinary tract and may prevent incontinence. The stems of horsetail, for example, can be taken in the form of juice, powder in capsules, or tincture. (The juice form can be difficult to find.)

Other beneficial herbs include buchu, saw palmetto, corn silk, plantain, and nettles. St.-John's-wort is also often added to an herbal remedy for urinary incontinence. Herbs can also be effective for ailments related to or precipitating incontinence, such as recurrent urinary tract infection, constipation, and diarrhea.

Here's a sample prescription for horsetail: Take 5 mL of juice three times a day. Or, if the juice in unavailable, take 30 drops of the tincture two to three times a day.

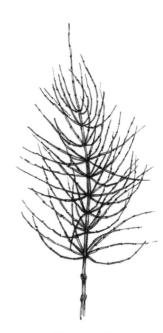

Horsetail

OTHER THERAPIES

ACUPUNCTURE—An acupuncturist can correct imbalances in the flow of vital energy, or qi. Urinary incontinence, for example, is thought to result from a deficiency of qi in the kidney.

HOMEOPATHY—Prescriptions can be tailored to individual symptoms to stimulate the body's peak performance.

NUTRITIONAL THERAPY—Dietary changes and supplementation can strengthen the body and avoid taxing the digestive tract. Fiber and water should be added to the diet, and several foods should be avoided, including coffee and alcohol. Food allergies may also play a role in incontinence.

Infertility

Infertility is the inability of a woman and man to conceive children. At any given time, approximately one in six couples is infertile. Infertile couples may become fertile later; the condition of sterility, however, has more finality.

CONVENTIONAL APPROACH

Allopathic medicine's treatment program for infertility begins with exhaustive examinations, tests, and counseling for both the woman and man. If there is an underlying condition, such as impotence (in men) or uterine fibroids (in women), then that must be treated. Otherwise, infertility treatment can include lifestyle changes (including stress reduction), drug therapy, or surgery. Only about half of the infertility cases that doctors treat result in pregnancies.

Men should avoid or reduce their use of alcohol, cigarettes, caffeine, and certain drugs, all of which can reduce sperm count. If not enough sperm are being produced, drug therapy may be effective. Commonly used medicines include clomiphene and gonadotropin hormones. Surgery is available if the passage for sperm is blocked.

If the woman is not ovulating (releasing mature eggs), some of the same drugs used for male infertility (clomiphene and gonadotropin hormones) may be helpful. Multiple births may result, and side effects of clomiphene can range from hot flashes to ovarian cysts. To correct hormonal imbalances related to the pituitary gland, the drug bromocriptine may be effective. Several surgical procedures are also available:

- Damaged fallopian tubes (which lead from the ovaries to the uterus) can be repaired.
- In artificial insemination, the sperm of the partner or a donor is injected into the woman's cervix.
- In vitro fertilization is a procedure in which one of the woman's eggs is surgically removed and then mixed with the man's sperm. After several days, the resulting embryos are injected into the woman's uterus.

ALTERNATIVE APPROACHES
TRADITIONAL CHINESE MEDICINE

In traditional Chinese medicine, the kidney system controls the reproductive system. Therefore, infertility is treated by rebalancing the flow of the body's energizing life force, or qi, through the kidney meridian. For example, a treatment for men with abnormal semen is Ju Jing Powder, which combines nine herbs and other substances including radix rehmanniae, fructus lycii, and radix polygoni multiflori. The mixture, made into a decoction to drink, is formulated depending on the exact problem with the semen. So, if the sperm swim slower than normal, the therapy includes more ingredients that warm and supplement qi. Typically, acupuncture, moxibustion, and dietary changes are also part of the treatment.

Regulations on who can practice acupuncture and other forms of traditional Chinese medicine vary from state to state. In addition to traditional Chinese physicians, some naturopathic physicians and medical doctors are trained in acupuncture. A practitioner can also instruct you on acupressure points you can use yourself and home exercises that can help.

MIND/BODY MEDICINE

Emotional stress can lower the level of fertility. For example, stress in a woman can affect the hormones being released from the brain's pituitary gland, interrupting ovulation (the release of mature eggs). If the stress is combined with another "fertility-lowering" condition, such as low sperm count or partially blocked fallopian tubes, then it can lead to infertility.

Several therapies can reduce stress and encourage relaxation, including
- guided imagery
- creative visualization
- meditation
- prayer
- support groups
- hypnotherapy

One proof that mind/body medicine is an effective part of infertility treatment is a University of Massachusetts study that showed that infertile couples who joined support groups were more than twice as likely to conceive children as couples who didn't participate in any groups.

Several times a day, set aside 15 to 30 minutes for relaxation exercises followed by guided imagery exercises related to the reproductive system. Have someone else read the script to you, or have it on tape nearby so you can play it right after finishing the exercises. Here's an excerpt of an imagery script:

On the stalk, imagine delicate buds swelling with color and energy and warmth, slowly opening, unfolding under nature's direction. Focus on the gentle wind carrying grains of pollen. Some grains float to the blossoming flower. Watch the blossom welcome the pollen, holding it and closing on it.

OTHER THERAPIES

AROMATHERAPY—Essential oils of rose maroc or rose otto may be prescribed.

ENVIRONMENTAL MEDICINE—Certain chemicals (from pesticides to hair sprays), molds, stress, infections—almost anything in the environment—may trigger infertility. Treatment involves removing these substances or lessening exposure to them.

HERBAL MEDICINE—Helpful herbs for women include blue cohosh and false unicorn root. For men, saw palmetto and damiana may be effective.

HOMEOPATHY—Remedies are personalized to the man or woman's state of health and may include natrum muriaticum and sepia.

HYDROTHERAPY—Cold sitz baths may help men increase their sperm counts. Alternating hot and cold sitz baths can improve pelvic circulation in both sexes.

NUTRITIONAL THERAPY—Supplements (such as zinc, vitamin C, and essential fatty acids) and special diets (such as one without the wheat protein, gluten) can be effective in treating male and female infertility.

MIND/BODY MEDICINE—Emotional counseling and meditative therapies play a major role in the treatment of infertility.

Influenza

Influenza, commonly known as the flu, is an infection of the respiratory tract. Many different viruses cause the sickness, and the particular strain dictates the severity of the symptoms. The flu strikes in outbreaks and epidemics, affecting a large group of people at once.

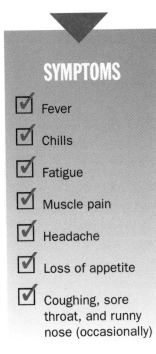

SYMPTOMS

- ☑ Fever
- ☑ Chills
- ☑ Fatigue
- ☑ Muscle pain
- ☑ Headache
- ☑ Loss of appetite
- ☑ Coughing, sore throat, and runny nose (occasionally)

CONVENTIONAL APPROACH

Allopathic medicine's treatment program for the flu consists of bed rest and medication. However, no drug can get rid of the virus. Doctors usually recommend painkillers, such as aspirin and acetaminophen, to lower the fever and ease aches and pains. The relief is temporary, and possible side effects range from stomach irritation to nausea. (Children younger than 18 years with fevers should not be given aspirin, which may lead to the potentially fatal disorder called Reye syndrome.)

Some people's state of health requires a more aggressive treatment of the flu. Elderly people or people with heart or lung diseases can take the drug amantadine, which can work to kill viruses. Side effects can include nausea and dizziness.

As a preventive measure, flu shots (or vaccines) are available. They must be taken at the beginning of each year's flu season to work. Their success rate, however, is hardly impressive: Up to 40 percent of people who receive the shots can still catch the flu.

ALTERNATIVE APPROACHES

Many alternative therapies hold that suppressing the symptoms of the flu may actually prolong the illness. Instead, they seek to bolster the body and its defenses, allowing the body to work through the illness. Usually the alternative therapies that are effective in the treatment of the common cold also work well on the flu, including nutritional therapy, herbal medicine, and aromatherapy.

HOMEOPATHY

Homeopathy can stimulate the body to overpower the flu virus. The therapy uses highly diluted, nontoxic doses of a natural substance that would produce flu symptoms if given in full strength to a healthy person. The substances are taken from plant, mineral, or animal sources.

To find a remedy for the flu, a classical homeopath would scrutinize the extent and nature of the patient's symptoms and the course of the illness. The treatment is then tailored to the individual's symptoms. (Combination remedies, available over the counter, are formulated for the most common flu symptoms. Because of this lack of individualization, they are less effective.) Many details are studied to get a full picture of the patient's case. The following are some factors to consider:

- Did the flu begin after a change in temperature?
- Is there a fever? Is it burning? Alternating with chills?
- Is the sickness accompanied by exhaustion?
- Are there body pains? Where?
- Is it accompanied by thirst?
- Does it cause a change in temperament?

The following are some typical remedies for the flu:

- arsenicum album for the flu that causes restlessness, anxiety, thirst for small sips of warm liquids, a desire for company (even fear of being alone), burning pains, burning discharge from the nose, wheezing cough, remittent fever, chills, and symptoms that are worst between midnight and 3:00 A.M.
- gelsemium for the flu characterized by dull, dizzy, droopy, dopey feeling; aches all over; chills down the spine; no thirst; and heavy eyelids
- baptisia tinctoria for the flu that causes putrid breath; severe dizziness, aches, chills; and serious illness with great prostration
- bryonia alba for the flu that causes irritability, a desire to be alone in the quiet and dark, bursting headache, and a thirst for large amounts of cold water
- eupatorium perfoliatum for the flu characterized by deep bone pain, thirst, sore eyeballs, sore skin, and symptoms that are worst between 7:00 and 9:00 A.M.

HYPERTHERMIA

A fever is a common symptom of the flu and is considered proof that the body is trying to eliminate infecting viruses. Many viruses can't withstand high temperatures. Hyperthermia treatment can give the body's defense system a helping hand, either by raising the body temperature (if a slight fever has already set in) or inducing a fever (if none is present).

In addition, practitioners of hyperthermia believe suppressing a fever—by taking acetaminophen, for example—may actually lengthen a bout with the flu. Hyperthermia treatment can be directed to the infected breathing passages or to the entire body.

Ways to use this therapy include
- soaking in hot baths
- inhaling steam (Be careful to avoid burns.)
- covering with layers of clothes and blankets
- drinking hot teas or broths

These methods are usually combined with herbal medicine, nutritional therapy, and detoxification therapy. Hyperthermia should be employed with great care. The patient's temperature should be taken frequently, and the

COVER THAT MOUTH

By coughing or sneezing, a person with the flu can spread the virus. The contagious period is thought to last from the time just before the symptoms start to up to ten days later.

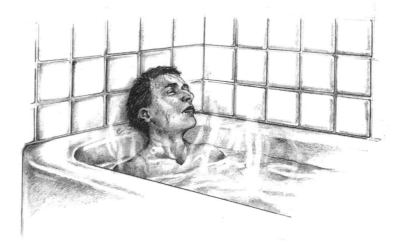

fever should not go higher than 104°F (as measured orally).

A sample hyperthermia treatment for the flu may be to soak in a bathtub full of hot water for about ten minutes. Keep these points in mind:

- It's important to take frequent readings of the body temperature. Get out of the tub if the fever is more than 104°F.
- The bathwater should be about 103°F. Add more hot water to keep the temperature constant.
- When finished, dry off thoroughly, stay warm, and get into bed right away.

AYURVEDIC MEDICINE

According to Ayurvedic medicine, a flu virus can only cause sickness in an unhealthy person, someone whose constitutional type is out of balance. This therapy works to bring the constitution back into harmony.

The Ayurvedic treatment for the flu is highly personalized for each patient, depending on both the current and ideal state of the constitution. For example, does kapha need to be calmed? Should pitta be strengthened?

The treatment can involve several approaches, including

- dietary alterations—eating certain foods and avoiding others to rebalance the constitution
- herbal therapy—taking a mix of herbs (in tea, tincture, powder, pill, or other form), also to rebalance the constitution
- nasal douching—rinsing the nose and mouth passages with salt water, to cleanse and detoxify
- meditation—calming and concentrating the mind
- breathing exercises—encouraging the body's flow of energy (prana)

An Ayurvedic physician may recommend the following breathing exercise:

- Sit up or lie down in bed.
- Inhale slowly and deliberately, sticking out your stomach as you draw in the breath.
- Exhale, bringing your stomach in.
- Repeat inhaling and exhaling, but focus on expanding and then bringing in the rib cage instead of the stomach.
- Repeat again, this time focusing on moving your shoulders up and then down.
- Finally, inhale, sticking out your stomach, expanding your rib cage, and then lifting up your shoulders.
- Exhale, bringing your shoulders down, the rib cage in, and the stomach in.

OTHER THERAPIES

BODYWORK—Techniques include massage and reflexology to increase blood circulation and stimulate the sinuses and lymphatic system.

HERBAL MEDICINE—Herbs to strengthen the immune system and ease flu symptoms include echinacea (or purple coneflower), hypericum, baptisia, and elderberry.

NUTRITIONAL THERAPY—Therapy can provide the body with needed nutrients and proscribe avoiding foods that weaken the defenses such as sugars and dairy products.

INSOMNIA IS THE INABILITY TO GET A GOOD NIGHT'S SLEEP. THE CONDITION HAS MORE TO DO WITH QUALITY OF SLEEP THAN QUANTITY; IN FACT, SOME PEOPLE NEED AS LITTLE AS FOUR HOURS PER NIGHT. THE CAUSES OF INSOMNIA INCLUDE MENTAL ANGUISH, BREATHING PROBLEMS, UNCOMFORTABLE OR ERRATIC SLEEPING ARRANGEMENTS, DRUG AND ALCOHOL MISUSE, DIGESTIVE DISORDERS, AND DEPRESSION, AMONG MANY OTHERS.

CONVENTIONAL APPROACH

Allopathic medicine's treatment program for insomnia depends on its causes. Sleeping troubles triggered by breathing problems or other physical disorders, as well as by psychological conditions such as anxiety or depression, require treatment. Drug therapy and lifestyle adjustments are recommended for most other types of insomnia.

DRUG TREATMENT

Several prescription and over-the-counter medicines encourage sleepiness, and many do this by cutting down on brain activity. These drugs may also cause daytime drowsiness and confusion and should only be used for short periods of time because of their habit-forming nature. They include

- antidepressants
- antihistamines with sedative effects
- barbiturates, such as secobarbital
- benzodiazepine drugs, including diazepam, flurazepam, temazepam, and triazolam
- chloral hydrate

OTHER TREATMENT

Certain measures can be taken to encourage better sleeping, including

- making the bedroom dark and quiet
- winding down before bed by taking a warm (not hot) bath
- keeping a regular sleeping schedule
- avoiding napping during the day
- avoiding caffeine in the evening
- exercising daily

ALTERNATIVE APPROACHES

Several alternative approaches stress the importance of identifying the cause of insomnia before deciding on a treatment. Whenever possible, the cause—which can range from depression and diabetes to restless legs—requires its own treatment. In the meantime, or if the cause is not readily apparent, several alternative therapies offer effective choices that go beyond sleeping pills and their side effects.

NUTRITIONAL THERAPY

According to nutritional therapists, taking supplements of certain hormones or nutrients—or adding them to the diet in food form, if possible—can effectively treat insomnia.

Perhaps the most exciting news about insomnia concerns melatonin, a hormone that's produced by the pineal gland in the brain. Researchers have found that supplementation with this hormone can help the body reset its internal clock (circadian rhythms) if it is out of pace, resulting in sounder, longer

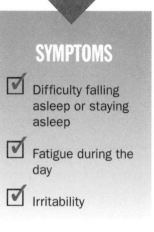

SYMPTOMS

☑ Difficulty falling asleep or staying asleep

☑ Fatigue during the day

☑ Irritability

sleep. However, melatonin should not be used for long-term sleep disorders. Because it can interact with hormones in the body, it should not be taken in high doses (over 3 mg) without the supervision of a naturopathic or other qualified health care practitioner.

Serotonin, a chemical messenger in the brain, plays a role in bringing on sleep and requires the presence of the amino acid tryptophan to work. Therefore, tryptophan supplements are ideal for people with insomnia, but they're unavailable in some countries. (The Food and Drug Administration banned the supplements after contaminated batches hit the streets and were linked to causing serious injury.) Eating foods high in tryptophan, such as soybeans, eggs, and turkey, may not be the best way to get the amino acid. Instead, high-carbohydrate foods can make it easier for any tryptophan in the body to travel to the brain.

Other supplements that may be helpful include magnesium, calcium, and vitamin B_6. Of course, good sleeping also depends on a sound diet and regular exercise. Avoid heavy meals, sugar, alcohol, and stimulants such as caffeine in the evening.

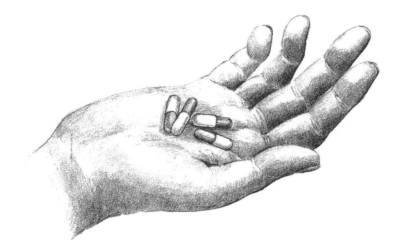

Here's a sample prescription for melatonin: For two weeks, take a 2-mg capsule one hour before bedtime. Maintain a regular sleeping schedule. If you're not getting a good night's sleep after two weeks, the prescription may need to be readjusted.

ACUPUNCTURE

Acupuncture views illness as an imbalance in the body's vital energy force, or qi. One possible explanation for insomnia is that it results from a deficiency of yin in the kidney system, which is causing fire in the heart system. (Together, yin and yang create harmony in the body.) There are many other explanations, all of which depend on the particular patient.

Acupuncture works to correct these qi imbalances with the use of tiny needles inserted in specific points on the body. Manual pressure (acupressure) can also be applied to these points. Auriculotherapy—a form of acupuncture that treats the entire body through specific corresponding points on the ears—is particularly recommended for insomnia.

One Chinese clinical study tested treatments on 160 people with insomnia. Eighty patients were instructed to apply pressure to certain auricular points nightly, and the other 80 took sleeping pills (diazepam). After one month, 65 of the acupuncture patients were cured or improved their sleeping patterns, while only 11 of the drug therapy patients improved.

Acupuncture treatment for insomnia may also be paired with herbal therapy, dietary changes, relaxation techniques, and certain exercises. An acupuncturist may recommend the following measures to people with insomnia:

- Eat small, light, easily digestible dinners.
- Avoid exciting prebedtime activities (such as reading a thrilling book or watching an action film).
- Wash feet in warm water just before going to bed.

 An acupuncturist, traditional Chinese physician, or naturopathic physician can perform acupuncture. For your first visit, be prepared to discuss the details of your insomnia, as well as your general health, diet, and lifestyle.

WAVE THERAPY

Wave therapy employs different forms of light and sound in the treatment of insomnia.

Light therapy aims to reset the body's internal clock, or circadian rhythms, by exposing the patient to very bright lights in the morning and during the day and dimmed lights and darkened eyeglasses to reduce light exposure in the evening. So far, research has shown that measures like these can have a significant positive effect on people with insomnia.

Sound therapy can also be helpful. This therapy uses certain types of music—often natural sounds like waves on a beach or wind rustling leaves—to ease tension and anxiety before bedtime.

 Here is some light therapy to use at home:

- Sit outside in the morning to soak up some sun.
- Turn on very bright lights at the breakfast table.

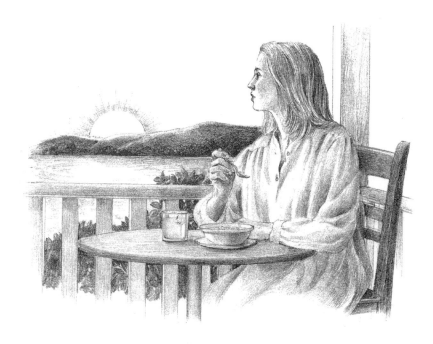

OTHER THERAPIES

BIOFEEDBACK TRAINING—Electromyographic and thermal biofeedback, together with relaxation exercises, are useful in treating insomnia.

GUIDED IMAGERY AND CREATIVE VISUALIZATION—Various techniques can bring on relaxation and deep sleep.

HERBAL MEDICINE—Valerian, passionflower, chamomile, lavender, and St.-John's-wort may be effective.

HOMEOPATHY—Specific remedies must be tailored to the individual, but common prescriptions include aconitum napellus, coffea cruda, nux vomica, and sulphur.

HYPNOTHERAPY—Treatments, including self-hypnosis, can reduce anxiety and make falling asleep easier.

QIGONG—The exercises and meditations can balance the flow of vital energy, or qi, and encourage relaxation.

Irritable Bowel Syndrome

Irritable bowel syndrome (IBS) is a disorder of the colon that involves irregular bowel movements and discomfort in the abdomen. With IBS (also called spastic colon or mucous colitis), the nerves and muscles in the colon overreact to normal functions of digestion. Its causes are unclear, but it's probably not related to a disease of the bowels.

SYMPTOMS

- ☑ Pain in the abdomen, which may be relieved by passing gas or stool

- ☑ Bloating and gas

- ☑ Bouts of diarrhea or constipation, or alternating between the two

- ☑ Mucus in the stool (occasionally)

- ☑ After bowel movement, a feeling that the bowels are still full

These symptoms may be triggered by stress, anxiety, or certain foods, but they often come and go without warning or apparent cause.

CONVENTIONAL APPROACH

Because there is no cure for IBS, allopathic medicine works to relieve its symptoms. Self-treatment measures include adding fiber to the diet (from food sources such as bran and vegetables) and reducing stress (by exercising and adopting regular sleep habits). Fiber can also be added in the form of bulking agents, including methylcellulose and psyllium. Taken with fluids, they can relieve diarrhea as well as constipation. If anxiety or stress are thought to play a role in the patient's IBS, then psychotherapy can be effective.

Medications can be effective for some patients. They may include:

- Anticholinergic drugs, such as propantheline, block the responses of nerves in the colon. Potential side effects are dry mouth, blurred vision, and difficult urination.

- Narcotics, including diphenoxylate and loperamide, can stop diarrhea by slowing the movement of stool through the intestine. They can lead to constipation and are potentially addictive.

- Antidepressants, such as amitriptyline, may be effective, whether the patient is depressed or not. They can, however, cause dizziness, hot flashes, and other side effects.

- Antianxiety drugs, such as chlordiazepoxide, fight off anxiety by decreasing nerve activity in the brain. If used regularly, they can become addictive.

- Barbiturates, including phenobarbital, bring feelings of calmness. Side effects can range from drowsiness to excitement.

Some conventional doctors have also recognized the benefits of the alternative approach of biofeedback training (see below).

ALTERNATIVE APPROACHES

Several alternative therapies can offer relief from the symptoms of IBS or even prevent them. These treatments are usually combined with a high-fiber diet, exercise, and stress-reduction techniques.

BIOFEEDBACK TRAINING

Biofeedback training has been shown to be very effective in the treatment of IBS. One way that biofeedback can help is by teaching people with IBS to manage stress in their lives, thereby lessening the chances of future attacks. Especially when combined with other relaxation techniques, this approach to prevention is effective enough to attract the attention of many conventional physicians.

To a lesser extent, people may use biofeedback training to gain control over some actions of the colon. The treatment uses monitors that "feed back" certain biological levels. Armed with this information, patients can learn to alter involuntary functions of the body.

Thermal biofeedback is often used to teach relaxation to people with IBS. Here's how it works:

- The biofeedback trainer tapes sensors to the patient, often on the finger, to measure skin temperature. Shown on the monitor, the temperature is used to gauge the level of blood flow.
- Next, the trainer leads the patient through various visualization and breathing exercises—all designed to bring a state of relaxation to the patient.
- The monitor shows whether there is any progress—a corresponding rise in skin temperature. The patient and trainer can then use the information to guide or intensify visualization efforts.

Several studies have shown positive results for people with IBS when biofeedback is combined with instruction in positive thinking or assertiveness and education on the link between stress and the bowels.

Biofeedback trainers will usually instruct their patients in progressive muscle relaxation, which can be done at home to reinforce the training sessions. Here is an example of progressive muscle relaxation:

- Wearing loose clothing, lie down on a firm but not hard surface.
- Close your eyes and imagine tightening the muscles in your feet.
- Then release these muscles.
- Next, direct your attention to your calves, tensing and then easing these muscles in the same fashion.
- Continue up the body, including your arms, until you end with your scalp.

NUTRITIONAL THERAPY

Nutritional therapists hold that altering the diet may prevent the symptoms of IBS. One well-established strategy is to increase your intake of fiber to help regulate the bowels. However, this should be done with caution. Excessive fiber, particularly insoluble fiber, can exacerbate IBS symptoms in a few people.

Several foods or specific ingredients seem to trigger IBS in some patients. In fact, food allergies and sensitivities may play a role in the condition. The common culprits include

- dietary fats
- corn
- wheat
- monosodium glutamate
- fructose
- caffeine
- dairy products
- tomatoes

Nutrient deficiencies can be a problem for some people with IBS because intestinal abnormalities make absorption of certain nutrients difficult. In these cases, supplementation may be helpful.

The best way to tell if a certain food is to blame for your bouts with IBS is to keep a food and symptom diary. Record the following in your diary:

- What you eat and when
- What symptoms you experience and when they occur
- How you're feeling each day (relaxed, stressed, excited, and so on)

After about a month, any correlations should be apparent. You can also bring your diary to your physician or practitioner; it may help them identify problems.

HERBAL MEDICINE

Herbs can be effective in easing disturbances in the digestive system and in reducing anxiety. Peppermint oil, which contains menthol, can reduce gas and abdominal pain and relax the intestinal muscles.

In a British study, tablets of peppermint oil worked better than a placebo in reducing the symptoms of IBS. The tablets had a special coating (called enteric) that allowed them to disintegrate in the small intestines, not the stomach. This coating also lessens the possibility of heartburn.

Other useful herbs include
- bayberry
- chamomile
- ginger
- marshmallow
- meadowsweet
- valerian

Here's a sample prescription for peppermint oil: Take two enteric-coated capsules (each containing 0.2 mL of oil) three times a day. Lower the dose as symptoms subside. Using enteric-coated capsules is very important to ensure that the oil is released at the proper time.

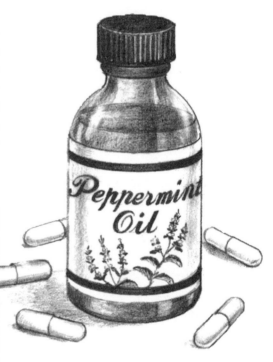

OTHER THERAPIES

HOMEOPATHY—Several remedies can be very helpful but an appropriate prescription requires an expert evaluation.

HYPNOTHERAPY—Certain techniques can teach people with IBS to relax and to imagine the easing of the bowel muscles. Several studies have shown that hypnotherapy reduces IBS symptoms in up to 85 percent of patients tested.

YOGA—Several aspects of yoga can be very effective relaxation tools.

KIDNEY STONES ARE HARD CRYSTALLIZED CLUMPS THAT ARE FORMED FROM CER- TAIN SUBSTANCES IN THE URINE. THEY RANGE IN SIZE FROM A GRAIN OF SAND TO A GOLF BALL. SOME ARE PASSED OUT OF THE BODY WITH URINE; OTHERS BE- COME BLOCKED IN THE URINARY TRACT. THEY MAY FORM BECAUSE OF A LACK OF FLUIDS IN THE BODY, REPEATED URINARY TRACT INFECTIONS, CERTAIN GENETIC DISEASES, OR OTHER FACTORS.

CONVENTIONAL APPROACH
TREATMENT

Depending on the size and location of the kidney stone, allopathic medicine's treatment program employs a combination of self-help measures, drug therapy, surgery, and ultrasound techniques. All patients are instructed to drink more fluids (at least four quarts daily) and to eliminate specific foods from the diet. For example, those who have the calcium oxalate type of kidney stones (the type that represents 80 percent of all kidney stones) should avoid foods high in oxalate, including

- peanuts
- chocolate
- coffee
- spinach and other leafy greens
- black tea
- rhubarb

If the stones are small enough, the patient can take painkillers (such as morphine or meperidine) until the hard mass passes through the urinary tract on its own. For larger stones, more aggressive treatment is used. The stones can be broken down or dissolved with drugs and then allowed to pass out of the body with urine.

One nonsurgical procedure (called *lithotripsy*) sends ultrasonic sound waves through the body to smash stones into smaller pieces so they can be passed. The crystals can also be surgically removed. Side effects and recovery periods vary depending on the procedure.

PREVENTION

Chances are good that people who have kidney stones will experience more in the future. Preventive measures typically include increased fluid intake, some dietary adjustments, and medication. Patients taking long-term courses of drugs should be monitored for side effects, such as low blood potassium.

ALTERNATIVE APPROACHES
NUTRITIONAL THERAPY

Nutritional therapists hold that many types of kidney stones are the result of an improper diet, and treatment and prevention require wholesale changes in eating habits.

A very common type of kidney stone, calcium oxalate, has been linked to a diet that's low in fiber and high in refined carbohydrates, animal protein (including meat and dairy products), and alcohol. Protein can cause problems by prompting the body to lose more calcium in the urine, making it available for stone formation. People who are prone to forming stones are advised to eat more vegetables, fruits,

SYMPTOMS

☑ Sharp, sudden, severe pain radiating from the lower back into the abdomen, groin, and thigh

☑ Nausea and vomiting

☑ Frequent urge to urinate

☑ Difficulty urinating or burning pain when urinating

☑ Smelly, cloudy, or bloody urine

☑ Fever, chills, and fatigue (occasionally)

Sometimes kidney stones exhibit no symptoms at all, particularly when they are still in the kidney and not moving down the ureter toward the bladder.

whole grains, and beans. A vegetarian diet, consisting of no beef, poultry, and seafood, is often recommended as an ideal way to meet these nutritional guidelines. As with the suggestions in conventional medicine, daily water consumption should be about four quarts. And specific foods, such as those high in oxalate listed above, should be cut from the menu.

Deficiencies in magnesium and vitamin B_6 may also lead to calcium oxalate stones. Several studies have shown that doses of these nutrients can prevent stones in many people who previously had them. Several other supplements may also be prescribed, including vitamin K.

For someone with the calcium oxalate type of kidney stones, a naturopathic physician might prescribe the following supplementation regimen: 300 mg of magnesium daily and 50 mg of vitamin B_6 daily.

HERBAL MEDICINE

In the treatment of kidney stones, herbs can be used to break them down and prevent their formation in the first place. Herbs can also encourage the flow of urine and relieve the irritated walls of the urinary tract. Gravelroot has long been used to dissolve kidney stones. The root is commonly taken in decoction or tincture form. Madder, hydrangea, and rumex can also help break up stones. Aloe vera juice may clear stones and prevent new ones from forming.

Other herbs, such as cornsilk and couch grass, can soothe the walls of the urinary tract. Juniper berries, often used to clear urinary tract infections, can be added to an herbal treatment for stones.

To dissolve kidney stones, an herbalist might recommend drinking a ½ cup of gravelroot decoction three times a day. Make the decoction by bringing 2½ cups of water and 20 grams of dried gravelroot to a boil. Simmer the mixture for about an hour. Strain out the gravelroot before drinking.

OTHER THERAPIES

AYURVEDIC MEDICINE—Typical kidney stone treatments involve dietary changes and herbal therapy.

BODYWORK—Reflexology is just one form of bodywork that can stimulate the organs and regulate bodily functions. Treatment can focus on the reflexes of the pituitary gland, thyroid and parathyroid glands, spleen, and kidney, among others.

HOMEOPATHY—Common remedies can include berberis, magnesia phosphorica, and sarsaparilla.

HYDROTHERAPY—Treatments, such as warm sitz baths, can be used to relieve the pain of kidney stones.

Lupus Erythematosus

SYSTEMIC LUPUS ERYTHEMATOSUS IS A DISEASE THAT CAUSES INFLAMMATION OF VARIOUS PARTS OF THE BODY, ESPECIALLY THE SKIN, JOINTS, BLOOD VESSELS, AND KIDNEYS. IT RESULTS FROM A MALFUNCTIONING IMMUNE SYSTEM, WHICH ATTACKS THE BODY INSTEAD OF PROTECTING IT. CONTRIBUTING FACTORS MAY INCLUDE GENETICS, INFECTIONS, ULTRAVIOLET LIGHT, EXTREME STRESS, AND THE USE OF CERTAIN DRUGS.

CONVENTIONAL APPROACH

No cure is available for lupus. Therefore, allopathic medicine treats its symptoms with drugs that reduce inflammation and suppress abnormalities of the immune system:

- Nonsteroidal anti-inflammatory drugs, such as aspirin, ibuprofen, and naproxen, are effective in fighting pain, but their side effects can range from nausea and diarrhea to stomach ulcers and ringing in the ears.
- Acetaminophen can also ease pain. It is less effective than aspirin yet carries fewer side effects.
- Corticosteroids reduce inflammation and suppress the activity of the immune system. With long-term use, they may cause weight gain, diabetes, and osteoporosis.
- Antimalarial drugs, such as chloroquine and hydroxychloroquine, can relieve skin rashes and swollen joints. They can take months to work, and their side effects may include diarrhea, stomach pain, muscle weakness, rashes, and various eye problems.
- Anticancer drugs, including azathioprine and cyclophosphamide, have effects similar to corticosteriods, and their side effects can be serious, including anemia, low white blood cell counts, reduced ability to fight off infections, and an increased risk of developing cancer.

Several factors can trigger a flare-up of lupus symptoms. Whenever possible, these guidelines should be followed:

- Minimize sun exposure and use sunscreen lotions.
- Exercise regularly.
- Maintain immunizations.
- Alleviate stress with support groups and counseling.

ALTERNATIVE APPROACHES
NUTRITIONAL THERAPY

Diet can aggravate the symptoms of lupus or contribute to its onset. Treatment may call for dietary alterations and supplementation for any nutrient deficiencies. Food allergies and sensitivities have been implicated as a possible trigger of the disease. Many believe alfalfa sprouts to be a common trigger of lupus symptoms; people that have had lupus symptoms may want to avoid them. An elimination diet can help to identify any other culprits. Here's how an elimination diet works:

- For two to three weeks, the patient's commonly eaten foods are eliminated from the diet. Common food allergens (such as wheat, eggs, milk, peanuts, and corn) are also avoided.

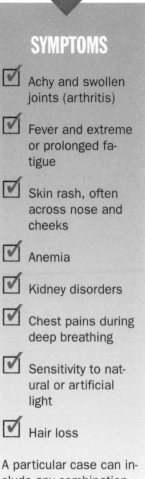

SYMPTOMS

- ☑ Achy and swollen joints (arthritis)
- ☑ Fever and extreme or prolonged fatigue
- ☑ Skin rash, often across nose and cheeks
- ☑ Anemia
- ☑ Kidney disorders
- ☑ Chest pains during deep breathing
- ☑ Sensitivity to natural or artificial light
- ☑ Hair loss

A particular case can include any combination of these symptoms, which also tend to come and go.

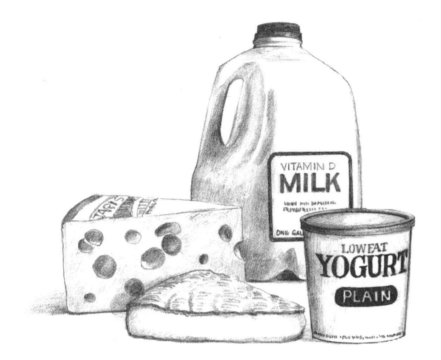

Milk, cheese, and other dairy products are common allergens that may play a role in lupus.

- If symptoms have subsided or not appeared by the end of this period, then the food challenges can begin. If the symptoms are still present, then more foods should be eliminated from the diet.
- Reintroduce one at a time, every two days, the commonly eaten foods and common food allergens that you eliminated noting if any symptoms appear.
- Continue in this fashion with the other foods.

It should be noted that lupus symptoms can go into remission for weeks or years. Linking a remission to an avoided food allergen may take some detective work.

Hydrochloric acid deficiency also has been linked with lupus and rheumatoid arthritis. The stomach normally secretes this strong acid, which helps digest proteins. If indicated, supplements in capsule form can be taken with meals.

To treat people with lupus, a low-protein diet is often prescribed. Large amounts of protein may be harmful for several reasons:

- It can tax weakened kidneys. (Half of the people with lupus have kidney disorders.)
- It has the ability to rob calcium from the bones. (People with lupus are often at higher risk for osteoporosis because of the drugs they take and their instructions to avoid the sun.)
- It may tax the immune system.

Besides being low in protein, the ideal diet should be low in fat and high in green leafy vegetables, such as bok choy, collard greens, and kale. These vegetables may help people with lupus to metabolize estrogen better.

Supplements may also be prescribed, including vitamin B_6, vitamin C, and essential fatty acids. Vitamin E, taken orally and applied to the skin, can help heal the skin rashes that sometimes accompany lupus. Supplements are often recommended instead of trying to get the vitamin from food sources because most of the food sources of vitamin E (such as vegetable oils) contain a lot of fat. Fish oil, especially EPA, is another effective supplement.

A sample prescription for the skin rashes associated with lupus might be to take 800 IU of oral vitamin E daily.

ENVIRONMENTAL MEDICINE

Like nutritional therapy, environmental medicine recognizes that diet can play a role in triggering lupus. But environmental medicine goes several steps further to implicate pollutants, pesticides, molds, stress, infections—

almost anything in the environment. The exact mix of triggers is different for every person with lupus.

These environmental factors do not trigger the disease in the same way that an allergy might. Instead, it is the repeated exposure to multiple offending substances over time that weakens the body's immune system. Eventually, an autoimmune disease like lupus strikes. An autoimmune disease is one in which the immune system, instead of protecting the body, begins to attack it.

Skin tests, rotary diversified diets, and other testing procedures can help pinpoint the environmental stressors. For example, one procedure checks for culprits by placing drops of certain substances (foods or chemicals) under the tongue. If symptoms develop, then the substance can be identified as a trigger. As an example, overexposure to the chemical formaldehyde has been suggested as a lupus trigger in some people. Formaldehyde can be found in dozens of home and office products, such as plywood paneling and nail polish.

Once an environmental factor is identified, treatment can include
- avoidance of the triggers (from installing air filters to changing the diet)
- immunotherapy in which minute drops of the offending substance are given under the tongue or in injections in amounts so small that they won't cause any symptoms but should build up the body's defenses and increase the body's tolerance to that substance
- nutritional adjustments
- generally, as few drugs as possible

 Keeping a diary with the details of your symptoms is an

OTHER THERAPIES

HERBAL MEDICINE—Echinacea, feverfew, goldenseal, and pau d'arco are just a few of the helpful herbs.

HYDROTHERAPY—Cold or hot compresses can be used for pain relief.

MIND/BODY MEDICINE—Creative visualization, spirituality, relaxation techniques, biofeedback, and other mind/body treatments can strengthen the immune system, as well as reduce joint pain and ease accompanying depression.

TRADITIONAL CHINESE MEDICINE—Treatment may involve acupuncture, herbal therapy, dietary alterations, and exercise.

important step in understanding your case of lupus and will also help your physician. Be as exhaustive in your note-taking as possible, mentioning
- which foods you ate
- the soaps you bathed with
- the rooms and buildings you stayed in
- how much time you spent driving

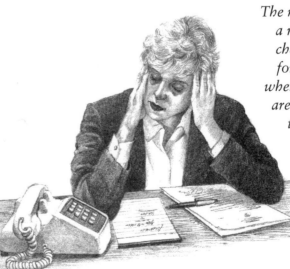

The modern office can be a repository of toxic chemicals, especially formaldehyde. Note whether your symptoms are worse during your time at school or in the office.

Menopause

MENOPAUSE—ALSO CALLED "THE CHANGE OF LIFE"—IS THE ENDING OF A WOMAN'S MONTHLY MENSTRUAL PERIODS AND OVULATION (THE PRODUCTION OF EGGS). IT ALSO SIGNALS OTHER CHANGES TO THE BODY AND MIND, BROUGHT ON IN PART BECAUSE THE BODY BEGINS PRODUCING SMALLER AMOUNTS OF THE HORMONES ESTROGEN AND PROGESTERONE (AMONG OTHERS). MENOPAUSE TYPICALLY OCCURS BETWEEN THE AGES OF 45 AND 55.

SYMPTOMS

The amount and severity of symptoms varies widely, but the following are all possible:

☑ Hot flashes (on the face and upper body) and night sweats

☑ Vaginal dryness, as well as dry skin and hair

☑ Reduced memory and concentration

☑ Mood swings and depression

☑ Insomnia

☑ Pain during sexual intercourse or altered sex drive

CONVENTIONAL APPROACH

Allopathic medicine relies on drug therapy to treat the symptoms of menopause and prevent some of the disorders, such as osteoporosis, that often follow this transition in life.

Hormone replacement therapy is a commonly prescribed cure-all for women going through menopause; however, its side effects can include
- headaches
- water retention
- breakthrough menstrual bleeding
- blood clots
- potentially increased risks of breast cancer and gallbladder disease

Beta blockers can ease hot flashes and migraine headaches for women who cannot take estrogen replacement therapy.

ALTERNATIVE APPROACHES

Alternative therapists often frown on widespread use of estrogen replacement therapy, citing its potential side effects and emphasizing that menopause is a natural occurrence, not a disease or a state of deficiency that requires aggressive treatment. Alternative treatments offer ways to ease or avoid some of the annoying symptoms of menopause. Additionally, osteoporosis and heart disease, whose risks increase with menopause, may be prevented with alternative methods (see osteoporosis, page 136, and heart disease, page 92).

HERBAL MEDICINE

Herbs that mimic female hormones or relieve symptoms ranging from fatigue to vaginal dryness offer a lot of promise to women with menopause. Several herbs contain natural plant estrogens (phytoestrogens) that are similar to but weaker than the estrogen hormone found in a woman's body. These herbs, including black cohosh, false unicorn root, and licorice, are often prescribed to ease the troublesome symptoms of menopause. Other phytoestrogens include alfalfa, dong quai, and soy.

Mexican wild yam, on the other hand, provides a substance similar to another female hormone, progesterone. A modified extract of the yam is used instead of synthetic progesterone to treat irritability and other menopausal symptoms and even increase bone density, with few if any reported side effects. It's available in capsules, as an oil, and as a cream. Most research now indicates that wild yam does *not* convert to progesterone in the body as was previously speculated, but the chemically converted extract seems effective.

From another class of herbs is Siberian ginseng (eleuthero)—a well-known energy tonic that can reduce irritability and fatigue associated with menopause. It's typically used in tincture or capsule form.

Evening primrose oil is often prescribed to lessen fatigue, hot flashes, and indigestion. The oil, made from evening primrose seeds, contains the essential fatty acid called gamma-linolenic acid, which is given credit for reducing those symptoms. It's available in capsule form.

Other helpful herbs include
- chamomile and valerian root for insomnia
- dandelion root, Oregon grape, and chaste tree (vitex) for hot flashes
- chickweed, cleavers, kava kava, and valerian root for mood swings
- aloe vera and calendula for vaginal dryness

An herbalist may prescribe one Mexican wild yam capsule three times daily to reduce irritability triggered by menopause. Dong quai, licorice (in the absence of high blood pressure), alfalfa, and chaste tree (vitex) may also be part of the prescription.

YOGA

Yoga delivers benefits to both the body and mind, alleviating menopausal symptoms such as insomnia, depression, hot flashes, and mood swings. It encourages deep breathing and relaxation, maintains muscle tone and flexibility, improves blood circulation, and increases the levels of mood-regulating chemicals in the brain, among other advantages.

Because menopausal women are concerned with osteoporosis and heart disease, yoga is doubly valuable. It provides weight-bearing exercise that encourages strong bones. And, as several clinical studies have shown, it can contribute to lower cholesterol and improve the efficiency of the heart. Yoga sessions normally last from 20 to 60 minutes and are performed three to seven times a week. They include a combination of breathing exercises, warm-ups, poses, and meditation.

The following pose might be part of a complete yoga routine that can help alleviate menopausal symptoms. It emphasizes good posture and breathing:
- Stand up straight with your feet together.

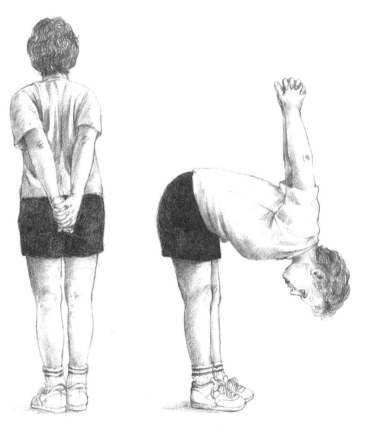

WORKOUT WONDERS

Regular aerobic and weight-bearing exercise is a smart move for preventing heart disease and osteoporosis. The workouts, ideally performed at least three times a week, can also induce relaxation (valuable in easing mood swings, hot flashes, and insomnia), stimulate blood circulation in the lower body (important for vaginal dryness and infections), and stimulate endorphin production (relieving hot flashes).

- Put your hands behind your back and clasp them together. Keep your arms straight.
- Inhale deeply.
- As you exhale, slowly bend forward, letting your arms extend straight up toward the ceiling and your head hang down gently. Try not to bend your knees.
- Inhale and slowly come back up to a standing position.
- Repeat two times.

NUTRITIONAL THERAPY

Nutritional therapists hold that certain foods or nutrient deficiencies can trigger or exacerbate symptoms. Still other foods may boost the body's tolerance for fluctuating hormone levels. Soybean products such as tofu contain natural plant estrogens (phytoestrogens) that may reduce menopausal symptoms. Japanese women, whose diet is typically high in soy foods, report few incidents of menopause-induced hot flashes. Phytoestrogens are also found in lima beans, berries, and several other foods.

Another preventive measure is drinking at least eight glasses of purified water per day to ease hot flashes and vaginal dryness.

Particular foods may trigger hot flashes, mood swings, vaginal discomforts, and other menopausal symptoms. These culprits include sugar, caffeine, alcohol, refined foods, and spicy foods. Keeping a diary that notes symptoms and food intake can be helpful in pinpointing which foods may be provoking which symptoms.

Vitamin E offers several benefits for women with menopause. Oral supplements of the vitamin can ease hot flashes (and perhaps also headaches, insomnia, nervousness, fatigue, and other symptoms), while vitamin E oil applied to the vagina may reduce dryness and relieve painful sexual intercourse. Another group of vitamins, the B complex, helps relieve hot flashes for some women. And magnesium deficiency may be to blame for menopausal symptoms such as fatigue. Other helpful supplements include

- vitamin A
- vitamin C

ACCENTUATE THE POSITIVE

Many practitioners of alternative medicine emphasize that half of the battle of menopause is maintaining an upbeat attitude. Women can better weather the accompanying emotional and physical stresses if they embrace and look forward to this change of life. After all, it is a perfectly natural part of a healthy life, not a disorder to endure.

- essential fatty acids (evening primrose oil, black currant oil, borage oil, flaxseed oil)
- bioflavonoids (especially hesperidin for hot flashes)
- calcium
- potassium
- boron

Here's a sample vitamin E treatment for hot flashes: Take 800 IU of the vitamin daily. (Women with diabetes, high blood pressure, or heart disease should not take such high doses of vitamin E.) As an alternative to supplements, good food sources of vitamin E include kale, wheat germ, almonds, vegetable oils, and egg yolks.

TRADITIONAL CHINESE MEDICINE

During menopause, a woman's body adjusts to the changing hormone levels. According to traditional Chinese medicine, a bothersome menopausal symptom will appear only if the body's vital life energy, or qi, (in particular the kidney energy) is out of balance. Treatment to correct this imbalance may involve any combination of herbal therapy, acupuncture, moxibustion, dietary changes, and qigong.

Chinese herbs are often prescribed in combination mixtures that are individualized to the patient's situation. Dong quai, for example, can be used to relieve the hot flashes, anxiety, and constipation that may accompany menopause. Other Chinese herbs commonly included in menopause treatments are

- ginseng
- licorice
- rehmannia

Acupuncture is particularly effective in easing annoying hot flashes and night sweats.

A traditional Chinese physician will tailor a menopause treatment program for the patient after performing an extensive examination, which often includes questioning, an analysis of the diet, feeling the pulse, and examining the tongue. It is not recommended that you use powerful herbs such as dong quai and ginseng without a practitioner's supervision.

OTHER THERAPIES

AYURVEDIC MEDICINE—Treatment involves dietary and lifestyle alterations, herbal therapy, meditation, and other therapies, all focused toward balancing the body's constitution.

BIOFEEDBACK TRAINING—Thermal biofeedback, together with relaxation techniques, can teach women to control their blood flow and relieve hot flashes.

BODYWORK—Massage is used to improve blood circulation and lower tension and stress.

HOMEOPATHY—Remedies tailored to the individual can treat hot flashes, mood swings, insomnia, and other symptoms.

HYPNOTHERAPY—Hypnotic trances can ease or eliminate hot flashes, insomnia, anxiety, and other accompanying disorders.

MEDITATION—Regular practice can clear the mind and bring lowered heart rates and blood pressure, thereby eliminating mood swings and other symptoms.

Muscle Pain

A SKELETAL MUSCLE THAT HAS BEEN MISUSED, OVERUSED, OR INJURED TYPICALLY PRODUCES PAIN. THE COMMON PAIN-INDUCING CULPRITS ARE STRAINS (TORN OR PULLED MUSCLES) AND CRAMPS (MUSCLES THAT EXPERIENCE PROLONGED CONTRACTIONS OR SPASMS). A STRAIN INVOLVES BLEEDING IN THE MUSCLE, RESULTING IN SCAR TISSUE.

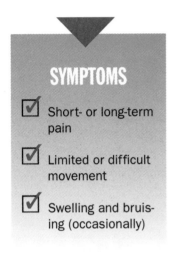

SYMPTOMS

- ☑ Short- or long-term pain
- ☑ Limited or difficult movement
- ☑ Swelling and bruising (occasionally)

CONVENTIONAL APPROACH

Allopathic medicine treats muscle pain with rest, drug therapy, and physical therapy. Several medicines can relieve pain and stiffness:

- Analgesics (painkillers) include aspirin and acetaminophen.
- Nonsteroidal anti-inflammatory drugs such as ibuprofen ease pain.
- Muscle-relaxant drugs include carisoprodol and diazepam.
- Quinine, used in low doses, can block leg cramps that occur at night.

Muscles that are cramped should be rested for a couple of minutes and then gently stretched or massaged. Strained muscles can be treated with ice packs, wrapped in snug bandages, and rested.

ALTERNATIVE APPROACHES
BODYWORK

Bodywork therapies can ease muscle pain and restore complete body function. Massage is particularly recommended to relieve muscle pain and tension and boost blood circulation to bring oxygen and nutrients to the affected muscles and carry away any toxic substances. In the case of strains, massage can lessen the amount of scar tissue and prevent the muscle from shortening as it heals.

Other useful bodywork therapies offer help for those affected by muscle pain:

- The Feldenkrais method offers new ways to move the body, helping to relax cramped or tense muscles.
- Reflexology applies pressure to certain reflex points on the feet and hands to help the body heal itself.
- Rolfing manipulates muscles and connective tissue to realign the body with respect to the field of gravity.
- Shiatsu involves finger pressure at certain points on the body's meridians, to ease pain and improve circulation.

A trained practitioner is needed to perform any of these bodywork therapies. (See chapter on Bodywork, page 192, for help finding a qualified practitioner in the field.)

AROMATHERAPY

Aromatherapy uses essential oils from certain plants and herbs to relieve pain and any accompanying spasms or inflammation. The oils can be applied with gentle massages or compresses. A few can also be added to bathwater. Commonly used oils for muscle pain include

- ginger
- helichrysum (Italian everlasting)
- marjoram
- peppermint
- thyme (linalol and red)

Here's a sample aromatherapy treatment for muscle pain: Mix 20 drops of commercially prepared essential peppermint oil with one ounce of massage oil (such as almond oil). Gently massage the mixture into the painful muscles.

BIOFEEDBACK TRAINING

Biofeedback training can be useful for muscle pain that refuses to go away. Depending on the injury and current status of the muscle, the therapy teaches people to relax or tense their muscles.

Electromyographic biofeedback is the technique typically used for muscle pain. In this therapy, electrodes are attached to the patient's skin and measure the electrical activity in the muscles. A special monitor displays the level of this activity, which reveals the amount of tension in the muscles. Armed with this information, the patient can learn to alter the tension with the use of relaxation exercises, guided imagery, and other methods. Along the way, the biofeedback monitor signals the progress.

Biofeedback also gives people a sense of control over their health, a significant plus when it comes to successfully managing pain.

Biofeedback trainers often teach progressive muscle relaxation to their patients so they can practice controlling muscle tension at home. Here are the steps:
- Wearing comfortable clothes, lie down on your back on the floor or a firm mattress.
- Close your eyes and breathe slowly and deeply.
- Tighten the muscles in your feet. Hold for a couple of seconds. Release these muscles.
- Next, tense the muscles in your calves. Again, hold and release.
- Continue up the body in this fashion. (Don't forget to include the arms and end with the scalp.)
- Remain lying down in a relaxed state until you are ready to get up

OTHER THERAPIES

ACUPUNCTURE—This therapy is particularly successful in easing or eliminating pain.

CHIROPRACTIC—Manipulation or adjustments can correct misaligned parts of the spine, eliminating pain and letting the body heal itself.

GUIDED IMAGERY AND CREATIVE VISUALIZATION—These techniques are effective in pain management and tension reduction.

HERBAL MEDICINE—Commonly used herbs, including arnica, comfrey, ginger, and kava kava, are all applied externally.

HYDROTHERAPY—Alternating hot and cold compresses can ease pain and speed healing. Warm Epsom salt baths are also an option.

NEURAL THERAPY—Injections of local anesthetics may bring relief for long-term muscle pain.

NUTRITIONAL THERAPY—Treatments are tailored to the type of muscle pain. For example, calcium and magnesium supplements may help treat nighttime leg cramps. Enzyme therapy with bromelain can also treat certain types of pain.

Nausea & Vomiting

THROWING UP, AS EVERYONE KNOWS, IS NOT PLEASANT. USUALLY, BUT NOT ALWAYS, IT'S PRECEDED BY A QUEASY SENSATION IN THE BELLY CALLED NAUSEA. THE TWO CONDITIONS CAN BE A SIGN THAT THE STOMACH IS IRRITATED (BY A CERTAIN FOOD OR MEDICINE, TOO MUCH FOOD OR ALCOHOL, OR AN INFECTION) OR A SYMPTOM OF A DISORDER (SUCH AS MOTION SICKNESS, APPENDICITIS, MIGRAINE, OR ULCER).

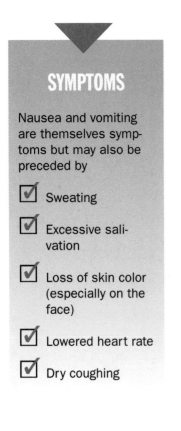

SYMPTOMS

Nausea and vomiting are themselves symptoms but may also be preceded by

☑ Sweating

☑ Excessive salivation

☑ Loss of skin color (especially on the face)

☑ Lowered heart rate

☑ Dry coughing

CONVENTIONAL APPROACH

The nausea and vomiting that happen once in a great while (such as during the flu or at the end of a wild New Year's party) are considered an inevitable fact of life by allopathic medicine. A few self-help remedies are available to offer some relief, but generally, these minor episodes are allowed to run their course.

On the other hand, nausea and vomiting that happen regularly (say, when traveling), continue without apparent reason, or involve blood receive close attention.

Over-the-counter remedies that contain concentrated simple carbohydrates (sugars) can settle the upset stomach associated with nausea.

For nausea and vomiting linked to motion sickness, vertigo, morning sickness, radiation therapy, and other conditions, allopathic medicine relies on the family of drugs called *antiemetics*. These medications focus their power on the inner ear or stomach to block nausea or vomiting. Some drugs that can be useful are

- antidopaminergics, such as chlorpromazine and metoclopramide
- antihistamines, such as dimenhydrinate, meclizine, and promethazine
- anticholinergics, such as meclizine and scopolamine

ALTERNATIVE APPROACHES
ACUPRESSURE

Acupressure holds that stomach disturbances happen when the body's energy flow, or qi, is blocked or unstable. The energy channel can be reopened and recovery stimulated by applying firm, deep pressure to certain points on the body with the fingers and hands. Acupressure can be performed during nausea but before vomiting. The following are some of the frequently used pressure points:

- P6 (also known as *HP6* or *PC6*)—on the pericardium meridian, on the inside of the forearm, about two inches above the wrist crease.
- LI4—on the large intestine meridian, the webbing between the thumb and index finger, on the back of the hand. (Pregnant women should never use this point without professional guidance.)
- ST44—on the stomach meridian, on top of the foot, the indentation between the tendons of the second and third toes.

Studies have shown that applying pressure to the P6 point can alleviate nausea in cases of motion sickness, morning sickness, surgery recovery, and chemotherapy. In many trials, the researchers used elastic wrist bands that apply pressure with plastic disks.

Here's a sample treatment using the pressure point P6:

- To find the point on one of the inner forearms, measure two thumb widths up from the wrist crease between the tendons.
- You or the practitioner can calm this point, massaging with gentle pressure for two minutes.
- Repeat the treatment on the other forearm.

NATUROPATHIC MEDICINE

Naturopathic medicine looks for what might be at the root of the nausea and vomiting. For example, why does the motion of a plane bring on an uneasy stomach, and what can be done to eliminate this susceptibility?

A naturopathic physician performs a detailed examination of the patient, looking over diet, lifestyle, emotional state, and when and how the nausea or vomiting happens. Herbal medicine, a change in diet, supplements, homeopathy, acupuncture, or other treatments may be prescribed.

Dried gingerroot, for example, can reduce or prevent nausea and vomiting, especially when the symptoms are related to motion sickness, morning sickness, or sickness reltaed to surgery recovery. Teas made from ginger or peppermint, when sipped very slowly, can usually ease the upset stomach of nausea.

If you're planning to travel by plane or boat, this remedy may be prescribed to prevent nausea: Drink 1½ teaspoons of dried, ground gingerroot dissolved in 2 cups of a hot or cold liquid half an hour before boarding.

AROMATHERAPY

Aromatherapy works to calm a fragile, irritated, or nervous stomach with essential oils from plants and herbs. The oils can be given on the tongue, massaged into the skin, or applied with a compress. Peppermint, a digestive aid, is considered one of the most effective essential oils for curbing nausea. Other oils used for their action on the digestive tract are chamomile, damask rose, fennel, and lavender.

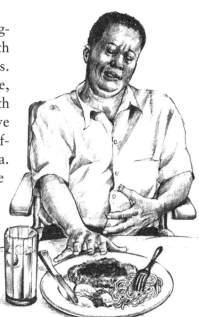

Here's a sample remedy: Mix four drops of essential peppermint oil with one tablespoon almond oil. Gently massage this mixture onto the belly.

OTHER THERAPIES

BODYWORK—Several therapies may offer relief, including reflexology and Therapeutic Touch.

DETOXIFICATION, FASTING, AND COLON THERAPY—A short fast or juice diet or a colonic irrigation can be used to address the possible causes of nausea and vomiting.

HOMEOPATHY—Common remedies include arsenicum album, ipecacuanha, and nux vomica.

HYDROTHERAPY—Alternating hot and cold compresses to the trunk can be effective.

MEDITATION—Regular meditation can reduce stress and clear the mind, which is helpful for nausea and vomiting brought on by tension and anxiety.

TRADITIONAL CHINESE MEDICINE—Several Chinese herbal combinations are very effective for nausea and vomiting, especially in pregnancy.

Obesity

OBESITY MEANS HAVING TOO MUCH BODY FAT. TO MEET THIS DEFINITION, ONE MUST WEIGH APPROXIMATELY 20 PERCENT OR MORE ABOVE ONE'S DESIRABLE BODY WEIGHT. AGE, HEIGHT, AND BODY FRAME HELP DETERMINE IDEAL BODY WEIGHT.

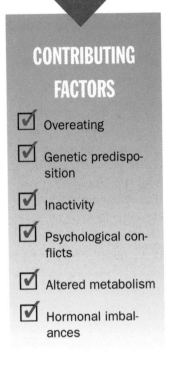

CONTRIBUTING FACTORS

☑ Overeating

☑ Genetic predisposition

☑ Inactivity

☑ Psychological conflicts

☑ Altered metabolism

☑ Hormonal imbalances

CONVENTIONAL APPROACH

Allopathic medicine treats obesity with dietary measures and exercise, which are often combined with drug therapy or surgery. Nonetheless, the success rate is less than ideal.

Low-calorie diets are typically recommended for people with obesity, so that the body will tap into its stored fat to meet its energy requirements. Nutritional counseling to establish good eating habits usually accompanies the dietary changes. A regular exercise program is also essential.

The most commonly used drugs for obesity are appetite suppressants, such as fenfluramine. In an effort to help the patient feel satisfied with less food, the stomach can be surgically stapled to make it smaller. The jaw can also be wired together, leaving only enough space so a liquid diet can be consumed.

Liposuction is a surgical procedure that involves sucking out fat cells. The long-term ramifications of this procedure are not yet known. This procedure is not generally performed for health reasons on obese people, but rather for cosmetic reasons on people slightly overweight.

ALTERNATIVE APPROACHES

Alternative therapies treat obesity without drugs or surgery. All emphasize proper diet and regular exercise.

NUTRITIONAL THERAPY

Of course, since food intake is so closely related to obesity, nutritional therapy has a great deal to say about the condition. In general, the treatment involves eating differently, not eating less. More than half of the calories eaten each day should come from carbohydrates, and less than a quarter should be derived from fats. The remainder of calories should come from proteins. Carbohydrates and proteins supply four calories per gram, while fat provides nine. Some of the foods that should be emphasized include

- high-fiber and unrefined complex carbohydrates, such as whole grains, because the body is less successful digesting these and feels full sooner than with refined carbohydrates, such as sugar and white flour
- raw or lightly cooked vegetables
- protein with low amounts of saturated fat, including dry peas and beans

---

NO EASY ANSWERS

Despite the billions of dollars spent every year on weight-loss efforts, there really is no one quick way to lose weight. A successful weight-loss program requires a long-term commitment to changing eating habits and increasing physical activity with a regular exercise program.

To reduce the amount of fat in a diet, many practitioners of nutritional therapy recommend limiting foods from animal sources to nonfat dairy products and egg whites. Other practitioners go further and suggest avoiding all animal products. Limiting sugar intake is also important.

Nutritional therapy's treatment program for obesity also calls for drinking plenty of purified water each day, altering eating habits, and exercising daily. Certain nutritional supplements may also be prescribed. Supplements of zinc, B vitamins, and chromium may prove useful.

A typical first step in devising a treatment program for obesity is keeping a food diary for at least one week. The following information can help a nutritional therapist assess the best treatment for you:

- What foods do you eat each day, including all snacks and portion sizes?
- When and where do you eat?
- Are you alone or with other people?
- What is your mood or stress level while eating?
- When are your bowel movements?

DETOXIFICATION, FASTING, AND COLON THERAPY

Detoxification therapy holds that certain toxins (from chemicals to pesticides) can build up in the body, particularly in fat cells. These toxins need to be cleansed away as part of a dietary and exercise treatment program for obesity. In addition, various detoxification regimens can help prevent obesity from returning. Treatments may include fasting, colonic irrigations, and several other measures.

Several herbs, such as dandelion root or burdock, can be used in conjunction with a detoxification and fasting regimen to boost the function of the liver, which cleanses toxins from the body.

A juice fast for detoxification might consist of carrot and green vegetable juices diluted with an equal amount of water. Consume one quart daily plus additional water if thirsty. Any fast should be supervised by a health care professional.

OTHER THERAPIES

AYURVEDIC MEDICINE—Treatment can include dietary changes and herbal therapy. One study showed that any of three Ayurvedic herbal remedies led to significant weight loss in patients when compared with a placebo.

GUIDED IMAGERY AND CREATIVE VISUALIZATION—Exercises can aid in weight loss by allowing people to envision how manageable lowering their weight is and what they would look like.

HERBAL MEDICINE—Possible herbal treatments include dandelion root, plantain, and garcinia.

HYPNOTHERAPY—Hypnotic trances dealing with eating habits and recognizing true hunger, coupled with a diet and exercise program, are particularly effective for obesity treatment.

TRADITIONAL CHINESE MEDICINE—Acupuncture (on points on both the ear and entire body), acupressure, herbal therapy, and hydrotherapy are typically used for weight loss.

Osteoporosis

OSTEOPOROSIS IS A DISEASE THAT CAUSES BONES TO BECOME THIN AND FRAGILE. IT CAN LEAD TO BONE FRACTURES, TYPICALLY IN THE HIPS, SPINE, AND WRIST. OVER A LIFETIME, BONES NATURALLY LOSE SOME OF THEIR DENSITY, BUT OSTEOPOROSIS IS AN EXAGGERATION OF THIS PROCESS. CONTRIBUTING FACTORS MAY INCLUDE A HORMONE DEFICIENCY (IN WOMEN), LOW-CALCIUM DIET, LACK OF EXERCISE, SMOKING, AND CERTAIN MEDICATIONS.

SYMPTOMS

☑ Unusually frequent bone breaks

☑ Back pain

☑ Stooped posture and loss of height (a sign of fractured spinal bones called a dowager's hump)

☑ Limited mobility

Often, there are no symptoms until the condition is fairly advanced.

CONVENTIONAL APPROACH

Allopathic medicine treats osteoporosis with a combination of dietary measures, an exercise regimen, and drug therapy.

Getting enough of the mineral calcium is of paramount concern to conventional practitioners. Vitamin D, needed by the body for calcium absorption, can be administered with supplements if needed. Regular weight-bearing exercise, such as walking or aerobics, is also vital.

Several medications are available:

• Hormone (estrogen) replacement therapy is used only for women after menopause and can help preserve the density of bones, but carries a potential increased risk of breast and uterine cancer.

• Alendronate sodium is also intended only for women after menopause. It may increase bone density. Side effects range from stomach pain to headaches.

• Calcitonin slows the loss of bone density.

• Biphosphonates also halt bone loss.

ALTERNATIVE APPROACHES
NUTRITIONAL THERAPY

Nutritional therapy, like allopathic medicine, recognizes that getting enough dietary calcium is important in treating and preventing osteoporosis. However, the dietary needs for this condition are more complex than calcium alone. Several nutritional factors either help or hinder the absorption and retention of calcium. It's interesting to note that people in parts of the world where calcium intake is low have some of the lowest rates of osteoporosis. The following factors may play a role in this fact:

• Excessive protein intake is linked to osteoporosis, because protein causes calcium to be excreted from the body with urine. In addition, meat contains high levels of phosphorus, which also competes with calcium for absorption. People who follow cereal-based diets with low to moderate levels of protein, such as vegetarians, require lower levels of calcium for healthy bones. In fact, several studies have shown that vegetarians have a lower rate of bone loss than nonvegetarians.

• Sodium (salt), refined sugar, and caffeine also encourage the loss of calcium through the urine.

• Too much saturated fat and unusually large amounts of fiber, iron, and zinc all limit the quantity of calcium that's absorbed in the digestive tract.

• Vitamin D, vitamin K, magnesium, and boron are among the nutrients

USE THEM OR LOSE THEM

Regular exercise is one of the essentials of an effective osteoporosis treatment or prevention program. Particularly important are weight-bearing exercises such as aerobics, walking, jogging, weight training, and Tai Chi. Research has shown that exercise helps build bone density, even for people in their 80s.

that support healthy bones. (Magnesium is extremely important for keeping calcium in the bones.)

So are milk and other dairy products a good thing? While they supply a lot of calcium, they usually also provide saturated fat and high levels of protein. Instead, practitioners of nutritional therapy typically recommend getting calcium from green leafy vegetables, dark-green vegetables, and certain types of beans as well as other foods, all of which provide little or no protein and fat.

Here's a sample of good calcium sources that are low in protein and fat:

- 1 cup bok choy (250 mg of calcium)
- 1 cup kale (200 mg)
- 1 cup broccoli (180 mg)
- 1 cup great northern beans (140 mg)
- 5 dried figs (135 mg)
- 2 corn tortillas (120 mg)

Note: The Recommended Dietary Allowance for calcium for menopausal women is 1000 to 1200 mg, although a practitioner of nutritional therapy may recommend less than that depending on the woman's typical dietary sources of protein.

HERBAL MEDICINE

Several herbs can be beneficial for preventing and treating osteoporosis when combined with a diet and exercise program.

Different herbs approach the problem differently; some provide dietary calcium, some regulate the body's use of calcium, and some increase the level of certain hormones in the body. For example, horsetail (silica) is recommended to boost the body's absorption of calcium. Once this plant, which often resembles a horse's tail, is dried, it can be used as a tea or in tincture or capsule form. Other helpful herbs include

- alfalfa, black cohosh, and wild yam, which are all phytoestrogens
- comfrey, which may cause liver toxicity if used continuously for long periods
- false unicorn root, which stimulates the ovaries
- oatstraw

An herbalist may prescribe taking one capsule of dried, powdered horsetail three times a day. A more comprehensive formula may also include daily doses of alfalfa, black cohosh, wild yam, vitex, and dong quai.

OTHER THERAPIES

AYURVEDIC MEDICINE—The treatment focuses on dietary changes, coupled with herbal therapy.

TRADITIONAL CHINESE MEDICINE—Treatment includes herbal therapy (including dong quai), acupuncture, and Tai Chi.

Pregnancy Discomforts

PREGNANCY BRINGS WITH IT A MENU OF DISCOMFORTS THAT CAN COME AND GO THROUGHOUT THE NINE MONTHS. HORMONAL CHANGES AND PRESSURE FROM THE EXPANDING UTERUS CAN HAVE MANY EFFECTS ON A WOMAN'S BODY. SOME OF THE MOST COMMON DISCOMFORTS ARE MORNING SICKNESS, WATER RETENTION, HEADACHE, BACK PAIN, FATIGUE, DIGESTIVE PROBLEMS, AND MOOD SWINGS.

SYMPTOMS

☑ Morning sickness—nausea and vomiting, often during the first three months of pregnancy

☑ Water retention—swollen feet, ankles, and legs

☑ Aches and pain typically on the head, back, buttocks, and legs

☑ Fatigue

☑ Digestive upsets—heartburn, constipation, or gas

Insomnia, high blood pressure, food cravings, hemorrhoids, varicose veins, and stretch marks may also accompany a pregnancy.

CONVENTIONAL APPROACH

Allopathic medicine emphasizes nonaggressive methods to treat pregnancy discomforts. The benefit of treatment to the mother must be measured against any risks to the fetus, especially during the early stages of pregnancy.

Several small meals, eaten throughout the day, may alleviate morning sickness and some digestive upsets. Also, eating crackers or rice cakes just before getting out of bed can prevent nausea. To prevent constipation, the diet should include a lot of fiber from sources such as fresh vegetables and fruits and whole grains, and more than five glasses of water per day. Avoiding spicy or rich foods can ease heartburn, as can sleeping with the head and chest propped up.

Taking naps throughout the day and eliminating some day-to-day activities can lessen fatigue. And regular, moderate exercise can improve moods, reduce back pain, lessen the instances of constipation and hemorrhoids, and provide other benefits. Swollen feet and legs should be elevated while sitting or lying. Mild exercise, such as walking in the cool part of the day, will reduce swelling.

Both over-the-counter and prescription drugs should be used infrequently and only with a doctor's advice. Some of the medicines may include

- acetaminophen, which can relieve pain and headaches
- low-sodium antacids, which neutralize stomach acid to treat occasional heartburn
- simethicone to ease gas
- mild laxatives to eliminate constipation

ALTERNATIVE APPROACHES
ACUPRESSURE

Acupressure offers the chance to relieve morning sickness, aches and pain, swollen feet and ankles, and several other pregnancy discomforts, with no side effects to the mother or fetus. Using the fingers and hands to apply moderate pressure to specific points on the body, this therapy rebalances the flow of vital life energy, or qi, in the body.

Each pregnancy discomfort calls for treatment of different acupressure points. The treatment can be performed several times a day or week as a preventive measure. Or, as in the case of nausea, it can be done whenever the symptom strikes.

Acupressure treatment of morning sickness has received special scrutiny from the scientific community. For example, a recent trial conducted in part by the University of California School of Nursing in San Francisco tested this treatment on expectant mothers. Half of the 60 patients tested were taught to apply pressure to the P6 point on the lower arm for ten minutes, four times a day. The other patients were instructed to use a "sham" acupuncture point. The women using P6 experienced significantly less nausea than the other women.

It's wise to consult a trained acupressure practitioner before performing self-treatments at home. Applying pressure to a few points, such as LI4 on the webbing between the thumb and index finger, may induce early labor.

Here's how to ease nausea and vomiting with P6:

- To locate the point on one of your inner forearms, measure two thumb-widths up from the wrist crease.
- Using your thumb on the opposite hand, apply moderate pressure to this point for two minutes. Meanwhile, breathe deeply.
- Repeat on the other forearm.

YOGA

Yoga can greatly reduce or eliminate many pregnancy discomforts and can prepare the body and mind for childbirth. Its benefits include

- better posture (important for avoiding back pain)
- improved breathing (boosting the flow of oxygen in the mother's body and placenta and releasing emotional tension)
- improved blood circulation (also good for both the mother and fetus and may lessen the chances of varicose veins and hemorrhoids)

- gentle exercising (important to strengthen back, eliminate constipation, and improve sleeping)

The yoga routines consist of poses and breathing exercises and can last from 20 to 60 minutes. Pregnant women should not perform any poses that are strenuous or require lying on the abdomen. Depending on the stage of pregnancy, certain other poses should also be avoided. A qualified yoga instructor can devise a personalized program.

Here's a sample pose, the "downward-facing dog," that is useful for pregnancy discomforts and may be included in your yoga session:

- Wear comfortable clothing and no shoes or socks.
- Get on your hands and knees, placing your hands shoulder distance apart and your knees hip distance apart. Keep your arms straight. Bend your feet so your toes and the balls of the feet are on the floor.
- Inhale deeply.
- Exhale deeply and slowly straighten your legs, raise your buttocks toward the ceiling, and gently hang

---

A WORD OF CAUTION

Just because your normal routine of alternative therapies (from daily nutritional supplements to herbs for a bout with the common cold) has worked for you in the past doesn't mean it's OK for a fetus in the womb. Many herbs, such as goldenseal, are unsafe during pregnancy. Check with your health care practitioner first.

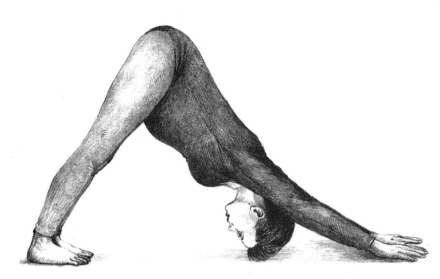

your head toward the floor. Your body should look like an upside-down *V*.

- Return to kneeling position.
- Repeat two times.

HERBAL MEDICINE

Herbs can be used to soothe the digestive tract, induce relaxation, act as an astringent, and encourage urination, among other actions. Gingerroot is one of the more frequently prescribed herbs for morning sickness. One clinical study reported that ginger eliminated all instances of nausea and vomiting for 75 percent of the pregnant women tested. Dried, powdered ginger is available in capsule form, or fresh ginger can be added to foods or made into a tea. Herbalists recommend that expectant mothers take no more than one gram of dried ginger or the equivalent per day.

Chamomile, lemon balm, peppermint, and raspberry leaf are also effective in treating morning sickness. Other helpful herbs for pregnancy discomforts include

- dandelion leaf for water retention
- lavender, mint, and slippery elm for heartburn
- butcher's broom, hawthorn, and yarrow, applied externally to varicose veins
- garlic for high blood pressure
- witch hazel, applied externally to hemorrhoids

To ease morning sickness, an herbalist might recommend taking one gram of dried, powdered ginger per day, as needed for symptoms. Powdered ginger is best tolerated in capsule form.

OTHER THERAPIES

AROMATHERAPY—Essential oils from clary sage or lavender mixed in bathwater can help insomnia. Other oils are beneficial for treating aches and pain, nausea, and tension.

CHIROPRACTIC MEDICINE—Adjustments and manipulation can treat back pain, headaches, constipation, and even nausea.

HOMEOPATHY—A variety of remedies are available for all pregnancy discomforts. They must be tailored for the individual and should be used at the lowest effective potency.

HYDROTHERAPY—Treatments include warm abdominal compresses for morning sickness, warm baths for insomnia, and cold sitz baths for hemorrhoids.

NUTRITIONAL THERAPY—Dietary adjustments are combined with nutritional supplements as needed.

OSTEOPATHY—Manipulations can help the body deal with the added weight that pregnancy brings, which may cause back and leg pain.

Premenstrual Syndrome

PREMENSTRUAL SYNDROME, OR PMS, IS A SERIES OF PHYSICAL AND EMOTIONAL SYMPTOMS THAT CAN OCCUR EACH MONTH BEFORE A WOMAN'S MENSTRUAL PERIOD. THE SYMPTOMS CAN START ANYWHERE FROM 2 TO 14 DAYS BEFORE MENSTRUATION AND USUALLY END AS THE BLEEDING BEGINS. ITS CAUSE IS UNKNOWN, BUT PMS IS PROBABLY RELATED TO CHANGES IN THE LEVELS OF HORMONES, ESPECIALLY ESTROGEN AND PROGESTERONE.

CONVENTIONAL APPROACH

Because the causes of PMS are not understood, allopathic medicine's treatment program focuses on relieving its symptoms. The most often prescribed treatment consists mainly of drug therapy, although lifestyle changes may also be suggested.

Several medicines can ease PMS symptoms:

- Diuretics, such as hydrochlorothiazide or spironolactone, remove retained water that may be causing swelling or bloating. Some diuretics may cause low levels of potassium in the blood, among other side effects.
- Analgesics, such as ibuprofen and acetaminophen, control aches and pains. Side effects can include nausea and intestinal bleeding.
- Oral contraceptives regulate hormone levels and alter the menstrual cycle. Depending on the type of pill, side effects range from bleeding between periods to increased risk of cervical cancer.
- Progestin or progesterone supplements are often given as vaginal suppositories or injections. Their side effects range from weight gain to ovarian cysts (with synthetic progestins).
- Benzodiazepine drugs (tranquilizers), such as alprazolam, control anxiety

and insomnia. Side effects may include daytime drowsiness and dizziness. These drugs can be habit-forming.

ALTERNATIVE APPROACHES

More and more, allopathic doctors are acknowledging the benefit of several alternative therapies—particularly nutritional therapy and relaxation therapies—in treating PMS.

NUTRITIONAL THERAPY

Nutritional therapists maintain that a nutritional deficiency or too much or too little of certain foods can trigger PMS in susceptible women. For many women, nutritional supplements and an appropriate dietary restrictions effectively eliminate the monthly onslaught of symptoms.

Vitamin B_6 (pyridoxine) is one of the more commonly prescribed supplements for PMS treatment. Clinical research has shown that the overwhelming majority of women who take vitamin B_6 supplements regularly significantly reduce their symptoms, including

- breast tenderness
- mood swings
- fatigue
- headache
- acne flare-ups

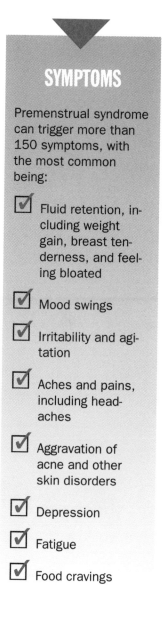

SYMPTOMS

Premenstrual syndrome can trigger more than 150 symptoms, with the most common being:

☑ Fluid retention, including weight gain, breast tenderness, and feeling bloated

☑ Mood swings

☑ Irritability and agitation

☑ Aches and pains, including headaches

☑ Aggravation of acne and other skin disorders

☑ Depression

☑ Fatigue

☑ Food cravings

This vitamin is thought to perform several functions that alleviate PMS symptoms, such as helping produce serotonin (a mood-regulating chemical in the brain) and blocking the manufacture of the hormone prolactin (which is linked to breast tenderness). In addition, women with PMS symptoms may be deficient in vitamin B_6.

Women with PMS also may have a magnesium deficiency. Supplementation with this mineral has been shown to relieve the symptoms of water retention and nervousness, among others. Other helpful supplements include

- calcium
- vitamin A
- vitamin C
- vitamin D
- vitamin E
- chromium

In general, a diet rich in vegetables (especially leafy green vegetables), fruits, whole grains (with lots of buckwheat, millet, and barley but not much wheat), and beans is least likely to encourage PMS symptoms for most women. Drinking at least eight glasses of water per day can actually reduce water retention. Meals should be small,

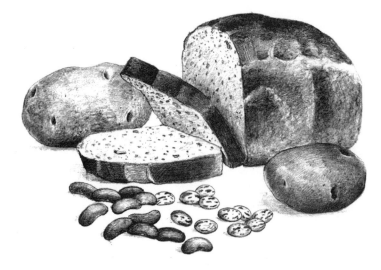

DO I HAVE PMS?

No lab test can confirm if you have premenstrual syndrome. The best way to tell is to keep a daily diary for three months, noting when your symptoms occur and the beginning and ending dates of menstruation.

frequent, and spaced throughout the day to keep blood sugar levels in check. The following are some other specific suggestions:

- Avoid sodium (salt) and alcohol, which deplete vitamins and minerals that keep PMS at bay and which also trigger water retention. Instead, eating asparagus and watermelon can encourage urination.
- Eliminate sugars, which can also lead to water retention, block the absorption of needed vitamins and minerals, and contribute to hypoglycemia.
- Limit dairy products, which inhibit the absorption of magnesium and contain arachidonic acids that can cause certain PMS symptoms.
- Cut down on saturated fats, which may promote cramps, among other symptoms.

A naturopathic physician may prescribe the following supplementation treatment:

- Take 500 mg of magnesium and 50 to 100 mg of vitamin B_6 daily (perhaps in conjunction with other B vitamins in a multivitamin).
- About three days before your PMS symptoms normally begin, start taking an extra 100 mg of vitamin

B$_6$ daily until a few days into your period.

Caution: Daily doses of vitamin B$_6$ over 500 mg may cause nerve damage.

HOMEOPATHY

Homeopathic treatments work to stimulate the body into righting any emotional or physical upsets that produce PMS symptoms. It uses highly diluted doses of natural substances that would cause PMS symptoms if given in full strength to a healthy person. The substances are from plant, mineral, and animal sources (including snakes). A remedy is individualized to each patient and depends on her particular mix of emotional and physical symptoms, as well as her general state of emotional and physical health. For example, if a woman with PMS easily becomes weepy, she may be prescribed one of several remedies, including

- pulsatilla nigricans, a perennial plant, if the weepiness is accompanied by symptoms such as diarrhea, a lack of thirst, desire for open air, desire for company, and cravings for creamy foods.
- sepia, a cuttlefish ink, if the tearfulness is matched with exhaustion, constipation, a sensitivity to cold, irritability, lack of joy, indifference or aversion to one's family, and cravings for sour foods.

Other common PMS remedies include ignatia amara, lachesis, lycopodium, and nux vomica.

For PMS characterized by lower-back pain, diarrhea, weepiness, depression, a lack of thirst, and other symptoms noted above, here's a sample homeopathic remedy: Take

---

A HELPFUL HERB

Evening primrose oil has gained a lot of attention lately for alleviating PMS symptoms. Credit for this action goes to the fatty acid called gamma-linolenic acid (GLA) found in evening primrose oil. Black currant seed oil and borage oil also supply GLA, although in smaller quantities. A recommended dose of evening primrose oil is two 500-mg capsules three times daily.

---

one dose of pulsatilla nigricans, 12c, every four hours. (The *12c* refers to the potency of the remedy.) Stop treatment as soon as the symptoms decline.

YOGA

Emotional stress can amplify any premenstrual fluctuations of hormone levels and the resulting PMS symptoms. Yoga seeks to clear the mind, induce deep breathing, and ease muscle tension and stiffness. It also satisfies the body's need for a good, regular workout. The yoga poses and breathing exercises should be done throughout the month, with less vigorous ones performed during the time of menstrual bleeding. The sessions usually last from 20 to 60 minutes and are performed three to seven times a week.

Here's a sample yoga pose, often called the butterfly or diamond pose, that can be performed while you are experiencing PMS:

- Sit on the floor with your knees bent pointing out to your sides and the bottoms of your feet flat against

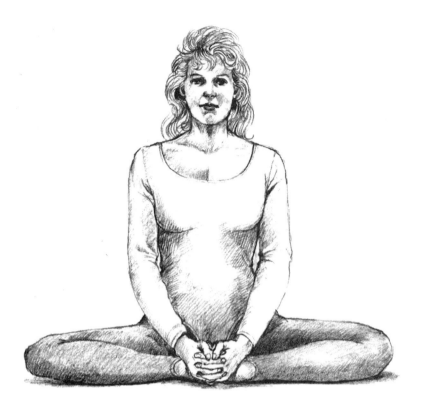

each other. Keep your spine straight while clasping your toes.
- Pull your feet as close to your groin as possible.
- Take several slow, deep breaths.
- Then, exhale and slowly lean forward from the hips, still clasping your toes and keeping the spine straight.
- Inhale and slowly lean back to your original position.
- Repeat this gentle rocking and breathing for one minute.

AROMATHERAPY

The essential oils of several herbs can relieve the symptoms of PMS gently and with fewer, if any, side effects. The typical treatments for PMS call for mixing several drops of an oil into a warm bath or into a carrier oil (such as almond or grape seed oil) that can be massaged into the skin, often around the abdomen or breasts. The oils are used by themselves or together to take advantage of their potentially synergistic qualities.

Depending on the symptoms, different oils are recommended. Here are some suggestions:
- For water retention, use grapefruit, fennel, or juniper.
- For stress and tension, use clary sage or lavender.
- For depression, use bergamot, chamomile, or geranium.

An herbalist may recommend soaking in a tub of water spiked with six drops of essential clary sage oil. Mix the oil in thoroughly before getting into the tub, and keep the bathroom door closed to retain the aromas in the room.

OTHER THERAPIES

AYURVEDIC MEDICINE—Treatment can involve dietary changes, herbal therapy, and meditation.

BODYWORK—Reflexology and massage can be effective in relieving emotional and physical tension.

HERBAL MEDICINE—Herbs can be used to control water retention (dandelion and parsley), stabilize hormone levels (dong quai), and perform other helpful functions.

MEDITATION—Daily exercises can reduce the stress and tension that exacerbate PMS.

TRADITIONAL CHINESE MEDICINE—Acupuncture, herbal therapy, and lifestyle changes are part of the treatment program.

Prostate, Enlarged

THE PROSTATE GLAND NORMALLY MEASURES ABOUT THE SIZE OF A WALNUT. FOUND ONLY IN MEN, THIS GLAND SITS UNDER THE URINARY BLADDER AND WRAPS AROUND THE TOP OF THE URETHRA (THE TUBE THROUGH WHICH URINE AND SEMEN FLOW OUT OF THE BODY). ENLARGEMENT OF THE PROSTATE IS A CONDITION THAT USUALLY AFFECTS MEN OVER 50. THE REASON FOR THIS ENLARGEMENT IS NOT ALWAYS CLEAR, BUT HORMONE LEVELS APPEAR TO PLAY A ROLE.

CONVENTIONAL APPROACH

Allopathic medicine often does not treat an enlarged prostate that has few or no symptoms. Instead, the condition is carefully monitored with regular visits to the doctor. (Of course, prostate cancer needs to be ruled out first, though.)

However, if the symptoms become severe and normal urination is disrupted, doctors may recommend draining the urine from the bladder with a flexible tube (catheter) to ease discomfort and avoid complications. Several types of drug therapy and surgery are also options for cases that cause severe symptoms.

An enlarged prostate can lead to bladder infection and kidney damage. Therefore, professional evaluation and monitoring are crucial even if no direct course of treatment is persued.

DRUG TREATMENT

The following drugs may be prescribed for cases causing annoying or dangerous symptoms:

- Finasteride treats enlarged prostate by blocking certain hormonal chain reactions. Its side effects can include decreased sexual sensation and the inability to have an erection (impotence).

- Terazosin can relax the muscles around the prostate to allow urination. It may also cause a sudden drop in blood pressure, dizziness, and blurred vision, so it must be used with caution.

SURGICAL TREATMENT

If drug therapy fails to produce results, the prostate can be totally or partially removed surgically. In a few cases, the operation may be followed by a short period of bleeding, requiring a blood transfusion, but this complication is becoming more rare. Most often, normal urination resumes after recovery.

Removing the prostate leaves most men sterile. As with medications prescribed for the condition, some men experience reduced sexual sensation or are unable to get or maintain an erection.

When the added risks of poor health or age prevents surgery, the urine can be drained with a permanently fitted catheter.

ALTERNATIVE APPROACHES

Alternative therapies approach the problem of an enlarged prostate much differently. Several therapies offer viable options beyond drugs and surgery.

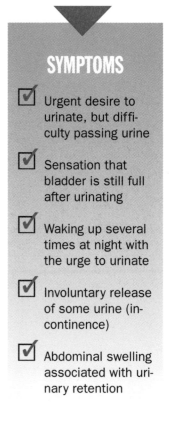

SYMPTOMS

- ☑ Urgent desire to urinate, but difficulty passing urine

- ☑ Sensation that bladder is still full after urinating

- ☑ Waking up several times at night with the urge to urinate

- ☑ Involuntary release of some urine (incontinence)

- ☑ Abdominal swelling associated with urinary retention

HERBAL MEDICINE

Herbal therapy has a lot to offer the treatment of prostate problems. Herbs can reduce the size of an enlarged prostate and even prevent one. Relief from the annoying symptoms is also possible.

First, it's important to understand the probable cause of this condition. The abnormal growth may be triggered by the presence of dihydrotestosterone, which is produced in the body by the male hormone testosterone and an enzyme.

An extract of saw palmetto berries can halt the body's manufacture of dihydrotestosterone, according to several studies, reducing the size of the gland, making urination easier and less frequent, and relieving any accompanying pain and discomfort. The berries come from a small palm tree that's native to the southeastern coast of the United States.

Panax ginseng can also offer relief from some of the symptoms of an enlarged prostate, postponing the need for drugs or surgery. This herb can be taken in the form of an extract or as a dried root.

Bark from the *Pygeum africanum* tree has received widespread use for treating enlarged prostate in some European countries. Researchers have found that it significantly lessens the symptoms.

Other helpful herbs include
- couch grass
- damiana
- hydrangea
- nettles

 Here's a sample herbal remedy: Take 160 mg of a standardized saw palmetto extract (with 85 to 90 percent fatty acids and plant sterols) two times daily. Don't be intimidated by the terminology; your herbalist or health food store will understand and can help you find the right prescription.

NUTRITIONAL THERAPY

According to nutritional therapy, diet and supplements can effectively treat an enlarged prostate.

High cholesterol levels have been linked with a larger than normal prostate and its accompanying symptoms. A diet low in fat, especially saturated fat, can help lower cholesterol. A vegetarian diet, eating no meat, poultry, or seafood, can be one way to achieve an overall reduction in dietary fat and saturated fat. According to The American Dietetic Association, vegetarians typically have lower total blood cholesterol levels and low-density lipoprotein cholesterol (the so-called "bad cholesterol") levels than meat-eaters.

Diet can have a direct effect on the health of the prostate, as well. Certain foods may irritate the prostate, causing symptoms to worsen. Some of the foods to be avoided include
- coffee (both caffeinated and decaffeinated)
- other caffeine sources (soda, chocolate, and tea)
- alcohol
- red pepper

Sometimes food allergies may be the source of some irritation in the urinary tract, thus exacerbating the problem of frequent urination. Potential allergens should be investigated and avoided (see page 22).

Zinc disables the enzyme that helps produce dihydrotestosterone and is, therefore, commonly recommended to men with prostate problems. Researchers have shown that patients can decrease their enlarged prostate symptoms by adding zinc to their diet. (Care should be taken with zinc supplementation, though, as large doses of zinc decrease the body's absorption of copper and may lead to copper deficiencies; a good ratio is 1 mg of copper per 15 mg of zinc with a daily maximum of 3 or 4 mg of copper.)

As an alternative to zinc supplements, try pumpkin seeds. They provide a lot of the mineral, as well as essential fatty acids, which are also beneficial to men who have enlarged prostates.

Other good sources of essential fatty acids include cold-pressed unrefined vegetable oils such as flaxseed oil. (Sunflower and sesame oil are also decent sources.) Vitamin B_6 supplements are typically prescribed along with zinc.

OTHER THERAPIES

DETOXIFICATION, FASTING, AND COLON THERAPY—A short-term cleansing diet may eliminate some of the causes of an enlarged prostate including constipation (possibly bowel toxicity) and waste products in the blood.

ENVIRONMENTAL MEDICINE—Pesticides and other chemicals have been linked to prostate growth. A whole-foods, organic diet can bolster the body against these toxins.

HOMEOPATHY—Several remedies can be helpful, but chronic problems with the prostate require a professional homeopath who can tailor the remedy to the individual's symptoms.

HYDROTHERAPY—Alternating hot and cold water sprays or sitz baths can offer pain relief.

YOGA—Breathing exercises and postures can reduce stress, provide exercise, and balance the energy flow.

To boost the levels of dietary zinc, a naturopathic physician may recommend eating about two ounces of raw pumpkin seeds per day. The equivalent amount of zinc can be obtained from daily supplementation with 50 mg of zinc picolinate, but the pumpkin seeds may contain other beneficial substances as well.

Psoriasis

Psoriasis is a chronic skin disease in which the skin cells divide 1,000 times faster than normal, resulting in a discomforting and unsightly pileup of cells. The lesions appear red and inflamed and are often covered with silvery scales. By some estimates, psoriasis affects 1 out of every 50 people.

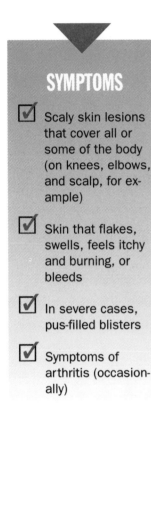

SYMPTOMS

- ☑ Scaly skin lesions that cover all or some of the body (on knees, elbows, and scalp, for example)

- ☑ Skin that flakes, swells, feels itchy and burning, or bleeds

- ☑ In severe cases, pus-filled blisters

- ☑ Symptoms of arthritis (occasionally)

CONVENTIONAL APPROACH

Because there is no cure for psoriasis, allopathic medicine focuses on temporarily easing the discomfort and reducing the size and severity of lesions. Dermatologists prescribe both treatments that are applied to the skin and medicataons that are taken internally. Their effectiveness depends on the severity of the disease, and these therapies may lose their effectiveness with repeated use.

Treatments include

- topical agents such as corticosteroids, anthralin (a derivative of petroleum), synthetic vitamin D, moisturizers, and refined coal tar in creams or shampoos (as a general rule, those therapies that are least complicated, least messy, and with the fewest side effects are the least effective.)

- prescription medications such as methotrexate (an anticancer drug), retinoids, and sulfasalazine, taken orally or by injection (All carry side effects that can be serious, from birth defects to liver damage.)

- exposure to artificial ultraviolet light, used by itself or with tar or a light-sensitizing drug such as psoralen (Sometimes patients are instructed to bathe in natural light, but they should be careful as sunburn aggravates psoriasis.)

ALTERNATIVE APPROACHES

When doctors at a university hospital in Norway surveyed psoriasis sufferers, they found that more than 40 percent had used some type of alternative therapy for their skin condition. The reason? Most turned to the therapies because conventional medicine failed to offer relief.

Alternative medicine aims to do two things for psoriasis patients: 1) lessen the pain and the lesions and 2) prevent the skin cells from malfunctioning in the first place.

One alternative therapy, light therapy, has met with some acceptance with conventional doctors.

NUTRITIONAL THERAPY

Nutritional therapy holds that the absence of certain foods and the presence of others trigger the overproduction of skin cells. Food allergies have also been implicated.

Foods, or specific nutrients, that have offered relief to some psoriasis patients include cold-water fish oils, vitamin A, zinc, vitamin E, and selenium. These can be taken in the form of whole foods or as supplements. Researchers in England found that psoriasis patients who each took ten fish-oil capsules a day for eight weeks greatly reduced their symptoms of itching, redness, and scaling, whereas similar sub-

HOME HYDROTHERAPY ENHANCEMENTS

Several household products can add to the effectiveness of hydrotherapy treatments. The following recipes are recommended by the National Psoriasis Foundation:

- Dissolve 1½ cups of baking soda in 3 gallons of water to use as an anti-itch compress.
- Add a handful of Epsom salts or Dead Sea salts to your bathwater. You can also add a squirt of mineral oil or baby oil to the water with the salts.
- Put 3 tablespoons of boric acid (available in pharmacies) in 16 ounces of water and use as a compress.
- Add 2 teaspoons of olive oil to a large glass of milk and use it as a soothing bath oil.
- Add 1 cup of white vinegar to the bath to ease itching.

jects who were given the placebo capsules filled with olive oil had no change in symptoms.

On the other hand, those things to eliminate from the diet include alcohol and excessive animal foods. One study done in Sweden showed that psoriasis sufferers who ate a vegan diet (no meat, fish, milk, or eggs) for three to four weeks experienced fewer symptoms than on their regular diet.

In addition to animal products, wheat and acidic foods (citrus, tomatoes, coffee, pineapple, and soda) also tend to aggravate psoriasis.

A sample supplement recommendation for fish oil (eicosapentaenoic acid, or EPA) might be 10 to 12 grams per day. Eating a little more than five ounces (150 grams) of a cold-water fish, such as mackerel, salmon, sardines, or herring, daily would give you the same amount of oil. Flax oil is a vegetarian alternative to fish oil.

HYDROTHERAPY

Water therapy can supply heat, moisture, and minute amounts of key minerals to the skin. Some types of hydrotherapy that offer relief from psoriasis include

- bathing in warm water, which stimulates blood circulation
- using a room humidifier, which eliminates dry air that can aggravate lesions
- bathing in water high in minerals (especially sulfur) that may seep through the skin and aid in healing

The Dead Sea, located between Israel and Jordan at the lowest point on Earth, has earned a great reputation with psoriasis sufferers from around the world. They go there to bathe in the mineral- and salt-rich waters and sunbathe under the unique natural ultraviolet spectrum of light. According

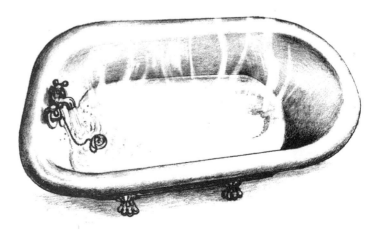

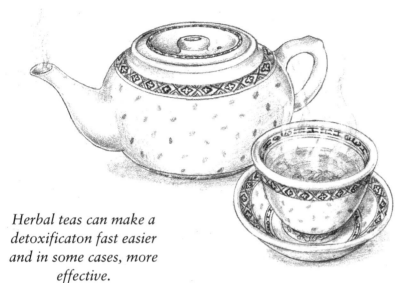

Herbal teas can make a detoxificaton fast easier and in some cases, more effective.

to a study, 88 percent of the patients at one Dead Sea psoriasis clinic experienced a significant or total reduction in their lesions.

Here are some helpful hints for psoriasis sufferers: When taking a bath, use warm (not hot) water. Never rub the skin dry. Instead, gently pat it with a soft towel.

DETOXIFICATION, FASTING, AND COLON THERAPY

Detoxification therapy works on the premise that getting rid of the body's lingering toxins and waste products can enable the skin cells to function properly again. Another theory of detoxification holds that psoriasis lesions are a sign that the body is trying to release toxins through the skin; people with psoriasis tend to have high levels of endotoxins (components of bacterial cell walls) in their intestines.

Some cleansing techniques include
- water fasting, which gives the body a chance to rid itself of toxins
- enemas, intended to empty the bowels and aid in the fasting process
- colonic irrigation, which gently pumps water in and out of the large intestine to wash out residue and excess gas

A cleansing program that includes colonic irrigation usually begins with a supervised water fast, which can last from three to seven days. If you feel hungry during the fast, try sipping herbal teas or clear vegetable broths. Supervision by a qualified practitioner such as a naturopathic physician is essential for a safe and effective water fast.

OTHER THERAPIES

HERBAL MEDICINE—Many herbs are important in the treatment of psoriasis, including sarsaparilla (which binds with endotoxins), *Coleus forskoli, Psoralen coryliforia,* and many others.

AROMATHERAPY—The essential oils of bergamot, calendula, or lavender can be mixed with carrier oils and massaged into the skin.

HYPNOTHERAPY—Hypnotic trances may be used to offer the subconscious mind suggestions regarding pain control, skin healing, and stress reduction.

TRADITIONAL CHINESE MEDICINE—Effective treatment may include herbal therapy and acupuncture directed toward the organ system that has the imbalance of vital life energy triggering the skin lesions.

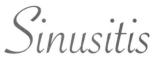

Sinusitis

SINUSITIS IS AN INFLAMMATION OF THE MUCOUS MEMBRANE THAT LINES THE SINUS CAVITIES (LOCATED AROUND THE NOSE). WHAT CAUSES IT? AN INFECTION (RESULTING FROM A COMMON COLD, TOOTH ABSCESS, OR OTHER AILMENT), ALLERGIES SUCH AS HAY FEVER, OR AN INJURY TO THE NOSE. ONCE SOMEONE HAS THE SINUS DISORDER, IT CAN GO AWAY, ONLY TO RETURN THE NEXT TIME A COLD HITS.

CONVENTIONAL APPROACH

Allopathic medicine strikes back at sinusitis with medications to fight the infectious organism and to restore free breathing:

- Antibiotics are prescribed according to the type of infection.
- Decongestants—available over the counter in tablets, nasal sprays, and drops—can provide relief by clearing the sinuses but should be taken only for very short periods.
- Antihistamines may be added to the decongestants.

If all else fails, surgery may be the answer. To drain the sinuses, the surgeon may open up any blocked passages from the sinuses to the nose or create a new passage.

ALTERNATIVE APPROACHES

Unlike conventional medicine, many alternative therapies believe that the symptoms and infectious organisms related to sinusitis are not the primary concern. Instead, these treatments try to uncover the causes of the sinus disorder.

CHIROPRACTIC

Chiropractic medicine holds a great deal of promise for people with sinusitis. Its treatments can target the bones and mucous membrane that surround the air-filled sinus cavities, as well as the joints and muscles of other parts of the body. Patients of chiropractic have reported improvements in their breathing, their postnasal drainage, their ability to sleep, and their sense of smell, as well as fewer headaches. Several treatment methods may be appropriate:

- Chiropractic manipulative therapy—adjusting joints beyond their normal limitations to correct a misalignment—allows the body to return to proper function and heal itself.
- Nasal-specific technique—inserting small balloonlike tools into the nasal cavity and gently inflating them—can expand the sinus openings. (This technique is often practiced by naturopathic physicians.)
- Trigger point therapy—applying pressure to a "trigger point" on the body (somewhere other than the sinus area)—can eliminate the sinus pain.
- Light-force cranial manipulation—involving adjustments of the skull bones and surrounding fluid—may also provide relief.

A typical chiropractic treatment for sinusitis may require 15 visits spread out over two months. Only a trained practitioner is qualified to perform spinal manipulation. Chiropractors specialize in treating the spine and other joints. Osteopaths and naturopathic physicians may also em-

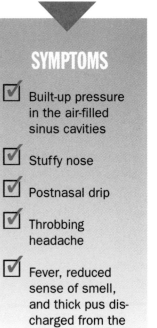

SYMPTOMS

- ☑ Built-up pressure in the air-filled sinus cavities
- ☑ Stuffy nose
- ☑ Postnasal drip
- ☑ Throbbing headache
- ☑ Fever, reduced sense of smell, and thick pus discharged from the nose (occasionally)

ploy these techniques, while physical therapists and massage therapists often incorporate elements such as trigger point therapy into their work.

HERBAL MEDICINE

Herbs can be used to stimulate the immune system and to reduce the production of mucus, dry out the sinuses, and reduce inflammation of the membranes. Both echinacea (also called purple coneflower) and goldenseal may strengthen the immune system, making it harder for future infections to trigger an attack of sinusitis. Goldenseal is also considered an effective reliever of sinusitis symptoms. The herb's root can be taken in capsule or tincture form or diluted with warm water and used as a nasal rinse. Teas made from elderflower, ginger, chamomile, ground ivy, or peppermint can clear out mucus. Other herbs that offer relief of sinusitis include eyebright, goldenrod, and marshmallow. (For suggestions on how to use purple coneflower, see Appendix 3.)

Here's a sample prescription for goldenseal: Take one 400-mg capsule of the powdered root three times a day during sinusitis flare-ups.

ACUPUNCTURE

According to acupuncture therapy, sinusitis can have several origins. It may result from a weakness in energy, or qi, in the lungs, which can leave the respiratory system in an unhealthy state. The disorder may also follow a disturbance in the intestines.

In assessing a patient with sinusitis, the acupuncturist looks beyond the symptoms to understand the health of the entire body. The acupuncturist may do a complete physical exam or make a pulse or tongue diagnosis and ask for your personal history. As needed, tiny needles are inserted in certain points on the body to replenish or disperse the energy, bringing it back to its ideal level. These points can also be stimulated with needles, electrical current, pressure, or heat. Herbal remedies and dietary alterations may also be prescribed.

An acupuncturist, a traditional Chinese physician, or a naturopathic physician can perform acupuncture. For your first visit to the practitioner, be prepared to discuss in detail your sinusitis symptoms, as well as your general health, diet, and lifestyle.

OTHER THERAPIES

AROMATHERAPY—The essential oils of eucalyptus, pine, or rosemary can be added to a steam inhalation treatment.

HOMEOPATHY—Common remedies include allium cepa, kali bichromicum, and sulphur.

HYDROTHERAPY—Alternating hot and cold baths or compresses can be beneficial.

NUTRITIONAL THERAPY—Recommendations include taking vitamins B_6 and C and avoiding dairy products and food allergens.

YOGA—Poses and breathing exercises can improve breathing, reduce tension and stress, and support the immune system.

Sore Throat

A SORE THROAT IS A RAW SENSATION IN THE BACK OF THE THROAT THAT MAKES SWALLOWING PAINFUL. IT CAN BE A SYMPTOM OF PHARYNGITIS (INFLAMMATION OF THE THROAT) OR STREPTOCOCCAL INFECTION (STREP THROAT); OFTEN IT'S THE INITIAL SYMPTOM OF A COLD, THE FLU, LARYNGITIS (INFLAMMATION OF THE VOICE BOX), OR ANOTHER CONDITION. A SORE THROAT CAN ALSO RESULT FROM OVERUSE (SUCH AS TOO MUCH SCREAMING) OR ABUSE (SMOKING), AND CAN, IN SOME INSTANCES, RESULT FROM PROBLEMS IN THE SINUSES, LUNGS, OR A DIFFERENT PART OF THE DIGESTIVE TRACT.

CONVENTIONAL APPROACH

To stop the pain of a sore throat, allopathic medicine suggests taking aspirin, acetaminophen, or one of the nonsteroidal anti-inflammatory drugs (such as ibuprofen and naproxen sodium).

For temporary relief, people with sore throats can also gargle with warm salt water or use commercially prepared saltwater nasal sprays. Over-the-counter throat sprays and lozenges, containing an antiseptic, may offer short-term help but should not be used for extended periods.

People with strep throat or bacterial pharyngitis are usually given antibiotics, such as penicillin, to treat their infections.

ALTERNATIVE APPROACHES

Many alternative therapies can provide ways to soothe and heal a sore throat—ways that don't disrupt the body's harmony in the process. Remember, though, if your sore throat is severe or persistent, be sure to have it checked out; strep throat should not be ignored or treated casually, as it can lead to kidney problems or rheumatic fever.

HERBAL MEDICINE

Herbs can soothe and heal the throat, ease inflammation of its mucous membranes, and help the immune system fight off infection. Garlic works against bacterial infections and promotes a strong immune system. Try to tolerate the taste and smell of lots of fresh garlic, which is considered more effective than commercially prepared capsules.

Several herbs can be taken for their astringent properties on the mucous membranes. Agrimony, loosestrife, and thyme are good examples. Tea made from these herbs can be gargled to provide relief.

Myrrh is especially helpful in sore throats, as are tonics such as goldenseal, cleavers, and marigold (calendula).

Echinacea (or purple coneflower) stimulates the immune system and can significantly shorten the duration of a sore throat. (For suggestions on how to prepare and use purple coneflower, see Appendix 3.)

Other herbs commonly used to treat rough and raw throats include cayenne pepper, licorice, red sage, and white horehound.

SYMPTOMS

☑ Pain felt from the back of the mouth to the top of the larynx (voice box)

☑ Hoarse voice

Occasionally, a sore throat can be accompanied by

☑ Congestion

☑ Coughing

☑ Sneezing

☑ Runny nose

☑ Headache

☑ Earache

☑ Fever

☑ Swollen lymph nodes in the neck

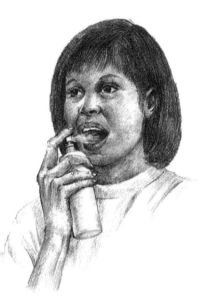

A mixture of six parts marigold (calendula) succus (plant juice) and one part bitter orange oil can be sprayed directly on the back of the throat. The marigold is very soothing and the bitter orange oil is a potent antibacterial.

NUTRITIONAL THERAPY

Nutritional therapy supplies the body with nutrients needed to boost the immune system and target infections. When used to treat sore throats, zinc gluconate lozenges may stop viruses from multiplying. A father in Texas discovered this benefit by chance after his young daughter, suffering with a cold, sucked on a zinc tablet instead of swallowing it; her symptoms went away. A study that tested the lozenges against a placebo confirmed zinc's ability to speed up recovery of raw and scratchy throats, as well as coughs, runny noses, and sneezing.

Supplements of vitamin C and bioflavonoids also can be taken for their ability to improve immune system functioning. These supplements may be able to shorten the course of a sore throat.

Liquids (decaffeinated and nonalcoholic, of course) can rehydrate the mucous membranes in the throat and should be consumed in large amounts. Herb teas, vegetable juices, and water are the preferred drinks. Fresh fruit juices (not bottled, canned, frozen, or packaged in any way) can cool the system if the sore throat is caused by a heat condition, and they also provide many important vitamins.

One possible sore throat remedy: Suck on one zinc gluconate lozenge (containing about 23 mg of zinc) every two hours, except during sleep. Discontinue as soon as the throat feels better, because long-term use can affect other nutrients in the body.

AROMATHERAPY

Inhaling or gargling the essential oil of certain plants and herbs can relieve pain. Commonly used oils include

- eucalyptus
- geranium
- sandalwood
- thyme

Depending on the oil, it can be added to hot, steaming water and inhaled or mixed with drinking water and gargled.

Here's an example of an aromatherapy remedy for sore throats: Mix five drops of commercially prepared eucalyptus oil with two cups of water. Shake or mix well. Gargle small amounts at a time.

OTHER THERAPIES

DETOXIFICATION, FASTING, AND COLON THERAPY—Water and herbal tea fasts and juice diets, lasting only a couple of days, can be helpful.

HOMEOPATHY—Specific remedies must be tailored to the individual, but common prescriptions include baptisia tinctoria, belladonna, causticum, and rumex crispus.

HYDROTHERAPY—A damp cloth wrapped around the neck and covered by a wool scarf helps bring the body's healing factors to the neck and throat area.

Temporomandibular Disorder

THE TEMPOROMANDIBULAR JOINT IS THE JAW JOINT ON BOTH SIDES OF THE HEAD THAT ALLOWS THE MOUTH TO OPEN AND CLOSE. WHEN THE JOINT AND SURROUNDING MUSCLES AND LIGAMENTS MALFUNCTION IN SOME WAY, IT'S CALLED A TEMPOROMANDIBULAR DISORDER, OR TMD. CONTRIBUTING FACTORS INCLUDE GRINDING THE TEETH, AN INCORRECT BITE, INJURY, OR OSTEOARTHRITIS.

CONVENTIONAL APPROACH

Allopathic medicine's treatment program for TMD focuses on easing pain, preventing spasms of the chewing muscles, and correcting any bite or jaw problems. Typical recommendations include

- eating foods that require little or no chewing
- applying moist heat or ice to the jaw area as needed
- massaging the muscles around the jaw, also as needed
- wearing a bite plate during sleep to prevent grinding the teeth

Several medications can relieve the symptoms of TMD: Aspirin, nonsteroidal anti-inflammatory drugs such as ibuprofen, and muscle-relaxant drugs such as diazepam can ease discomfort, but all carry the potential for side effects.

The teeth may be ground down or fitted with orthodontic braces if an incorrect bite is causing the pain. Finally, if other treatments fail to bring relief, surgery is an option. The joint can be cleared of scar tissue or other tissues and repositioned or fitted with artificial implants.

ALTERNATIVE APPROACHES
BIOFEEDBACK TRAINING

Biofeedback training can greatly benefit people with TMD by teaching them to relax the jaw muscles and reduce overall stress, eliminating the need for such habits as clenching the teeth. Electromyographic biofeedback, which measures muscle tension, is commonly used to treat TMD. Electrodes are attached to the patient's skin in the area of the jaw joint to measure the electrical activity in the muscles. A special monitor "feeds back" the level of this activity, which reveals the amount of tension in the muscles. Using this information, the patient can learn to lower the tension with the use of relaxation exercises, guided imagery, breathing exercises, and other methods.

Here's an excerpt of a guided imagery exercise that may be used during biofeedback training:

- Close your eyes and take several deep, slow breaths, focusing on each inhalation and exhalation.
- Imagine something soft and cushionlike (such as a pillow, cloud, or balloon) sitting in the space where the lower jaw hinges with the skull on each side of the head. See how much room these cushions have.
- Picture slowly inflating these soft cushions, allowing in as much air as needed.
- Feel these cushions relaxing your muscles. See how easy and freely your jaw can move.

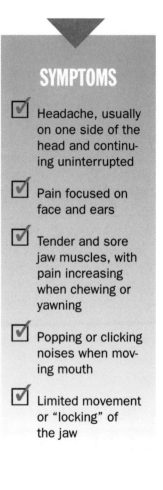

SYMPTOMS

☑ Headache, usually on one side of the head and continuing uninterrupted

☑ Pain focused on face and ears

☑ Tender and sore jaw muscles, with pain increasing when chewing or yawning

☑ Popping or clicking noises when moving mouth

☑ Limited movement or "locking" of the jaw

ACUPRESSURE

Acupressure operates on the principle that TMD results when the body's flow of vital life energy, or qi, is disrupted or unbalanced. Applying manual pressure to certain points can rebalance the flow through the body's energy channels or meridians. The acupressure points typically used to treat TMD include

- SI19—on the cheek directly in front of the ear canal
- ST6—between the lower jaw and skull
- GB20—at the base of the skull, on either side of the spine
- Taiyang—on the temples between the hairline and eyebrow.

ST36, located a couple of inches below the kneecap (on the stomach channel), is commonly treated to relieve headaches focused on the front of the head.

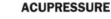 Self-treatment can include a program of several acupressure points performed two or three times a day. Here's a sample treatment that is focused on the acupressure point ST6:

- To find the point, clench your molar teeth and feel for the tightened jaw muscle, located between your lower jaw and skull.
- With your fingers, firmly press the point on both sides of the head while breathing slowly and deeply. Apply pressure on both sides simultaneously for two minutes.

CRANIOSACRAL THERAPY

Craniosacral therapists hold that TMD can result from misaligned bones in the skull. This misalignment blocks the flow of cerebrospinal fluid—a clear, watery liquid that cushions the brain and spinal cord from their encasing bones.

Treatment involves palpation (examination with the hands) to check for any skull and spinal bones out of their ideal placement and to assess whether the flow of the cerebrospinal fluid is adequate. Any adjustments needed to correct misalignments are also performed with the hands.

Many chiropractors, osteopaths, and naturopaths are trained to perform craniosacral therapy. Treatment would involve manipulation of the bones of the head and neck and pressure to points inside the mouth.

OTHER THERAPIES

BODYWORK—Massage can relieve stress and ease muscle tension.

CHIROPRACTIC—Treatment can include spinal manipulation as well as craniosacral therapy. Often people with TMD also experience back pain.

HERBAL THERAPY—Many herbs can be helpful. Examples include white willow bark for pain relief and chamomile and peppermint to soothe tension.

HYPNOTHERAPY—Hypnosis can teach people to reduce tension and control habits (such as teeth grinding).

A PEPTIC ULCER IS AN OPEN SORE THAT OCCURS ON THE MUCOUS LINING OF THE STOMACH OR THE DUODENUM (THE FIRST SECTION OF THE SMALL INTESTINE). IT IS LINKED WITH AN OVERPRODUCTION OF STOMACH ACID, AN UNDERPRODUCTION OF MUCUS, OR IRRITANTS (SUCH AS ALCOHOL, CAFFEINE, ASPIRIN, AND BACTERIA). STRESS ALSO PLAYS A ROLE IN CAUSING ULCERS.

CONVENTIONAL APPROACH

Allopathic medicine relies on drugs to heal ulcers. Once recovered, patients sometimes continue taking lower doses of certain drugs to prevent future attacks. In severe cases, surgery is used. Some lifestyle changes are also recommended to relieve pain and eliminate future ulcers.

DRUG TREATMENT

Several medications are used to relieve the pain of ulcers and promote healing:

- Antacids work to neutralize stomach acid.
- Histamine$_2$-receptor antagonists, such as cimetidine, famotidine, and ranitidine, cut down the production of stomach acid.
- Sucralfate forms a paste that coats the ulcer.

In recent years, the role of a certain bacteria—*Helicobacter pylori*—has been recognized in the formation of ulcers. Antibiotics (including tetracycline and amoxicillin) can fight off the bacteria. These drugs are often combined with the antibacterial bismuth subsalicylate.

SURGICAL TREATMENT

If drugs do not improve an ulcer condition, the ulcerated part of the stomach can be surgically removed. Another procedure involves cutting the nerve that regulates the production of stomach acid.

OTHER TREATMENT

People with ulcers can usually find some relief if they avoid ulcer irritants such as coffee, alcohol, aspirin, and cigarette smoking. Also, symptoms are usually milder if one eats several small meals throughout the day rather than three big meals.

ALTERNATIVE APPROACHES
NUTRITIONAL THERAPY

Nutritional therapists hold that the wrong diet can be a major cause of peptic ulcers. For example, a diet rich in highly processed grains (such as white flour) deprives the body of fiber and protein, which can shield the digestive lining from stomach acid. People with ulcers should eat as many unrefined and high-fiber plant foods as possible.

Some cases of ulcer are thought to be a symptom of a food allergy. An elimination diet can help to determine if any specific food triggers an increase in symptoms. An elimination diet involves avoiding frequently eaten foods and common food allergens for two to three weeks, then reintroducing them one by one, and taking note of which ones trigger symptoms.

SYMPTOMS

☑ Burning or aching pain in the abdomen (Depending on the location of the ulcer, eating may ease the pain.)

☑ Nausea and vomiting

☑ Persistent belching

☑ Reduced appetite and weight loss

☑ Traces of blood in stool or vomit (rarely)

Sometimes ulcers cause no noticeable symptoms, but if they perforate they can cause severe bleeding and death.

Like conventional medicine, nutritional therapy also recommends avoiding ulcer irritants such as coffee and alcohol. Several foods can aid the healing process of ulcers. Most notably, cabbage juice is prescribed for its ability to soothe the digestive lining and heal ulcers. Studies done in the 1950s showed the juice to be an effective ulcer treatment. Several supplements can promote healing, including

- vitamin A
- vitamin E
- zinc

Here's a green cabbage juice treatment that a naturopathic physician might prescribe: Drink an eight-ounce glass of fresh juice three times a day. For some variety, carrot or celery juice can be added to the cabbage juice.

OTHER THERAPIES

AYURVEDIC MEDICINE—Ulcers are often linked to an imbalance in pitta. Treatment includes dietary and lifestyle changes.

GUIDED IMAGERY AND CREATIVE VISUALIZATION—Because stress has been linked to ulcers, various "mind exercises" that bring relaxation can be helpful. Hypnotherapy, meditation, and yoga are also good stress-busters.

HOMEOPATHY—Common remedies include anacardium, argentum nitricum, and nux vomica.

TRADITIONAL CHINESE MEDICINE—Massage therapy that focuses on balancing qi in the stomach, spleen, and/or liver meridians can be effective. Other

HERBAL MEDICINE

Herbal medicine targets its efforts at relieving the symptoms of peptic ulcers and healing the walls of the digestive tract. Herbs should be combined with measures such as stress reduction and dietary changes that eliminate the causes of ulcers.

The bark of slippery elm is used for its ability to soothe the mucous membranes that line the stomach and duodenum. It's often taken in powdered form. Licorice (in particular, licorice with its glycyrrhizinic acid removed), which comes in chewable tablet form, can also soothe the membranes, and it can strengthen them (thereby preventing future ulcers). Several studies have confirmed deglycyrrhizinized licorice's ability to treat ulcers. In fact, some conventional ulcer drugs are made from derivatives of licorice.

Another treatment for an irritated digestive tract is Robert's Formula, a well-known naturopathic herbal remedy. It usually contains slippery elm, marshmallow root, comfrey, echinacea (purple coneflower), goldenseal, other herbs, and cabbage powder. (For the recipe, see Appendix 3.)

Herbal therapy may also incorporate minerals. For example, bismuth salts, such as bismuth subcitrate, have antibacterial properties and can be effective in treating ulcers that are attributed to the *Helicobacter pylori*. Again, some common conventional drugs for ulcer are made with bismuth.

An herbalist may recommend taking about one teaspoon of powdered slippery elm bark (added to one cup of warm water to form a gruel-like substance) three times a day.

Uterine Fibroids

FIBROIDS ARE NONCANCEROUS TUMORS IN THE MUSCULAR WALL OF THE UTERUS. FIBROIDS CAN BE AS SMALL AS A PEA OR AS LARGE AS A GRAPEFRUIT. THE BODY'S LEVEL OF THE ESTROGEN HORMONE SEEMS TO PLAY A ROLE IN THE CONDITION AS FIBROIDS TEND TO GROW DURING PREGNANCY AND SHRINK AFTER MENOPAUSE.

CONVENTIONAL APPROACH

Allopathic medicine tends to ignore fibroids that are small and relatively symptomless. In addition, some doctors recommend adopting a wait-and-see attitude for fibroids in older women, because the tumors usually shrink in size after menopause (when estrogen levels drop). However, many menopausal women take estrogen replacement drugs, which can encourage the tumors to grow.

If menstrual bleeding is heavy, anemia may occur. In this case, iron supplements are prescribed.

Certain drugs that inhibit the ovary's ability to produce estrogen can be helpful in select cases.

If the symptoms, such as pain or constipation from pressure on the intestines, become severe or the fibroids grow significantly in size, surgery is typically recommended. (In rare cases, removal is performed in fear of cancer, but according to one estimate, less than one-half of one percent of all fibroids become cancerous.)

A hysterectomy (removal of the uterus) is usually the treatment for women who are experiencing symptoms and no longer plan on having children. Hysterectomy is major surgery and recovery can take weeks or months. Depression is common after a hysterectomy.

If a woman with fibroids wants to become pregnant in the future, a myomectomy (removal of the tumor) is a possibility. The fibroids must not be too large or too numerous to qualify for this procedure.

ALTERNATIVE APPROACHES

Several alternative therapies offer ways to reduce estrogen levels naturally. The hope is to forestall or eliminate the need for a hysterectomy.

MIND/BODY MEDICINE

For women with fibroids, mind/body medicine focuses on significantly reducing stress. This is vital because stress can interrupt the development and release of eggs (a process called ovulation). When this process doesn't happen, the body's level of estrogen remains unnecessarily high, precipitating fibroid development. Mind/body medicine offers many therapies that teach relaxation and how to lower stress levels, including

- forms of guided imagery and creative visualization
- meditation
- yoga (including breathing exercises and stretches)
- biofeedback
- dance therapy
- hypnotherapy
- spirituality

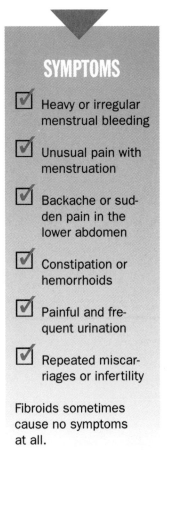

SYMPTOMS

- ☑ Heavy or irregular menstrual bleeding
- ☑ Unusual pain with menstruation
- ☑ Backache or sudden pain in the lower abdomen
- ☑ Constipation or hemorrhoids
- ☑ Painful and frequent urination
- ☑ Repeated miscarriages or infertility

Fibroids sometimes cause no symptoms at all.

Here's a sample relaxation breathing exercise that would be part of a guided imagery regimen:

- Wearing loose clothing, lie down or sit in a comfortable chair.
- Slowly close your eyes. Begin breathing deeply and slowly.
- When exhaling, imagine tension effortlessly flowing out of your body with each breath.

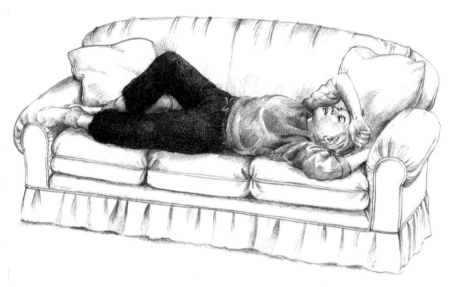

- As you inhale, picture yourself filling your body with fresh air and energy.
- Continue the slow, deep breathing for as long as you are comfortable.

HYDROTHERAPY

Hydrotherapy directed at the lower abdomen can stimulate blood circulation, which delivers nutrients and other beneficial substances to the cells and cleans away waste products. These treatments can also provide pain relief. Castor oil, made from the leaves of the castor-oil plant, is commonly applied to the lower abdomen as a warm pack.

The cold-pressed oil contains a substance that boosts the action of cells important to the immune system. Alternating hot and cold sitz baths can also be effective.

When symptoms flare up, a naturopathic physician may recommend applying castor oil packs to the lower abdomen (see Appendix 3 for instructions).

NUTRITIONAL THERAPY

According to nutritional therapy, diet and supplements can stabilize or even lower the levels of estrogen in the body. As estrogen amounts drop, existing fibroids should shrink and new ones can be prevented. Diet and supplements may also reduce some of the symptoms of fibroids.

One of the liver's roles in the body is to break down estrogens. Therefore, the diet should allow the liver to do its work and not include foods that can tax this organ. These taxing foods to be avoided include

- sugar
- meat
- dairy products
- alcohol

In addition, meat and dairy products can be a source of hormones (including estrogen) from livestock. Because they are also high in fat and estrogen is stored in fat cells, these foods may cause additional problems for women with fibroids. Instead, focus on eating fresh vegetables and fruits, whole grains, nuts, and raw seeds. These steps should also result in a diet that's high in fiber and low in fat.

The B vitamins also aid the liver and are recommended. They can be added in the form of whole foods (such as lentils, rice bran, and blackstrap molasses) or supplements. Vitamin B_6, in particular, enhances the breakdown and removal of estrogen from the body.

Natural plant estrogens, called phytoestrogens, can actually compete with human estrogen in the body, resulting in an overall lower level of estrogen. Soybeans are a good food source of this substance and can be used as a whole cooked bean or in its other forms, including tofu, tempeh, and soy milk.

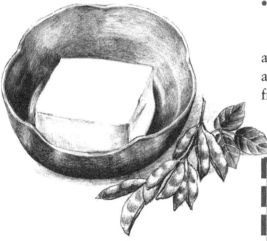

Researchers have linked heavy menstrual bleeding with low levels of vitamin A in the blood. One study gave women doses of vitamin A for 15 days, after which time menstrual bleeding was reduced in about 90 percent of the patients. To achieve proper levels of vitamin A in the body, most practitioners of nutritional therapy recommend eating foods rich in beta-carotene (such as carrots and sweet potatoes) or taking beta-carotene supplements (25,000 to 50,000 IU daily).

 A naturopathic physician may recommend a program of several supplements to normalize estrogen levels. A high-potency multivitamin-mineral supplement prescribed for uterine fibroids might include

- 100 mg of each B vitamin except B_{12}, which should be at 100 µg (These levels are typical in "stress formula" multivitamins.)
- 400 IU of vitamin E
- 25,000 IU of beta-carotene
- cysteine, methionine, choline, inositol (to help the liver metabolize estrogen and other substances more efficiently)
- iron (if the fibroids cause heavy menstrual bleeding and anemia)

Dietary recommendations include adopting a low-fat, high-fiber diet and avoiding meat, dairy products, eggs, refined sugar, and caffeine.

OTHER THERAPIES

ACUPRESSURE—Points along the liver and spleen channels are often targeted for symptom relief.

HERBAL MEDICINE—Some herbs that can ease the symptoms of fibroids are blue cohosh, dong quai, and wild cherry.

HOMEOPATHY—Remedies for short-term relief of symptoms can be very effective, but a careful diagnosis by a professional is necessary to tailor a long-term remedy for fibroids.

DETOXIFICATION, FASTING, AND COLON THERAPY—Several types of treatments can remove toxins and prevent certain organs (such as the liver) from being overworked. These therapies can also alleviate constipation and hemorrhoids related to fibroids.

Varicose Veins

VARICOSE VEINS ARE SWOLLEN AND DISTORTED BLOOD VESSELS, APPEARING COMMONLY ON THE LEGS. THEY OCCUR IF THE VEINS DEVELOP WEAKENED WALLS OR POORLY FUNCTIONING VALVES (WHICH REGULATE THE FLOW OF BLOOD). OBESITY, PREGNANCY, MENOPAUSE, AND LONG PERIODS OF STANDING MAY TRIGGER THE CONDITION, WHICH MAY ALSO BE INHERITED.

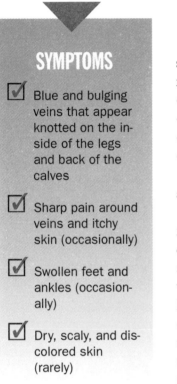

SYMPTOMS

- ☑ Blue and bulging veins that appear knotted on the inside of the legs and back of the calves

- ☑ Sharp pain around veins and itchy skin (occasionally)

- ☑ Swollen feet and ankles (occasionally)

- ☑ Dry, scaly, and discolored skin (rarely)

CONVENTIONAL APPROACH

For most cases of varicose veins, a series of self-help measures is all that is recommended, including
- wearing special elastic stockings
- minimizing standing
- elevating the legs while sitting
- exercising

Over-the-counter painkillers may also be used to ease some symptoms.

Severe cases of varicose veins receive more drastic actions. In the procedure called sclerotherapy, the twisted veins are injected with strong chemicals, which greatly damage the veins. The hope is that the varicose veins will seal off and nearby veins will take over the transport of blood. Another surgical technique (called stripping) involves removing the malfunctioning veins.

ALTERNATIVE APPROACHES

Several alternative therapies offer ways to reduce the swelling and discomfort of varicose veins and several ways to prevent them. Most of these therapies recommend the same self-help measures as conventional medicine does. Of particular importance is adding an exercise regimen, which can improve blood circulation in the legs. Try walking, bicycling, or swimming, activities where the legs are not pounded against the ground or floor but exercised nonetheless.

HYDROTHERAPY

Several forms of hydrotherapy can stimulate blood circulation and shrink swollen veins. Because varicose veins result when pools of blood form in the veins, improving and promoting circulation is the key to preventing or minimizing them.

Alternating hot and cold leg baths can be used to improve circulation. Cold compresses applied to the legs may also encourage circulation and can reduce the swelling of veins. An astringent such as apple cider vinegar or witch hazel may be added to the wet compresses to help ease the swelling of veins.

Here's a sample hydrotherapy treatment: (This treatment is not appropriate for people with diabetes. If you have diabetes, check with your physician before applying any treatment to your extremities.)
- Fill two large basins or buckets with water, one as hot as you can tolerate (not hot enough to scald your skin), the other as cold as you can tolerate.
- Put your legs in the hot water for three minutes.
- Remove and then immediately put your legs in the cold water. Hold for one minute.
- Repeat four times, ending with the cold water.

NUTRITIONAL THERAPY

Certain foods and supplements have the potential to heal and prevent varicose veins. Vitamin C and flavonoids are recommended for their ability to rejuvenate the blood vessels. These substances are found in oranges and grapefruits (eaten with the white inner rind intact). Dark red and purple berries are also rich in flavonoids. In addition to the whole fruits, extracts may also prove helpful. Supplements of vitamin E may provide benefits to the vessels as well.

Foods and spices that work with the blood to break down the substance called fibrin can also be helpful. That's because people with varicose veins have an abnormal tendency to store fibrin, which can disrupt the action of the blood vessels. Garlic, onions, cayenne pepper, ginger, and bromelain (derived from fresh pineapple) all help to dissolve fibrin.

Just as straining to have a bowel movement can lead to varicose veins in the anus (more commonly known as hemorrhoids), it can also lead to varicose veins in the legs. To prevent this straining, softer, bulkier stool is needed. Here are some ways to boost your fiber intake:

- Increase your intake of fiber by eating more vegetables, unrefined grains (such as brown rice, oatmeal, rye, and buckwheat, not white bread), beans, and fruits.
- Drink at least eight 8-ounce glasses of water daily.
- Add fiber-rich psyllium seed husks to the diet.

Excess body weight can also increase the susceptibility to varicose veins, so weight loss is recommended.

A naturopathic physician may recommend eating several servings of flavonoid-rich berries a day, including

- cherries
- blackberries
- black currants
- blueberries
- grapes

OTHER THERAPIES

ACUPRESSURE—Points on the legs along the spleen channel are often targeted (use the leg other than the one with the varicose vein, if possible).

AROMATHERAPY—Gentle leg massages with the following essential oils can be helpful: cypress, lavender, lemon, and rosemary. Massage toward the heart and avoid the varicose veins themselves.

BODYWORK—Reflexology may relieve the pain of varicose veins.

DETOXIFICATION, FASTING, AND COLON THERAPY—A short fast and enemas can bring the return of regular bowel movements, important in preventing varicose veins.

HERBAL MEDICINE—Some effective herbs are butcher's broom, comfrey, horse chestnut, marigold, and stone root.

HOMEOPATHY—Common remedies include carbo vegetabilis, ferrum metallicum, hamamelis virginica, and pulsatilla nigricans.

YOGA—Certain postures, especially those done with the legs above the head, can improve circulation and serve as a form of exercise.

Yeast Infection

THE FUNGUS CANDIDA ALBICANS IS ALWAYS PRESENT IN THE VAGINA. HOWEVER, WHEN THE FUNGUS MULTIPLIES OUT OF CONTROL, A YEAST INFECTION RESULTS. ANTIBIOTICS, BIRTH CONTROL PILLS, WEARING TIGHT UNDERGARMENTS, AND A SUPPRESSED IMMUNE SYSTEM ARE JUST A FEW FACTORS THAT CAN TRIGGER THE OVERPRODUCTION OF FUNGUS.

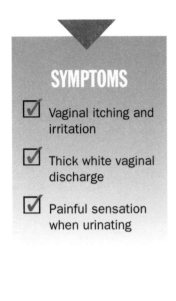

SYMPTOMS

☑ Vaginal itching and irritation

☑ Thick white vaginal discharge

☑ Painful sensation when urinating

CONVENTIONAL APPROACH

Drug therapy is at the center of allopathic medicine's treatment program for yeast infections. Typically, one of several antifungal drugs is used to interrupt the normal growth process of fungus. These medications can be taken as vaginal suppositories or creams or as regular pills, ranging from a single dose to doses spread out over a week. Possible medications include

- clotrimazole
- econazole nitrate
- fluconazole
- miconazole
- nystatin

These drugs carry potential side effects such as increased vaginal irritation, headaches, nausea, and stomach pain.

Often, the patient's sexual partners are also given the medications. Once treated, yeast infections may return later. In some cases, long-term treatment with antifungal drugs is prescribed. Some patients are taken off antibiotic treatment or birth control pills to eliminate the possibility of future infections.

ALTERNATIVE APPROACHES

Several alternative therapies place the emphasis of yeast infection treatment on the elimination of the causes, rather than eliminating the fungus.

NUTRITIONAL THERAPY

Nutritional therapy employs dietary changes and supplements to treat and prevent yeast infections. If you have problems with vaginal yeast infections, there are some foods that you should avoid and other foods that you should be sure to include in your diet.

Eating certain foods can contribute to a yeast infection in one of two ways: by encouraging the growth of the *Candida albicans* and by taxing the body's immune system. These bothersome foods may contain yeast or mold or trigger the symptoms of food allergies or sensitivities. Foods you may want to avoid include

- sugars (including honey, fruit juices, and maple syrup)
- artificial sweeteners
- cheese
- dried fruit
- alcohol
- mushrooms
- meat, poultry, and milk (which can have traces of antibiotics in them)

An elimination diet can help pinpoint any foods that trigger allergy symptoms: Frequently eaten foods and common food allergens (such as wheat and milk) are avoided and then reintroduced one by one, taking note of which ones bring on symptoms.

Some items can introduce "good" bacteria that keep fungus growth in check. They include live yogurt and the bacteria *Lactobacillus acidophilus* and certain species of *Bifidobacterium*, which can be taken orally or used as a douche. (Beware of sweetened yogurt and, for people with milk intolerance, lactose.)

Nutrient deficiencies may also contribute to an overabundance of fungus. Supplements that can be helpful include vitamin A, vitamin B_6, zinc, magnesium, and essential fatty acids, among others. (If taken, these should be yeast-free.)

Garlic can be added to the diet for its fungus-blocking properties and may prevent infections. (Cloves of garlic are also sometimes inserted into the vagina and then removed after a short time.) Caprylic acid, grapefruit seed extract, and undecenoic acid also have strong antifungal properties. In general, good nutrition that comes from eating a varied, whole-foods diet contributes to a strong immune system—one that can ward off infections.

As part of a tailored dietary regimen, a naturopathic physician may prescribe taking three garlic capsules three times a day. Fresh garlic should also be added freely to the diet.

HERBAL MEDICINE

Several herbs have the ability to knock out excess fungus, bringing the levels back to a healthy normal. Others can be effective in strengthening the immune system.

The bark of the pau d'arco tree has achieved folk-remedy status as a treatment for fungal infections, including vaginal yeast infections and athlete's foot. Researchers have examined its infection-fighting powers and have pinpointed lapachol as being the bark's possible active ingredient. It can be taken in the form of capsules, extract, or tea.

Goldenseal is one of the most commonly used herbs for its immune-boosting properties, and it is also believed effective in stabilizing the overgrowth of fungus. It's often administered as a douche. (Women who are pregnant should not use this herb.)

The following herbs also offer promise in the treatment of yeast infection. They can be taken in the form of capsules, extracts, or teas, and some may be used in douches. They include

- calendula
- echinacea (purple coneflower)
- German chamomile
- ginger
- rosemary
- tea tree
- thyme

(For suggestions on how to prepare and use purple coneflower, see Appendix 3.)

THE BIG PICTURE

Some alternative therapies consider yeast infection a much more extensive problem than conventional medicine does. The fungus overgrowth can affect the skin and the internal organs, and its symptoms may be as unexpected as fatigue, memory loss, irritability, headaches, and depression. Treatment in these disciplines requires a complete strengthening of the immune system and much more.

An herbalist may prescribe the following: Add one ounce of aged pau d'arco bark to one pint of boiling water. Simmer 45 to 60 minutes. Strain. Drink one cup three times a day.

HOMEOPATHY

Homeopathic medicine can stimulate the body to overpower the yeast infection. The therapy uses highly diluted doses of a natural substance that would produce the same infection symptoms if given in full strength to a healthy person. To tailor a remedy for yeast infection, a classical homeopath questions the patient on the symptoms and assesses the general state of physical and emotional health. Using these clues, the remedy is then individualized to the patient. Here are some yeast infection characteristics to consider:

- Is there any vaginal discharge? What is its color, consistency, and smell?
- Does walking or lying down increase the amount of discharge?
- Is there any discomfort around the vagina?
- Is urination difficult or uncomfortable?

Some typical remedies for yeast infections include

- borax veneta
- calcarea carbonica
- kreosotum
- mercurius solubilis
- pulsatilla nigricans
- sepia

Combination remedies, available over the counter, are formulated for the most common yeast infection symptoms. Because of this lack of individualization, they are considered less effective.

For a yeast infection characterized by a smelly yellowish discharge and itching and burning pains, among other details, here's a sample homeopathic remedy: Take one dose of kreosotum, 12c, every three hours. (The *12c* refers to the potency of the remedy.) Stop treatment as soon as the symptoms go away.

OTHER THERAPIES

AROMATHERAPY—Douches of water and essential tea tree or marigold oils can eliminate excess fungus in the vagina.

AYURVEDIC MEDICINE—Treatment, focusing on digestion and the immune system, often includes dietary changes and herbal therapy.

DETOXIFICATION, FASTING, AND COLON THERAPY—Colonic irrigation and enemas can cleanse the intestinal tract and contribute to a healthy balance of normal flora in the body.

HYDROTHERAPY—A hot sitz bath (perhaps spiked with calendula or thyme tea or vinegar) may relieve itching.

MIND/BODY MEDICINE—Guided imagery, meditation, and other treatment forms can reduce stress and strengthen the body's immune function.

OXYGEN THERAPY—Hydrogen peroxide treatment is used to give the immune system a boost, to assist it in controlling the overgrowth of fungus.

TRADITIONAL CHINESE MEDICINE—Acupuncture, herbal therapy, and diet and lifestyle changes offer ways to correct energy imbalances and enhance the body's defenses.

In this part, you'll find 28 chapters each dealing with an alternative therapy or, more accurately, 28 medical disciplines. These vary from treatments such as chelation therapy based on certain aspects of modern biochemical theories and technologies to systems such as Ayurvedic medicine and qigong that go back for millennia.

At times it seems there are as many treatment options in the world of alternative medicine as there are illnesses you can come down with. The number is, of course, not that huge, but the number of therapeutic variations is significant. Different practitioners emphasize different aspects of a therapy, and older therapies are constantly being updated as new techniques and technologies are discovered.

Another reason there seems to be so many therapies in alternative medicine is the treatment approach many alternative therapists use. Unlike allopathic medicine's one-size-fits-all approach to a certain disease, many alternative therapies are based on the notion that every individual's condition is specific to the patient and the whole person requires healing. Given the many variations of people in the world, it's easy to see how varied the alternative practitioner's palette must be.

To help you use the information in this section, here are some of the features you'll find in a chapter:

History—Each discipline has its own unique history. Some are marked by their time-honored traditions, others by their struggle to be recognized. The history of a therapy can often give you an idea of its place in contemporary healing practices.

Given the many variations of people in the world, it's easy to see how varied the alternative practitioner's palette must be.

What It Is—Before you venture into a therapy, it's natural to want to know what treatment in a certain medical discipline is like. Here you'll find what techniques are used, what equipment is involved, and generally what to expect from a visit to a practitioner.

Uses—For most of the therapies discussed, it would be impossible to discuss—or even list—every health condition that they can address. Many of these alternative therapies, such as Ayurvedic medicine and traditional Chinese medicine, are themselves medical systems no less complete than modern allopathic medicine. Therefore, the uses that are discussed were chosen to reflect either the therapy's most common applications or its particularly convincing therapeutic successes. When appropriate, clinical research studies that back up these uses are noted. (When you see a number in [ ], you can go to Appendix 1: References to find where the research was published.)

Who Does It—Because so many alternative therapies are based on highly individualized treatments and because of the intimate nature of the doctor– patient relationship in general, finding a good practitioner is vital. Here you'll find information on state and local requirements and licensing (if any), what a practitioner's training is like, and what to look for and ask.

Resources—There is no way to answer every question about every therapy, but most disciplines have professional- and consumer-oriented organizations that can address your specific concerns and guide you to a qualified practitioner. The address, phone numbers, fax number, e-mail address, and World Wide Web site (when available) are all listed.

Acupressure

STRICTLY SPEAKING, ACUPRESSURE IS A FORM OF ACUPUNCTURE, BUT INSTEAD OF INSERTING FINE NEEDLES INTO SPECIFIC POINTS ON THE BODY, ACUPRESSURE USES MANUAL PRESSURE ON THE POINTS TO ACHIEVE THE SAME RESULT. ALTHOUGH COMPLICATIONS FROM ACUPUNCTURE ARE EXTREMELY RARE, INFECTION IS A POSSIBILITY IF NEEDLES ARE REUSED AND IMPROPERLY STERILIZED. ACUPRESSURE, HOWEVER, CARRIES NO RISK FROM INFECTION BECAUSE NO NEEDLES ARE USED. ACUPRESSURE HAS MANY OTHER BENEFITS AS WELL: IT CAN BE EASILY TAUGHT AND, THEREFORE, SELF-ADMINISTERED.

WHAT IT IS

Acupressure has many similarities to acupuncture (see pages 173–177). Instead of inserting needles, though, acupressure uses pressure to stimulate points that can relieve nausea and pain, and treat certain ailments.

This pressure is usually applied with the fingers, but practitioners may also use small seeds or devices that contain little bumps that provide pressure to the specific point. For example, smoking cessation may be treated with either acupuncture or acupressure. In acupressure, tiny seeds or small metal pellets like ball bearings may be taped to the appropriate points on the ear, and the patient can press these spots when the urge to smoke occurs.

Some widely used bodywork techniques also use acupressure. Based on traditional Chinese medicine, these techniques involve applying pressure with the fingers to manipulate the body's meridians, or pathways for vital energy. Some of these related disciplines include shiatsu and tsubo, described under pressure point techniques (see page 210), and jin shin jyustu and jin shin do, described under polarity therapy (see page 209).

USES

Acupressure is used to promote general health and to treat a wide variety of ailments. Some of the many uses of acupressure include

- arthritis
- headache
- nausea
- pain

Most of the research and publicity concerning acupressure in the West has centered around its use to prevent or control nausea. Western doctors visiting China observed that pregnant

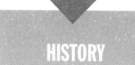

HISTORY

Acupressure is as old as peoples' tendency to rub a sore joint. The science of acupressure is based on traditional Chinese medicine and uses the points often used in acupuncture to stimulate meridians, or pathways for the body's vital energy.

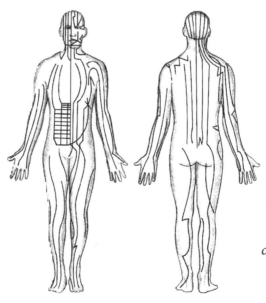

Vital energy, or qi, flows through certain pathways in the body called meridians.

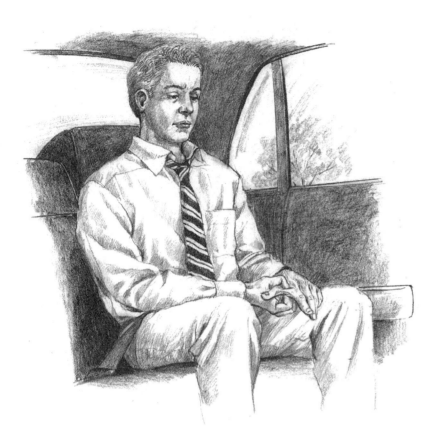

Pressure to the LI4 point in the webbing between the thumb and forefinger can ease motion sickness.

women were instructed to press a point on their wrist to control morning sickness. Intrigued, they began conducting studies of this point when they returned home.

Since then, a number of studies have looked at acupressure and its ability to control nausea and vomiting associated with a variety of conditions.

CANCER CHEMOTHERAPY

The use of noninvasive electrical stimulation along the P6 point has also been shown to be effective in controlling vomiting associated with cancer chemotherapy. A study of 100 patients with nausea and vomiting found that more than 75 percent achieved considerable benefit from the technique [1].

PREGNANCY

Morning sickness occurs in as many as 88 percent of pregnant women in the early stages of pregnancy. Because of the severe birth defects caused by the antinausea drug thalidomide in the 1960s, many pregnant women and physicians alike are reluctant to undertake any drug therapy for nausea during pregnancy. Acupressure represents an effective, harmless way to control nausea associated with pregnancy.

A study of 350 women in early stages of pregnancy compared P6 acupressure with "dummy" acupressure (pressure on a fake pressure point) and no treatment at all. Troublesome sickness was significantly less severe in women who received acupressure than in those using the dummy point, or those who received no treatment at all [2].

Another study of 60 women in early pregnancy comparing real acupressure to the P6 point to dummy acupressure found that women who received real acupressure had a 60 percent reduction

SEA BANDS

Based on acupressure's effectiveness in relieving nausea, sea bands were developed to provide continuous pressure to the P6 pressure point on the wrist—the point that combats nausea. These elastic wrist strips contain a small bump that presses on the point. Sea bands are widely available and are popular among professional sailors to combat motion sickness and with pregnant women to combat morning sickness.

POINTS OF INTEREST

Here are some acupressure points that can come in handy for treating common ailments.

GB20 is located on the back of the head at the base of the skull. There is one on either side of the spine. These points can be pressed simultaneously for relief of headaches and certain symptoms associated with temporomandibular disorder (TMD) and the common cold (see pages 63–64).

LI4—called the Hoku point—is located on the back of either hand in the webbing between the thumb and index finger. These points can be effective for nausea and headaches. (Pregnant women should not use this point without professional guidance because pressure here can induce early labor.)

LI11—called the Quchi point—is located at the top of the elbow crease on either arm. Pressure on these points can be used to treat colds with headache and fever (see pages 63–64).

P6—called the Neiguan point—is located on the inside surface of the wrist three finger-widths above the wrist crease. It can be used in cases of stomach upset such as nausea and vomiting.

S41 is located at the front of either ankle joint. Pressure to these points can be used to relieve heartburn (see page 97).

SI19 is located in front of the ear canal on either side of the face. These points can be used to treat TMD (see page 156).

SP6 is located approximately four finger-widths above the ankle on the inside of either leg. Pressure applied to these points can be useful for cases of menstrual cramps.

ST6 is located between the jaw and skull beneath either ear. These points can be useful for facial pain including TMD.

ST36 is located a few inches below the kneecap on the front of either leg. These points are useful for pain located in the front of the head. They appear to be effective for headaches focused in the front of the head and for some cases of TMD.

ST41 is located in the webbing between the tendons of the second and third toes (counting from the big toe) on the top of either foot. Pressure on these points can be useful for alleviating nausea and vomiting.

in morning sickness compared with only 30 percent of the control group [3].

POSTSURGICAL NAUSEA

After surgery, nausea and vomiting caused by anesthesia or painkillers are common. A study of 162 surgery patients compared acupressure using sea bands with fake acupressure bands and the use of antinausea drugs given along with each injection of painkiller. Nausea was less in patients who wore the real bands, and these patients needed fewer antinausea drugs than the other groups [4].

DENTAL PAIN

Toothache? Try ice—on your hand. Dental pain can be relieved by massaging your hand with ice. Scientists at

> **CAUTION**
>
> Acupressure has been shown to be a safe and effective way to relieve morning sickness associated with pregnancy. However, not all acupressure points are safe for use by pregnant women. For example, stimulation of the Hoku point on the webbing between the thumb and index finger could result in premature contractions of the uterus. Check with a knowledgeable practitioner or an authoritative guide to make sure the acupressure points for a specific condition are safe for use during pregnancy.

McGill University in Toronto found that rubbing ice on the Hoku acupuncture point (the LI4 point) on the back of the hand resulted in as much as a 50 percent reduction in pain in 36 patients with acute pain from cavities, abscesses, and other dental problems. Ice wrapped in gauze was used to massage the web of the hand gently between the thumb and index finger on the same side as the pain. The massage was performed for seven minutes or until the area felt numb [5].

This point should not be used by pregnant women. Stimulation of the Hoku point could result in premature contractions of the uterus. (See Caution at left.)

WHO DOES IT

Different forms of acupressure are performed by a variety of practitioners, including acupuncturists and practitioners of pressure-point techniques, such as shiatsu, or polarity therapy, such as jin shin (see pages 209–212).

RESOURCES

- Acupressure Institute
  1533 Shattuck Ave.
  Berkeley, CA 94709
  510-845-1059
  800-442-2232

The Acupressure Institute provides general information on acupressure, offers training and certification in acupressure, and sponsors classes and workshops in many geographic areas.

Acupuncture

USED IN CHINA FOR THOUSANDS OF YEARS AND IN WESTERN EUROPE FOR SEVERAL HUNDRED YEARS, ACUPUNCTURE CAME TO AMERICA IN THE LATE 1800S. SIR WILLIAM OSLER'S PRINCIPLES AND PRACTICE OF MEDICINE—AN EARLY AMERICAN MEDICAL TEXTBOOK, FIRST PUBLISHED IN 1892—RECOMMENDED ACUPUNCTURE FOR THE TREATMENT OF LUMBAGO, OR LOWER-BACK PAIN.

WHAT IT IS

Acupuncture is the insertion of tiny, hair-thin needles into specific points of the body. The Chinese believe that qi (pronounced chee), or vital energy, is responsible for health, and that an imbalance of qi results in illness. Acupuncture is used to correct the flow of qi, so to restore health and vitality.

Chinese medicine recognizes 12 major meridians, or pathways, for qi. Each of the 12 major meridians is associated with a vital organ or vital function. These meridians form an invisible network that carries qi to every tissue in the body. Acupuncture stimulates specific points along these pathways to rebalance a person's energy, or qi, by redirecting or stimulating it. Instead of needles, acupuncturists sometimes apply pressure to the points (acupressure), heat (moxibustion), or suction (cupping).

HOW IT WORKS

Western medicine has no direct parallels to the Chinese meridian system. Chinese practitioners believe that meridians provide links from the outside of the body to the organs, and that stimulation of these points can directly affect what is going on inside the body.

Chinese medicine is holistic, that is, it focuses on the entire patient. Physical exams concentrate on detecting a pattern of disharmony or imbalance, and treatment seeks to restore balance through the use of techniques such as acupuncture, diet, or herbal medicine. Modern Western medicine focuses on finding a specific cause for an illness or disease and directing treatment toward its eradication.

In recent years, an increasing number of scientists have tried to discover how acupuncture works from the viewpoint of Western science, and now a number of theories exist. Some believe acupuncture stimulates the release of endorphins, painkilling substances produced naturally by the body. Others say that stimulation from the needles interferes with normal nervous system pathways so that pain signals can't reach the brain. Still other studies suggest that acupuncture points have electrical properties that, when stimulated, alter chemical neurotransmitters in the body. Acupuncture may also alter the body's natural electrical currents or electromagnetic fields.

The science and terminology of conventional medicine may never be able to describe the workings of a system such as acupuncture. However, acupuncture does appear to be effective for treating a variety of ailments, including chronic conditions that are often not responsive to treatment by Western medicine.

HISTORY

Acupuncture is an integral part of traditional Chinese medicine that has been practiced for more than 2,000 years. Its use is recorded in the ancient Chinese medical text, *The Yellow Emperor's Classic*, written around 200 B.C. Some say acupuncture grew out of the observation that warriors wounded by arrows found that their symptoms from chronic ailments went away. While its origins may be unclear, acupuncture continues to be used to treat a wide variety of illnesses in China and an increasing number of disorders in the United States as well.

Alternative Medicine 173

FREQUENTLY ASKED QUESTIONS

Many people are uneasy about trying acupuncture for the first time. To Westerners used to conventional medicine's approach, the whole idea may seem a little strange. Some straightforward answers to the obvious questions should ease anxiety.

DOES IT HURT?

Most people feel only minimal pain as the needles are inserted. The tiny needles have smooth points and cause less pain than an injection with a hypodermic needle, which has a sharp cutting edge. Also, the needles are inserted into specific points on the body that are not the most sensitive areas.

HOW MANY NEEDLES ARE USED?

A minimum of two needles are used, with the average number being six to eight. Sometimes, such as in the treatment of substance abuse, very short needles with a special circular end are covered with tiny specks of adhesive and left in place in the ear so patients can stimulate the point when they experience withdrawal symptoms.

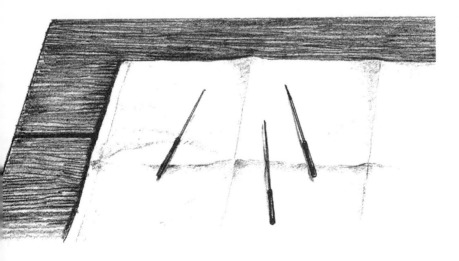

ARE NEEDLES ALWAYS INVOLVED?

Acupuncturists may also use very mild electrical energy to stimulate the meridian points further (electroacupuncture). These electrical stimulation points may involve current passed to the points via small electrodes placed on the skin or through needles already inserted.

In addition to needles, acupuncturists may also use moxa sticks—made from the herb *Artemisia vulgaris*—burned on or near the acupuncture sites to help increase stimulation. This is known as moxibustion, and is described in more detail in Traditional Chinese Medicine (see pages 246–353).

HOW MANY TREATMENTS ARE NEEDED?

The number of treatments required varies from person to person, and with the condition being treated. Complex or chronic conditions may require one to two treatments a week for several months.

USES

In the United States, acupuncture is widely used to treat lower-back pain and chronic pain. Its effectiveness in treating substance addiction has led some localities to mandate its inclusion in court-ordered rehabilitation programs. Some other promising uses of acupuncture include arthritis and nausea. Acupuncture not only treats existing problems, but can also be used to promote health and well-being and to prevent illness.

Acupuncture is one of the most thoroughly researched and documented alternative medical practices in use today. A number of clinical studies have shown compelling evidence that it is an effective treatment for a variety of conditions.

After the Chinese Revolution in 1949, government officials intent on "modernizing" China took a hard look at acupuncture and other elements of traditional Chinese medicine. The state sponsored a staggering array of studies and analyses, some involving thousands and thousands of patients, before determining that acupuncture and traditional Chinese medicine deserved equal status with conventional Western medicine. Most physicians trained in China today learn both systems.

Many studies of acupuncture are in Chinese or other foreign languages and have not been translated into English. Despite this limitation, a number of well-designed studies have been published in English and show the promise of acupuncture for a variety of conditions.

ALCOHOLISM AND ADDICTION

Acupuncture is often used for the treatment of alcohol and drug abuse. Research studies and clinical experience strongly suggest that acupuncture can play an important role in substance abuse programs for persons addicted to alcohol, cocaine, heroin, nicotine, and other harmful substances. In fact, acupuncture's high degree of success in these hard-to-treat areas has led some localities, such as New York City, to include the practice in its drug treatment programs.

One example of acupuncture's effectiveness in addiction treatment is a 1989 Minnesota study of 80 severe alcoholics. The patients who received "sham" acupuncture (not given at the correct points) were twice as likely to drink and be hospitalized for detoxification than those who received real acupuncture [1].

A study of 100 heroin addicts comparing real acupuncture to sham acupuncture found that persons who received real acupuncture attended the detoxification clinic more days and were more likely to continue beyond the 21-day detoxification period [2]. Clinical reports suggest that acupuncture may also be a useful adjunct to detoxification treatment for cocaine-addicted adults and infants and for persons addicted to prescription drugs.

ARTHRITIS

A Danish study of 32 patients awaiting knee-replacement surgery found that those treated with acupuncture showed improvement in knee function and had a 50 percent reduction in the use of pain medicine. In fact, 7 patients responded so well that they decided to not have the surgery at all [3].

NAUSEA

Acupuncture can be an effective way to stop nausea and vomiting caused by anesthesia, cancer therapy, motion sickness, and pregnancy. A study of 500 patients undergoing general anesthesia found that those who received acupuncture treatments not only responded better than those who received no treatment or sham acupuncture, but had slightly better results than those treated with the standard antinausea drugs [4].

Acupuncture controls nausea and vomiting by stimulating the P6 point above the wrist. A study of 130 patients undergoing cancer chemotherapy found that electrical stimulation of this point lessened symptoms of nausea in 97 percent of those treated [5].

The effectiveness of acupuncture, or acupressure, to this point has led to the development of sea bands—elastic wrist bands that contain a button that presses on the P6 point. Originally designed to eliminate seasickness, the bands have also been found to reduce morning sickness in pregnant women and nausea after surgery (see Acupressure, pages 169–172).

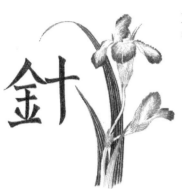

The Chinese character for acupuncture is made up of the characters for gold *(left) and* needle *(right).*

PAIN

Among patients with chronic lower-back pain, a study of 50 patients found that 83 percent of those treated immediately with acupuncture improved and took significantly fewer pain pills than those who were not treated. Only 30 percent of the group that was not treated reported improvement [6].

A study of 43 women suffering from dysmenorrhea (painful menstrual periods) found that 91 percent of those who received acupuncture showed improvement, compared with only 36 percent of the sham group. Patients who received acupuncture also used 41 percent less pain medication than the control group [7].

Acupuncture may also help sufferers of migraines. A study of 30 migraine sufferers found that patients who received real acupuncture reported 43 percent less pain and used 38 percent less pain medication than those who received sham acupuncture [8].

Patients with chronic neck pain may benefit as well. A study of 30 patients with chronic neck pain (pain that lasted an average of eight years) found that after 12 weeks of treatment,

80 percent reported improvement and took 54 percent less pain medication than before. Among patients who did not receive acupuncture, only 13 percent improved, and 60 percent worsened [9].

A study of 38 patients experiencing pain from kidney stones found acupuncture to be as effective as pain medication but without its accompanying side effects [10].

WHO DOES IT

There are an estimated 7,000 acupuncture practitioners in the United States, more than half of whom are certified by the National Commission for the Certification of Acupuncturists. In addition to that number, naturopathic and chiropractic physicians often practice acupuncture, and more than 3,000 medical doctors and osteopaths have training in the practice as well. Americans make an estimated 12 million visits per year for acupuncture treatment.

There are more than 40 schools and colleges of acupuncture and oriental medicine in the United States, 20 of which are approved by or in candidacy status with the Accreditation Commission for Schools and Colleges of Acupuncture and Oriental Medicine.

Currently, 32 states and the District of Columbia regulate acupuncture practitioners.

RESOURCES
ORGANIZATIONS

- American Association of Acupuncture and Oriental Medicine
  433 Front St.
  Catasauqua, PA 18032
  610-266-1433

Provides lists of state-licensed or NCCA-certified providers, and fact sheets on acupuncture.

- National Acupuncture and Oriental Medicine Alliance
206-851-6896

Operates a referral service for certified practitioners, provides lists of national organizations and information on health insurance organizations. Sponsors annual conferences and conventions, and an ongoing list of events.

- National Commission for the Certification of Acupuncturists
P.O. Box 97075
Washington, DC 20090
202-232-1404

Certifies practitioners in both acupuncture and Chinese herbology.

- National Acupuncture Detoxification Association
3220 N St. NW, Ste. 275
Washington, DC 20007
503-222-1362

Trains and certifies practitioners in the use of acupuncture for the treatment of substance abuse. Also operates a literature clearinghouse, at 360-254-0186.

ONLINE RESOURCES

- Acupuncture Online
http://www.acupuncture.com

CAUTION

Most professional acupuncturists in the United States use sterile, disposable needles. Improperly sterilized needles can lead to infection and the transmission of blood-borne infections such as hepatitis and AIDS. Check with your practitioner.

Over the years, there have been a few reports of broken needles that have later been found in the body. A rarely used technique in Japan intentionally leaves tips of the needles in place to provide continued stimulation. Responsible acupuncturists examine needles after extraction to make sure they are intact. And special short needles with a circular base that prevent entry into the body are used when prolonged stimulation is desired.

Even the American Medical Association, which considers acupuncture to be an unproven therapy, notes that there are remarkably few serious complications reported from its use.

Resources on acupuncture and other components of traditional Chinese medicine. Includes frequently asked questions about acupuncture; a variety of information at the consumer, student, and practitioner level; and links to other alternative medicine servers.

Aromatherapy & Essential Oils

REAL ESTATE AGENTS KNOW THAT PUTTING SOME CINNAMON TO SIMMER ON THE STOVE OR IN THE OVEN OF A HOUSE FOR SALE MAKES PROSPECTIVE BUYERS THINK "HOME." THE SCENT EVOKES MEMORIES OF APPLE PIE BAKING IN THE OVEN AND CONTRIBUTES TO A SENSE OF COMFORT, SECURITY, AND WARMTH. THE POWER OF AROMA TO EVOKE A VARIETY OF EMOTIONAL SENSES AND PHYSICAL RESPONSES HAS BEEN KNOWN FOR THOUSANDS OF YEARS. THIS POWER CAN BE USED FOR MORE THAN SELLING HOUSES; IT CAN PROMOTE HEALTH AND HEALING.

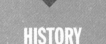

HISTORY

The term aromatherapy was coined by French chemist Rene-Maurice Gattefosse in the 1920s. A perfumer who discovered that lavender oil prevented scarring when he burnt his hand, Gattefosse then went on to explore the use of other oils.

Oils distilled from plants are reported to have been prepared as long ago as 3000 B.C. Aromatherapy was practiced by the ancient Egyptians, Greeks, and Romans. A variety of essential oils are used in the ancient Indian medical system known as Ayurveda. The Indian state of Kerala is reported to produce more than 100 different varieties of medicinal oils.

WHAT IT IS

Aromatherapy is the use of essential oils and hydrosols (suspensions) to promote personal health. Essential oils are made by distilling plant materials by heating them with water in a still. Aromatherapy is not just the use of products that contain fragrance but is the use of pure essential oils from plants, not synthetic preparations.

HOW IT WORKS

Smell is one of the most basic of human senses. Humans are able to detect thousands of different odors. The memory of a smell may evoke certain emotions, which in turn can create a certain response in the body. Even smells for which a person has no conscious memory association can help relax or stimulate.

Aromatherapy uses several methods for delivering the aroma to the senses.

BATHS

Baths are a popular method of using aromatherapy, especially for relaxation. Add a few drops of an essential oil to the surface of bathwater. Do not add other substances, such as bath oils. Soak for 10 to 20 minutes, allowing the heat of the water to help absorb the oil through your skin while you inhale the vapor. Essential oils can also be used in the shower. Add a few drops to a washcloth and rub briskly over your whole body. Then breathe the aromatic steam in deeply.

DIFFUSION

A variety of devices are used to fill a room with essential oils. Diffusers often use heat to evaporate essential oils and spread their molecules throughout a room. These include candle diffusers and ceramic rings placed on lightbulbs.

INHALATION

Essential oils may be inhaled from a handkerchief or be spritzed in the air or on the face and body and inhaled. Inhalation can be done simply at home by adding a few drops of essential oil to a bowl of steaming water, then placing a towel over your head and the bowl and inhaling the vapor for a few minutes. Be careful not to scald your face by getting too close.

MASSAGE

Massage is one of the most effective and popular ways of using essential oils. This incorporates the therapeutic power of touch while allowing absorption of the oils by blood capillaries close to the surface of the skin, immersing the whole body in the oils' aromas.

Dilute essential oils in an odorless carrier oil, such as almond, grape seed, or peach kernel. Start with a dilution of 1 to 3 percent essential oil to carrier oil (about one to three drops per teaspoonful) for adults, less for infants. Some people are more sensitive to the oils than others, so experiment with the concentration that works best for you.

THE ESSENTIAL OILS

Although the word *aromatherapy* suggests that this field is limited to the inhalation of essential oils, it also includes the topical use of essential oils.

One of the best studied essential oils used in Western medicine is tea tree oil, which is known for its antibacterial and antiseptic properties. An essential oil of the Australian native tree *Melaleuca alternifolia*, tea tree oil has been used in Australia since the early 20th century in the treatment of wound infections and bacterial and fungal infections of the skin.

Chamomile oil is best known for its calming properties. Add five or six drops to a hot bath to calm your nerves. A massage oil can be made by adding two drops of chamomile oil to five teaspoons of vegetable oil.

Melissa (lemon balm) and neroli (orange blossom) can have profound effects on mood. A few drops of melissa in a hot bath is said to soothe and help relieve depression. Add five drops of neroli to two teaspoons of oil to make a massage oil to help reduce anxiety.

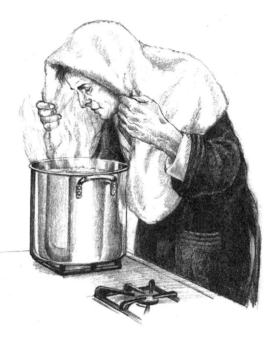

USES

ANXIETY

Relieving anxiety, reducing stress, and promoting relaxation are perhaps the most well known of the uses for aromatic essential oils. Several different essential oils are especially useful in this regard.

Lavender—A double-blinded study of the use of two essential oils of two different species of lavender on 28 intensive care unit patients, who had undergone cardiac surgery, found that massage with one lavender oil was almost twice as effective in alleviating anxiety than the other.

The essential oils were diluted in cold-pressed almond oil and about two teaspoons containing five drops of lavender were given for each patient. Patients were massaged with the oil for 20 minutes on specific areas of the body, such as arms, feet, forehead, and legs, for two consecutive days.

The study found that the hybrid lavender (*Lavandula burnatii*) was al-

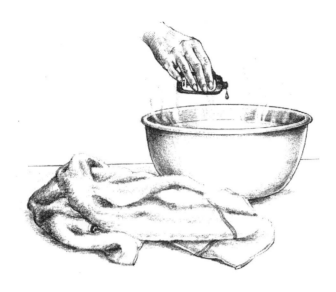

most twice as effective in alleviating anxiety as the naturally occurring lavender (*Lavandula angustifolia*). The investigator believes the different results disprove the hypothesis that aromatherapy is effective purely because of factors such as touch, massage, or placebo effect [1].

Neroli (Orange Blossom)—A British study of 100 patients who had undergone cardiac surgery found that those who had foot massage with neroli (orange blossom) had less anxiety than those who had foot massage with plain oil or no massage.

Patients were divided into four groups: One had no treatment, the second received a 20-minute chat, the third received a 20-minute foot massage with plain vegetable oil, and the fourth received a 20-minute foot massage with neroli (orange blossom) essential foot oil. Neroli was chosen because it is reported to calm the nervous system, help insomnia, relieve anxiety, calm palpitations, and have an anti-inflammatory effect.

Patients who received foot massage had significantly better short-term psychological results than the two control groups, although no difference was noted between the two massage groups. After five days, however, patients in the neroli group had a marked reduction in anxiety compared with the plain oil group and reported finding the effects more relaxing, calming, and restful [2].

HEADACHE

Peppermint oil and eucalyptus oil are used in a variety of traditional treatments for pain, including headaches. A German study found that a preparation of peppermint and eucalyptus oil applied to the forehead and temples significantly reduced tension in the temporal muscle of the head. The study of 32 healthy men found that it did not reduce sensitivity to pain, whereas a combination of peppermint and ethanol did [3].

SMOKING CESSATION

Aromatherapy may be very helpful for people who wish to quit smoking. A North Carolina study of cigarette smokers found that those who puffed on a device that delivered a vapor from essential oil of black pepper had significantly reduced craving for cigarettes. Persons who inhaled the vapors from the pepper also had reduced emotional and physical symptoms of anxiety compared with a control group [4].

ACNE

Tea tree oil can have powerful effects on dermatologic conditions. In some cases it can be used to treat acne. The gel state is best for this purpose because

CAUTION

Do not use undiluted essential oils. Never take essential oils internally. Store in a cool dark place. Never store essential oils in plastic bottles. Keep essential oils out of the reach of children. Toxicity has been reported in children who have ingested tea tree oil and eucalyptus oil.

Essential oils may also cause skin reactions in some people—try testing a small patch of skin with a highly diluted preparation when trying any new oil. For example, when making a massage oil, start by using one drop of essential oil to one teaspoon of carrier oil.

Persons with high blood pressure should avoid rosemary, sage, and thyme oils.

Pregnant women should exercise special caution. The use of some oils may be dangerous during pregnancy. Consult with a health care practitioner who is familiar with the use of essential oils before you use any of the following:

- peppermint
- rose
- rosemary
- chamomile
- lavender
- arnica
- basil
- clary sage
- cypress
- jasmine
- juniper
- marjoram
- myrrh
- sage
- thyme

other media can be very irritating and painful. A trial of 124 patients with mild to moderate acne found that 5 percent tea tree oil gel was effective in reducing the number of acne lesions. Although the tea tree oil worked more slowly than a lotion with 5 percent benzoyl peroxide, patients using the tea tree oil gel had significantly fewer side effects [5].

INFECTIONS

Onychomycosis—nail fungus—is the most frequent cause of nail disease. It can be caused by the fungi *Trichophyton rubrum* or *Candida albicans* and occasionally by certain kinds of molds.

A study of 117 patients found that twice daily applications of 100 percent tea tree oil solution to the affected toenail was as effective as treatment with a 1 percent clotrimazole solution (an antifungal drug) [6].

Tea tree oil has also been used to treat vaginal infections such as vaginitis. For this purpose, the oil should be very diluted—in the ratio of approximately one to ten. More concentrated solutions can be very irritating [7].

WHO DOES IT

A number of health care professionals incorporate the use of aromatherapy into their practice. Many naturopathic physicians, massage therapists, chiropractors, and sports medicine therapists occasionally rely on aromatherapy. Currently there are no certification standards for practitioners, but the National Association for Holistic Aromatherapy is working to establish certification standards and guidelines.

RESOURCES

- National Association for Holistic Aromatherapy
  P.O. Box 17622
  Boulder, CO 80308
  800-566-6735
  fax 415-564-6799

Ayurvedic Medicine

AYURVEDA IS BELIEVED TO BE THE OLDEST MEDICAL SYSTEM IN EXISTENCE, DATING BACK AT LEAST 5,000 YEARS TO ANCIENT INDIA. LITERALLY TRANSLATED FROM SANSKRIT AS "THE SCIENCE OF LIFE," AYURVEDA IS THE MOST PREVALENT FORM OF TRADITIONAL MEDICINE PRACTICED IN INDIA TODAY. OTHER SYSTEMS STILL IN USE INCLUDE EMCHI, PRAKRITKA CIKITSA (NATUROPATHY), SIDDHA, AND UNANI.

HISTORY

Many modern medical discoveries were chronicled in Ayurvedic medicine long before they were noted by Western science. The circulation of blood was described before 700 B.C., as was plastic surgery and the secretion of gastric juice and its role in digestion. Smallpox vaccination is also an ancient practice in India.

WHAT IT IS

Indian tradition holds that good health is necessary to fulfill the four primary objectives of human life:

- Dharma—to perform religious rites
- Artha—to acquire wealth
- Káma—to satisfy worldly desires
- Moksa—to attain salvation

Ayurveda believes that the body is governed by three basic biological principles, or doshas, that control the body's functions. These doshas and the functions they govern are

- vata—movement
- pitta—heat, metabolism, and energy production
- kapha—physical structure and fluid balance

Each individual has a combination of doshas. Imbalance of these doshas is the cause of disease. Ayurvedic practitioners seek to achieve health through the balancing of the three doshas. Treatment, therefore, centers on the entire person rather than just the affected part or the organism that causes the disease.

For example, an herbal product that has antibiotic activity may be prescribed to someone suffering from a respiratory ailment. A Western (or allopathic) physician is likely to prescribe an antibiotic to kill the organism responsible for the infection. Ayurvedic treatment, however, is intended to reduce the imbalance in the body—the excessive kapha dosha—that allows organisms to multiply and thrive in the respiratory tract in the first place.

Ayurvedic practitioners know that it is not possible to live in a world that is totally free of germs, so they try to make the body less susceptible to their ill effects. They believe that when the body is in balance, these organisms cannot produce illness.

As the nature of this approach to a specific disease suggests, prevention is a key element in Ayurvedic medicine. Ayurveda believes that the major factors in disease are

- dosha imbalance
- mental disorder
- unhealthy lifestyle
- accumulation of toxins in the body

DOSHAS

Evaluation of the doshas is performed largely by a pulse reading and a careful case history, among other investigations. This evaluation determines the type of therapy to be prescribed, such as what herbs should be used to balance the doshas.

MENTAL FACTORS

Ayurveda does not consider diseases to be exclusively psychological or somatic (physical). Imbalance and disease in the body is believed to begin with imbalance or stress in the consciousness of the individual. Mental techniques such as meditation are considered essential to prevention and to promote healing. Ayurveda also emphasizes the interdependence of individual health and that of society; therefore social attitudes and behavior often come into play in an Ayurvedic evaluation of an individual's health.

LIFESTYLE

Lifestyle interventions are a major approach to both prevention and therapy in Ayurvedic medicine. Patients may be prescribed an individualized diet, exercise, and rest program to help rebalance their doshas.

Practitioners use a variety of body postures from yoga, as well as breathing and meditation techniques to create individual self-care programs to improve physical health and personal consciousness (see Yoga, pages 360–364).

Herbal preparations are often used to treat specific conditions and for prevention and rejuvenation.

ACCUMULATION OF TOXINS

Ayurveda also seeks to cleanse and remove metabolic by-products and toxins that accumulate in the body's tissues. Panchakarma, a type of Ayurvedic physical therapy, consists of treatments to remove impurities from the body. These include herbalized oil massage, herbalized heat treatments, and therapies to improve bowel movements.

One practice said to promote health and longevity is the use of sesame oil retention enemas for several days each season. The beneficial effect of such treatment is suggested by a study of human colon cancer cells grown in a laboratory and then treated with sesame oil. Sesame oil was shown to inhibit the growth of cancerous cells.

Some of the agents used in panchakarma therapy are believed to have free-radical scavenging, or antioxidant effects. Naturally occurring molecules that are highly reactive with anything they come into contact with, free radicals may play a role in causing a wide range of disorders, including cancer and heart disease. Research in rats suggests that the Ayurvedic herbal agents maharadis amrit kalash 4 and 5 (MAK-4 and MAK-5) may protect against free radicals and therefore ameliorate cell damage.

Ayurveda also employs aspects of aromatherapy (see page 178) and sound therapy (see page 354).

MAHARISHI AYURVEDA

Most Ayurveda practiced in the United States today is Maharishi Ayurveda, brought to this country by Maharishi Mahesh Yogi. First in the international eye as the spiritual advisor to the Beatles in the 1960s, the Maharishi may be as well or even better known for bringing Transcendental Meditation to the United States. Transcendental Meditation is a form of mantric meditation involving the repetition of, or focusing on, a sound.

Advanced practitioners of one of its programs are taught to use their mental powers to levitate a few inches above the ground and are said to do other feats that Western thought considers beyond the possible. (One well-known practitioner of Maharishi

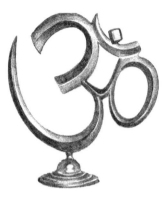

The Om symbol represents the life force in Ayurvedic medicine and can be used as a focus for meditation.

Ayurveda is the best-selling author Deepak Chopra.)

While Maharishi Ayurveda has done much to bring Western attention to this ancient system of healing, critics abound. When an article appeared on Maharishi Ayurveda in the *Journal of the American Medical Association* in 1991, a flurry of letters ensued in response. The sharpest critics charge that the Maharishi's Transcendental Meditation movement is a cult. Others say that the Maharishi's Ayurveda revival is an overpriced, commercialized version of the traditional health care practices of India.

Despite, or perhaps because of, the controversy, however, both traditional and Maharishi Ayurveda have been receiving increasing attention by Westerners in recent years. And the ancient practices of Ayurveda are gaining a new look by some of the most critical minds in the Western medical and scientific establishment.

For example, the National Cancer Institute, often a target of criticism from alternative practitioners for what many see as its narrow focus on sometimes harsh allopathic interventions such as chemotherapy, has funded research into the cancer-preventing properties of two important Ayurvedic herbal compounds, maharadis amrit kalash 4 and 5 (also known as MAK-4 and MAK-5).

USES

Ayurveda has an extensive array of uses, from prevention of disease to the treatment of a myriad of conditions. Ayurveda's classic eight branches parallel those of Western medicine, and include

- internal medicine
- surgery
- treatment of diseases of the head and the neck
- toxicology
- management of seizures by evil spirits and other mental disorders
- pediatrics
- geriatrics, including rejuvenation therapy
- science of aphrodisiacs

Despite its ancient origins, Ayurveda was almost unknown in the West until recently. The long history of foreign rule in India is blamed by some for the suppression of Ayurvedic institutions and dissemination of knowledge about this important medical system. As the following studies show, various aspects of Ayurveda have generated considerable interest and have been the topic of a number of scientific publications in the West in recent years.

AYURVEDIC HERBAL PREPARATIONS

Cholesterol—A study of 35 men found that supplementing the diet with raw Indian gooseberry led to decreases in cholesterol levels but that levels returned to their initial levels two weeks after therapy was stopped [1].

Hepatitis—A preliminary study of 60 hepatitis B carriers found that 59 percent of those treated with the herb phyllanthus lost the virus compared with only 4 percent of those who received a placebo [2].

Scabies—Scabies is caused by microscopic mites that burrow their way under the skin, causing itching and infection. Scabies is highly contagious and is easily spread in institutions such as barracks, camps, schools, and nursing homes. In the United States, stan-

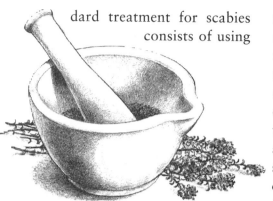

dard treatment for scabies consists of using lotions and shampoos that contain ingredients related to the banned pesticide DDT. While generally considered safe, these products in high doses may cause neurologic damage.

An Indian study looked at the use of two traditional Ayurvedic compounds, neem and tumeric, combined into a paste to treat 814 people with scabies. The study found that the paste cured 97 percent of the cases without any noticeable side effects or toxicity [3].

Cancer—Ayurvedic herbal preparations have been shown to have a variety of potentially beneficial effects for the treatment of certain cancers. For example, the National Cancer Institute has funded research into the cancer-preventing properties of the two Ayurvedic herbal compounds, maharadis amrit kalash 4 and 5 (MAK-4 and MAK-5). Animal studies of Ayurvedic herbal agents have shown that such compounds can reduce the incidence of experimentally induced mammary tumors in rats and reduce lung cancer metastasis in mice.

Antioxidant Properties—Ayurvedic herbal preparations such as MAK-4 and 5 are reported to contain a variety of substances known to act as antioxidants, such as alpha-tocopherol, ascorbate, beta-carotene, catechin, flavinoids, polyphenols, and tannic acid. Found in certain foods and vitamins, antioxidants scavenge dangerous free radicals and reduce the amount of damage they may cause. Laboratory experiments and studies in rats suggest that these Ayurvedic preparations act as antioxidants and should be further studied for their potential impact on conditions such as atherosclerosis (clogging of the arteries) and free-radical induced injury.

MEDITATION

Anxiety and Stress—A number of scientific studies have shown that yoga and meditation techniques can help reduce anxiety and relieve pain and stress (see Yoga, pages 360–364). In recent years, many studies have been conducted about the effects of Maharishi Ayurveda's Transcendental Meditation technique.

Aging—Proponents of Transcendental Meditation and other meditation techniques assert that it can help extend life and modify the aging process. A study of 73 nursing home residents compared Transcendental Meditation, mindfulness training (a technique in-

---

CAUTION

The use of metals in some Ayurvedic preparations has a long history in India. Advocates say they are processed so as to be nontoxic, but case reports do occasionally appear in the medical literature about cases of metal poisoning (such as lead poisoning) from herbal tablets purchased by visitors to India.

---

volving constant awareness of one's feelings and actions), relaxation, and no treatment. Participants were evaluated on learning, cognitive flexibility, mental health, blood pressure, behavioral flexibility, aging, and treatment effectiveness. Those in the TM group improved most, followed by mindfulness training. After three years, the survival rate was 100 percent for the TM group and 87.5 percent for the mindfulness training group, compared with lower rates for the other groups [4].

Heart Disease—Like any other alternative or conventional therapy, meditation works best when part of an overall lifestyle that includes proper diet, exercise, and avoidance of bad habits such as smoking. When these positive lifestyle practices are combined, they not only can help prevent illness but may even reverse disease.

High Blood Pressure—A study of 111 older African-American men and women with mild hypertension compared the effects of mental and physical stress reduction approaches (Transcendental Meditation or progres-

sive muscle relaxation) with a lifestyle-modification education program and with each other. The group that practiced Transcendental Meditation had a significantly greater decrease in blood pressure than either the other two groups [5].

Another study of 112 people who regularly practice Transcendental Meditation found that they had significantly lower blood pressure than people in the general population who did not practice meditation. In addition, blood pressure readings were lower for those who had practiced five or more years than those who had practiced less [6].

General Physiology—Transcendental Meditation has also been shown to increase cardiac output (the heart's blood-pumping ability), affect neuroendocrine function (hormone-related nervous system function), and may increase blood flow to the brain [7,8].

Substance Abuse—Other studies suggest that Transcendental Meditation may be helpful in addressing factors that contribute to substance abuse and chemical dependency. Transcen-

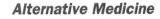

AVOID PREPARATIONS THAT CONTAIN HEAVY METALS

Commonly used Ayurvedic herbal preparations in the United States contain botanical and herbal compounds. Some may contain heavy metals such as lead. As with anything you ingest, make sure you know what the ingredients are in any herbal preparation you are taking.

dental Meditation can help provide relief from distress and can precipitate long-term improvements in well-being, self-esteem, personal empowerment, and other areas of mental and physical health.

WHO DOES IT

In India, Ayurvedic physicians undergo five years of training. Although a number of Indian-trained physicians practice in the United States, many Ayurvedic practitioners are trained in the Americanized version, Maharishi Ayurveda. The Raj (see below) can direct you to a practitioner in your area.

When looking for an Ayurvedic physician, the Raj recommends that you ask:

- How long did the physician study Ayurveda?
- How long has the physician been practicing Ayurveda?
- What percentage of practice is Ayurveda?

RESOURCES

- The Raj
  1734 Jasmine Ave.
  Fairfield, IA 52556-9005
  515-472-9580
  800-248-9050
  fax 515-472-2496

The center offers a spa and clinic services and referrals to Ayurvedic physicians. Call the toll-free number for a list of Maharishi Ayurvedic doctors in North American.

Biofeedback

BIOFEEDBACK THERAPY USES MONITORING EQUIPMENT TO "FEED BACK" TO PEOPLE PHYSIOLOGIC INFORMATION OF WHICH THEY ARE NOT NORMALLY AWARE. BY WATCHING THE MONITORING DEVICE, INDIVIDUALS CAN LEARN TO ADJUST THEIR THINKING AND OTHER MENTAL PROCESSES TO CONTROL BODY PROCESSES SUCH AS BLOOD PRESSURE, BRAIN-WAVE ACTIVITY, GASTROINTESTINAL FUNCTIONING, AND BODY TEMPERATURE.

HISTORY

When experimental psychologist Neal Miller proposed in 1961 that the autonomic nervous system—the part of the nervous system that we don't use consciously—was trainable, he was met with considerable skepticism. Prevailing thought was that autonomic responses, such as blood pressure and heart rate, could not be controlled. In fact, medical dictionaries of the time defined autonomic as "not subject to voluntary control." Miller's groundbreaking work showed that these responses could indeed be controlled through instrumental learning.

WHAT IT IS

Biofeedback is based on the principle that any function that can be monitored and displayed (or "fed back") to a person can then be regulated by that person. Modern electronic equipment can monitor internal responses and convert them to visual or auditory information that can then be used to regulate the response.

Biofeedback enables individuals to see how their breathing, posture, and thinking affect certain responses, such as heart rate. For example, when a person takes slow, deep breaths, the heart rate decreases. Thinking relaxing thoughts can also slow the heart rate. When people think about a stressful situation, however, the heart rate increases.

EQUIPMENT

The monitoring device used depends on what condition the patient is being treated for and the response to be regulated. For example, the biofeedback technician may use electroencephalogram (EEG) feedback to measure brain-wave activity. The resulting information relayed back to the patient is used to help him or her achieve a relaxation response.

A common form of biofeedback involves the measurement of muscle tension via electromyographic, or EMG, feedback. Electrodes are attached to the involved muscles to measure electrical energy from the patient. Information from the electrodes is fed into a small monitoring box that registers the results either through sound or sight. For example, sound may vary in pitch as the function being monitored decreases or increases. Visual meters may vary in brightness as the response decreases or increases.

There are a number of other biofeedback tools for a variety of purposes, including skin temperature (known as thermal feedback) and electrical conductance or resistance of the skin (electrodermal feedback).

Increasingly sophisticated measurement devices now allow a number of other responses to be measured and then fed back to the patient. These include

- esophageal motility—the muscular action involved in swallowing
- stomach acidity—the amount and concentration of secretions in the stomach
- activity of the detrusor muscle of the bladder—used to treat urinary incontinence
- activity of the internal and external rectal sphincters—used to treat bowel incontinence

TECHNIQUES

Biofeedback works best when patients can achieve a meditative state of deep relaxation. Many patients like biofeedback because it puts them in control and provides a sense of self-reliance over their health.

Biofeedback therapists teach patients mental exercises to reach the desired result, such as muscle relaxation or contraction. Through trial and error, patients learn to control their inner responses. Training time varies from person to person and depends on the disorder being treated. Training for some disorders requires eight to ten sessions before the patient can control his or her response without the help of a monitoring machine.

USES

Biofeedback is used to treat some 150 conditions, and its use for some conditions has already gained widespread acceptance. For example, the American Medical Association has endorsed the use of EMG biofeedback training for treating muscle-contraction (tension) headaches.

The effectiveness of biofeedback has been demonstrated in a number of conditions, including
- alcohol and other addictions
- anxiety
- asthma
- bowel and urinary incontinence due to muscle spasms
- epilepsy
- headaches
- heart irregularities
- high blood pressure
- irritable bowel syndrome
- migraines
- muscle dysfunction

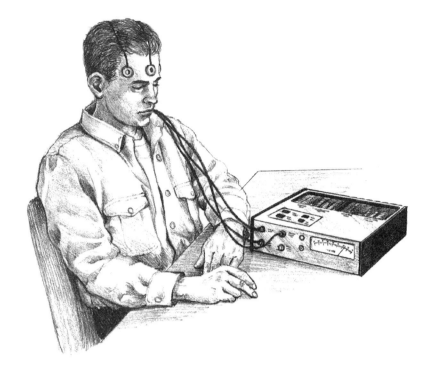

- neuromuscular disorders
- Raynaud disease
- respiratory problems
- sleep disorders
- vascular disorders

Since 1961, there have been more than 3,000 articles and 100 books published describing biofeedback and its many uses. While biofeedback has been demonstrated to be effective for a wide variety of disorders, it is more useful for some conditions than others.

Biofeedback is the preferred method of treatment for certain types of bowel and urinary incontinence, as well as Raynaud disease, which is a painful and potentially dangerous spasm of the small arteries.

Biofeedback is one of several preferred treatments for certain patients with attention deficit disorder, epilepsy, asthma, headaches, high blood pressure, and irritable bowel syndrome (also known as spastic colon).

BOWEL INCONTINENCE

A number of studies from across the world have shown biofeedback to be a highly effective therapy for adults and children who suffer from bowel incontinence. Patients learn to squeeze their anal sphincter through feedback from a monitor that measures sphincter pressure.

A study of 13 children who had not responded to conventional therapy found biofeedback to be effective in 12 after one course of therapy [1]. In adults, a study of 15 patients with bowel incontinence found that biofeedback helped 73 percent [2]. Another study of 28 patients with bowel incontinence found that 46 percent achieved excellent results, 28 percent had good results, but 25 percent did not improve after biofeedback therapy [3].

CONSTIPATION

Other studies show that biofeedback can also help people who suffer from severe constipation by teaching them to relax their anal sphincter. For example, a study of 26 children with chronic severe constipation compared standard medical care of enemas followed by laxative therapy and diet modification to standard medical care and biofeedback. Sixteen months later, parents of the children treated with biofeedback reported that the children had significantly less constipation and fewer painful bowel movements and used fewer laxatives than those who received standard care alone [4].

HEADACHES

A study of 25 patients with migraine headaches compared biofeedback therapy with relaxation techniques not aided by biofeedback. The group trained in biofeedback had significantly less pain and used less pain medication than the other group [5]. Another study of 10 women with migraines found a significant decrease in migraine episodes after 16 semiweekly sessions. The decreases continued after therapy as well [6]. Among children with migraines treated with biofeedback, another study found 80 percent showed clinical improvement [7].

Thermal biofeedback is commonly used for migraine therapy. And research suggests its effectiveness can be improved through regular practice of thermal biofeedback techniques such as hand warming. A study of 17 women who regularly experienced migraines compared those who received biofeedback training twice a week with those who received the training in addition to practicing hand warming at home. Persons who practiced hand warming at home had greater decreases in headaches and the use of pain medication [8].

Tension (or muscle-contraction) headaches can also be treated by biofeedback using EMG feedback. A study of 26 tension-headache sufferers found EMG biofeedback to decrease headaches in 50 to 100 percent of those treated compared with only 37 percent of persons in a relaxation control group. The variation among the patients who received biofeedback therapy reflects the finding that the success rate may depend on where exactly the electrodes are placed [9].

HIGH BLOOD PRESSURE

A study of 19 patients with high blood pressure found a significant decline in blood pressure among patients who received biofeedback therapy and muscle relaxation therapy compared with a tendency for increased blood pressure among those who received muscle relaxation therapy alone [10].

PAIN

A study of 57 patients with chronic back pain and 21 patients who suffered from temporomandibular (jaw) pain and dysfunction found that patients who received biofeedback training had significant reductions in pain [11].

Another study of 44 patients with chronic lower-back pain found biofeedback to be effective in reducing pain and improving functioning [12].

REHABILITATION

Stroke patients commonly experience difficulties in walking due to alterations in their gait cycle and foot-drop on the affected limb. A study of 16 stroke patients studied how electromyographic biofeedback treatment augmented conventional physical therapy. The patients who received biofeedback had significant improvements in their walking [13].

A review of eight studies including 192 stroke patients determined that the use of EMG biofeedback is an effective method for neuromuscular reeducation. Other research suggests that biofeedback may also help patients who have difficulty swallowing (dysphagia) after a stroke [14].

RESPIRATORY FUNCTION

Biofeedback has also been shown to improve breathing and lung function in patients with cystic fibrosis. A study of 26 persons with cystic fibrosis found that those who underwent eight sessions of biofeedback to learn breathing retraining and relaxation techniques had significant improvements in lung capacity and expiration [15].

URINARY INCONTINENCE

A study of 64 women with urinary incontinence found that alternating biofeedback and intravaginal electrical stimulation resulted in complete recovery for 21, recovery sufficient to avoid other forms of treatment for 20, and no success in 23, for an overall success rate of 64 percent [16].

WHO DOES IT

Biofeedback is used in many health care fields, including dentistry, internal medicine, pain management, physical therapy and rehabilitation, and psychology and psychiatry. There are more than 10,000 biofeedback practitioners in the United States. The Biofeedback Certification Institute of America, created in 1981, maintains standards and certifies those who meet those standards. Candidates must have a relevant degree from an accredited institution of higher education and have had at least 200 hours of formal training in biofeedback.

RESOURCES

- Biofeedback Certification Institute of America
  10200 West 44th Ave., Ste. 304
  Wheat Ridge, CO 80033
  303-420-2902
  The Institute certifies practitioners in the field. Publishes registers of certified practitioners in biofeedback and in stress-management education, and can provide lists of practitioners in your

Bodywork

In today's busy society, we tend to carry stress within our bodies. We have an argument or exchange cross words, and we can feel the tension creeping up our neck and into our head. A bad day at work, and our shoulders feel stiff and sore. Unnatural postures, such as sitting over a computer keyboard all day, bring even more tension to our already tense neck.

HISTORY

Touch is one of the oldest forms of healing, probably predating even the ancient Chinese and Indian medicine texts dating back thousands of years. It is instinctual, like stroking to comfort a sick child, and until the advent of modern Western medicine, it was also the physician's greatest and most important diagnostic and therapeutic tool. The importance of human contact and touch is vastly underrated in this day and age where we are more likely to get our money from an automated teller machine than a human behind the counter. Thousands of years of wisdom have been replaced by a love for technology and modern techniques.

Running around trying to take care of everything we need to do, we are often too busy to take the time necessary to care for ourselves until a problem presents itself. Athletes, musicians, and other performers who know that physical well-being is integral to their careers are more likely to take the time to care for their bodies. For the rest of us, it often takes the debilitating pain from an accident or illness to make us aware of how we are using our body and the adverse effects of improper use or stress on our physical and psychological functioning. Occupational injuries take their toll as well, whether it is lower-back pain from improper lifting or carpal tunnel syndrome from typing at a keyboard that is not aligned properly with our bodies.

Bodywork therapies are frequently used for rehabilitation after injury and illness, and for relief of stress and tension. Although many of these techniques are "delivered" by a practitioner to a patient suffering from a specific illness or injury, individuals can use other bodywork techniques on their own to feel and perform better.

THE POWER OF TOUCH

We all know that touch feels good and is comforting, but in modern medicine, measurements made by machines have become the norm. The link between emotions and the body has been cast aside; touch has been replaced by laboratory tests or even machines that can perform the tasks of physical therapists so they don't have to touch and spend time with their patients.

Modern clinical science sometimes writes off the positive effects of bodywork and therapies such as Therapeutic Touch (see page 197) to a placebo, or "sugar pill," effect in which the patient is helped solely by the caring presence of a healer. Anyone who can remember being comforted as a child by the touch of a parent or loved one can tell you that this caring may have done more good than the cod-liver oil they were given, or whatever the trend of the day was. Ask any mother or caregiver who has comforted a sick child or an elderly parent. They may not be able to explain why, but they know that touch is effective. To say otherwise is to run contrary to our basic instincts as well as thousands of years of experience throughout the world.

Modern Western medicine remains reluctant to acknowledge the importance of the link between body and mind. But, thanks to the reemergence of alternative and traditional therapies in recent years, their "scientific" value is being rediscovered. A growing number of researchers are demonstrating in carefully controlled scientific studies that many of these bodywork therapies are effective in treating a number of different conditions.

SELF-AWARENESS

While bodywork alone may help physical functioning, a key thing to remember is that alternative medicine is holistic. That is, these therapies are most effective when combined with overall changes in self-awareness, diet, exercise, and other interventions, such as meditation or relaxation techniques. Ideally, bodywork is not just something that someone does to you. It can help you become more aware of how you use your body, how to use it more effectively, and how to function at your best. The goal of all alternative therapies is to reintegrate the body with the mind, so that the mind works with the body.

For example, increased self-awareness can allow people to become observers of how they use their body, how they sit at the computer, or when they need to take a break. This self-awareness is a kind of preventive maintenance for the body. Improved self-awareness can help individuals take early corrective action when they recognize a mild discomfort.

Many of the techniques described in this section help people learn how to become aware of how they use their bodies and ways to use them more efficiently. This focus on learning how to use one's body more efficiently is important for both the prevention and treatment of postural and orthopedic problems and for general well-being.

Self-awareness is also an important principle in yoga (see pages 360–364) and other therapies described in the mind/body section (pages 282–293). It can help release emotional stress and its accompanying muscle tension, and help you relax, think more clearly, and deal more effectively with stress and change.

A RANGE OF THERAPIES

A wide variety of bodywork techniques are in use in the United States today to help people achieve peak performance, prevent injury, and recover from illness or trauma.

Many of these interventions could also be described under the category of mind/body therapies. The therapies described here as bodywork are those that focus primarily on the physical functioning of the body or its functioning in combination with the flow of vital energy, or qi, in the body.

Some of the best known and most popular forms of bodywork are described below. There is a good chance that you will hear of a method not described here. For example, there are an estimated 80 forms of massage alone, about 60 of which have been developed within the past 20 years. Instead of being a cause for despair and confusion, this really reflects the tremendous increase in interest in massage and other methods of bodywork in recent years.

Some of these methods were developed recently but are based on age-old wisdoms and experience that has been literally handed down over thousands of years. As bodywork practitioners experimented and expanded their practice to include a variety of techniques from different disciplines, many found themselves unable to describe their work along a strict line and coined their own terms for what they do.

Don't ignore combinations of bodywork, exercise, and meditation, such as yoga and qigong, found elswhere in this book, either. After all, your body is where you dwell. Make it a comfortable place.

APPLIED KINESIOLOGY

Applied kinesiology, and a closely related technique "touch for health," use the meridian qi (vital energy) and connections between the neurologic and muscular systems to make diagnoses and provide therapy. Applied kinesiology includes its own diagnostic method of determining dysfunctional states of the body in combination with standard medical diagnostic tests.

WHAT IT IS

Applied kinesiology evaluates the chemical, mental, and structural aspects of individuals through muscle testing and standard medical diagnostic tests. A wide variety of therapies—acupressure, diet, education, exercise, manipulation, and nutrition—are used to help restore balance and maintain well-being throughout life.

The functional assessment measures used in combination with standard medical tests include

- posture and gait analysis—evaluating the way a person stands and walks as an indicator of internal imbalances
- manual muscle testing as functional neurologic evaluation—testing the strength of individual muscles to examine neurologic function
- range-of-motion testing—determining the extent to which joints can move to check for joint fixation
- static palpation testing—assessing the muscles and joints while they are motionless to find muscle spasms or atrophy and joint misalignments
- motion analysis—feeling muscles and joints as they move to assess the adequacy of joint mechanics

Practitioners use these findings in combination with standard methods of diagnosis, such as clinical history, physical examination findings, and laboratory tests.

Applied kinesiology recognizes a close association between specific muscle dysfunction and related organ or gland dysfunction. This relationship can be a source of muscle weakness, and when combined with other diagnostic input, it can help the physician consider organs that may be part of the patient's health problem.

Sessions start with various muscle tests to determine the state of the flow

---

HISTORY

Applied kinesiology was developed in the 1960s by George Goodheart, a chiropractor who found that postural imbalances could be corrected by focusing on weak muscles instead of tight muscles as the majority of therapies did. Dr. Goodheart was also the first nonmedical practitioner to serve as a member of the U.S. Sports Medicine Committee of the U.S. Olympic Team during the 1980 winter games in Lake Placid, N.Y.

CAUTION

Some laypersons and professionals use a form of manual muscle testing without the necessary expertise to perform specific and accurate tests, warns the International College of Applied Kinesiology. These practitioners may also fail to coordinate muscle testing findings with other standard diagnostic procedures, leading to improper treatment. The college recommends that the practice of applied kinesiology be limited to health care professionals licensed to diagnose.

of qi (vital energy) through the meridians (see Qigong, pages 342–345). These muscle tests give an indication of the area to be worked on and are an integral part of applied kinesiology treatment. The final diagnosis relies on muscle testing and other standard medical tests and observations.

USES

In its early days, applied kinesiology focused on correcting postural imbalances caused by weak muscles. This goal later expanded from restoring normal function to the broader goal of maintaining robust health into old age.

Today, health maintenance is a primary goal of applied kinesiology. Practitioners believe it can help delay the onset of diseases, such as arthritis, cancer, diabetes, and heart disease, caused by degenerative processes. The therapy's goals include

- to restore postural balance, correct gait impairment, and improve range of motion
- to restore nerve conduction
- to balance endocrine, immune, digestive, and other visceral functions
- to prevent or delay the onset of diseases caused by degenerative processes

WHO DOES IT

Thousands of doctors—from professions such as chiropractic, naturopathic medicine, dentistry, general medicine, osteopathy, and podiatry—practice applied kinesiology. Applied kinesiology encompasses diagnostic procedures that should only be done by practicing doctors and individuals trained in diagnosis and applied kinesiology, says the International College of Applied Kine-

siology, which only offers courses to practitioners licensed to diagnose and students enrolled in accredited programs that will enable them to obtain a license to diagnose.

RESOURCES

- International College of Applied Kinesiology
  6405 Metcalf Ave., Ste. 503
  Shawnee Mission, KS 66202-3929
  913-384-5336
  fax 913-384-5112

BIOFIELD THERAPEUTICS

Often called *energy healing* or *the laying on of hands*, biofield therapeutics is one of the oldest healing practices. Cultures throughout the world have independently discovered and used this vital energy or life force method of healing, and have tried to characterize its nature. (See sidebar "Names of Biofields Around the World." on page 196 for a sampling of the many names.)

WHAT IT IS

Because biofield therapies mix concepts of physics and metaphysics, or ancient and modern wisdoms, it is not easily defined. Major hypotheses are that the biofield is metaphysical (outside the dimensions of space and time), an electromagnetic field effect, or a field effect in physics that is presently undefined.

Practitioners of biofield therapeutics believe that healing force comes from a source other than themselves, such as God or a universal life force. They also believe that the human biofield can be directed, enhanced, or modified by a practitioner.

HISTORY

Biofield therapeutics appear in the ancient Chinese medical text *The Yellow Emperor's Classic*. Western evidence of its use dates back to hieroglyphics and depictions of biofield healings from Egypt's Third Dynasty. In ancient Greece, Hippocrates (the "Father of Medicine") observed it, as did many of his successors. In the United States, it was popularized as "magnetic healing" by Austrian physician Franz Mesmer in the 1830s, and later by Andrew Still, the founder of osteopathy, and Daniel Palmer, the founder of chiropractic medicine.

NAMES OF BIOFIELDS AROUND THE WORLD

In..	It's called...
Ancient Egypt	Ankh
Ancient Greece	Pneuma
Ashanti	Ntoro
Australian aborigine	Arunquiltha
Bantu	Ntu
China	Qi
Ghana	Mulungu
Hawaii	Tane
India	Prana
Japan	Ki
Native American Cultures	
Algonquia	Manitou
Huron	Oki
Inuit	Sila
Iroquois	Orenda
Lakota	Wakan
Polynesia	Mana
South America	Gana

Practitioners often center themselves or meditate before beginning treatment. They then place their hands on or near the person being treated. Practitioners engage the biofield from their hands with that of the recipient to promote general well-being or to treat a specific disorder.

Sessions last from 20 minutes to more than one hour, and a series of sessions may be needed to treat some ailments. Practitioners say that the ability to perform biofield healing is universal and can be learned with instruction and practice.

The external portion of an individual's biofield (also known as the aura) extends outward from the body for several inches. Therefore, it is not necessary to physically place the hands directly on the body. This has actually made it possible for researchers to conduct blinded studies in which the subjects and the evaluators do not know who received treatment. For example, one study that showed therapeutic touch accelerates wound healing was performed by having patients put their arm into an opening so they could not see if they received therapeutic touch or not.

Some practitioners combine biofield therapeutics with mental healing (also known as psychic healing, absent healing, distant healing, and nonlocal healing). Some, such as Qigong masters (see pages 342–345), may also try to extend their biofield into the recipient's body from a distance of up to several feet.

DIAGNOSIS

Practitioners assess the patient's general health and disorder by using touch to sense subtle alterations in the biofield and the pattern of energy in the body. For example, they may detect areas of tension or sense blocked or congested energy flow.

TYPES

The following are the main types of biofield therapies currently used in the United States:
- Healing Science
- Healing Touch
- SHEN
- Therapeutic Touch

Other forms of biofield therapeutics in use include Huna (an ancient Hawaiian healing system), Natural Healing, and Mari-el. Reiki (see page 213) is sometimes also described as a biofield therapy.

Healing Science—Healing Science was established in 1978 by Barbara

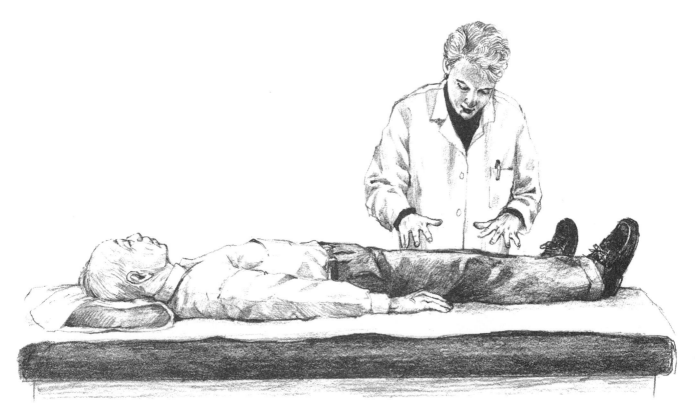

Brennan, a physicist, psychotherapist, and healer. The technique is based on the structure and function of the human energy field—the underlying energy-consciousness field that supports and energizes the body with life force. Practitioners believe that balance must be maintained within the human energy field as well as between it and nature to maintain health. Specific dysfunctions and the underlying causes of disease are diagnosed through "high sense perception," the ability to extend normal senses.

Therapeutic Touch—Therapeutic Touch is based on the assumption that energy fields are the fundamental units of humans and their environments. Therapeutic Touch uses a standardized technique that includes centering and focusing on the intent to heal, and using the hands to assess the patient's energy field to balance the patient's energy flow and transfer life energy into depleted areas.

Therapeutic Touch was developed in 1972 by Dora Kunz, a gifted healer, and Dolores Krieger, a professor of nursing at New York University. Today, its use is discussed as a nursing intervention in most basic nursing textbooks.

Therapeutic Touch has been extensively studied, and its effectiveness for a variety of conditions is often cited by practitioners of other methods of biofield therapeutics.

The technique is widely taught to health care professionals, primarily nurses, in colleges and in continuing education programs in universities and health care agencies. It has been taught to tens of thousands of nurses in 44 countries.

Healing Touch—The Healing Touch program was developed and piloted in 1981 by nurse Janet Mentgen. In 1989, it was incorporated into the American Holistic Nurses' Association, which offers a four-level certification program. Healing Touch builds upon the foundation of Therapeutic Touch. The practice includes techniques from a number of other biofield therapies as well, so that techniques are individualized by each practitioner.

Healing Touch practitioners may also use techniques from a variety of other energy-based interventions, including chakra connection, magnetic unruffling, chakra spread, etheric vitality, lymphatic unruffle, energetic back techniques, and other special techniques.

Healing Touch has been reported to assist with pain reduction, relaxation, and to enhance wound healing.

SHEN—Developed in 1977 by Richard Pavek, SHEN therapists believe that the biofield conforms to the laws of physics, and that a flux pattern can be discerned throughout the body. SHEN uses a sequence of paired-hand placements, usually one on top and one underneath, directly on the body. Placement is arranged according to the flux patterns of the patient. Comparing paired-hand placements and reversed paired-hand placements by trained and untrained practitioners, Pavek found that one arrangement produced feelings of relaxation and well-being, whereas the other resulted in agitation and anxiety.

SHEN is often used for emotional disorders and in alcohol and drug abuse and codependency recovery programs in some hospitals. In addition to tactile cues from the patient's body, SHEN practitioners use conventional medical and psychotherapy techniques that ask questions to uncover repressed emotional states.

Unpublished research by its founder suggests that SHEN therapy may be useful in other conditions such as anorexia, bulimia, irritable bowel syndrome, posttraumatic stress syndrome, premenstrual syndrome, and chronic migraine.

USES

Biofield therapeutics have been shown to be helpful for a variety of conditions, including
* anxiety
* pain
* wound healing
* high blood pressure

Although biofield therapies have undergone the test of time, most have not been extensively subjected to the rigorous scientific evaluation used in modern Western medicine. Therapeutic Touch is the most extensively studied of these therapies. Because the general process of Therapeutic Touch is similar to that used in other biofield therapies, it is often used to support the effectiveness of other techniques.

Practitioners say that Therapeutic Touch is effective in producing relaxation, reducing pain and the need for pain medication, accelerating the rate of healing, reducing nausea caused by chemotherapy, and promoting a general feeling of well-being, both emotional and spiritual.

Most of the formal research in the field has been done by nurses trained in research methods and considered experts in the technique. These studies show that Therapeutic Touch significantly speeds wound healing, decreases anxiety in hospitalized heart patients, and decreases the pain after surgery.

Dr. Krieger conducted her first pilot study of Therapeutic Touch in 1971 on 30 patients, and found that the hemoglobin levels of those who received Therapeutic Touch increased, but remained the same in persons who received no therapy. Subsequent studies in the early 1970s with more patients confirmed her findings.

Anxiety—A study of 90 patients hospitalized in a cardiac unit of a large medical center in New York compared the use of Therapeutic Touch to casual touch and no touch. Researchers found that patients who received Therapeutic Touch had significantly less anxiety than the other group [1].

Pain—A study of 60 persons with tension headaches found that 90 percent of those who received Therapeutic Touch had reduced pain [2]. Another study of 108 patients who had just undergone surgery found that those who received Therapeutic Touch waited longer to request pain medication than those who did not [3].

Relaxation—Open-heart surgery patients who received Therapeutic Touch had lower blood pressure than those who did not [4].

Wound Healing—A double-blinded study (neither patients nor evaluators knew who received treatment) found that the wounds of those who received Therapeutic Touch healed significantly faster [4].

WHO DOES IT

Overall, there are an estimated 50,000 biofield practitioners in the United States, about 30,000 of whom are trained in Therapeutic Touch. More than 90 colleges and universities around the world train student nurses in biofield therapeutics, and Therapeutic Touch is routinely included in nursing school curricula. In addition to nurses, a number of acupuncturists and massage therapists are trained in the technique as well.

At present, no states have licensure for biofield practitioners. The field is widely accepted and practiced in other countries, however. For example, the United Kingdom had more than 8,500 registered healers in 1993 and its use is approved at the government's 1,500 hospitals.

RESOURCES

- The Nurse Healers' Professional Associates
  The SHEN Therapy Institute
  Sausalito, CA
  415-332-2593

MASSAGE THERAPY

Massage is the use of manual techniques to achieve or increase health and well-being. Massage therapy encompasses a wide variety of techniques based on methods that have been around for thousands of years. All use touch to help the body heal itself.

One of the oldest therapies in existence today, massage has been practiced for thousands of years. It is a major component of traditional Chinese medicine and is included as a therapy in the ancient Indian medical system known as Ayurveda. Its use in Western medicine dates back to the time of Hippocrates in the fourth century B.C.

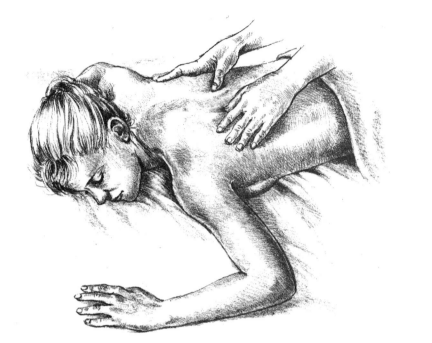

Western massage traces its origins back to the days of ancient Greece. In addition to Hippocrates, many other early physicians advocated its use, including

- Celsus (25 B.C.–50 A.D.) His *De Medicinia*, an encyclopedia of Roman medicine, dealt extensively with prevention and therapeutics using massage.
- Galen (131–200). The most influential physician in the ancient, medieval, and Renaissance worlds, he included techniques and indications for massage in his *De Sanitate Tuenda*, which translates as The Hygiene, or prevention.
- Avicenna (980–1037). His *Canon of Medicine,* considered the authoritative medical text in Europe for several centuries, includes extensive writings about massage.

Other prominent advocates of massage include

- Ambrose Pare, the father of modern surgery
- William Harvey, the discoverer of the circulation of blood
- Herman Boerhaave, the physician who introduced the clinical method of teaching medicine

Modern massage was introduced to the United States in the 1850s by two New York physicians who had studied in Sweden. The first massage therapy clinics were opened here after the Civil War by two Swedes. Early clients included U.S. Presidents Benjamin Harrison and Ulysses S. Grant.

The word massage is said to have entered the American medical vocabulary in 1873. Between then and 1939, more than 600 articles on its use appeared in mainstream English-language medical journals. As the American health care system began to focus on biomedicine and technology, however, physicians relegated massage to nurses and physical therapists. Although massage has continued to be a component of physical therapy, it came under increased attention in the 1970s, often under the auspices of alternative health care.

WHAT IT IS

Massage therapy is the systematized manipulation of soft tissues for the purpose of normalizing them. Practitioners use a variety of physical methods including applying fixed or movable pressure, holding, or causing movement to the body. Therapists primarily

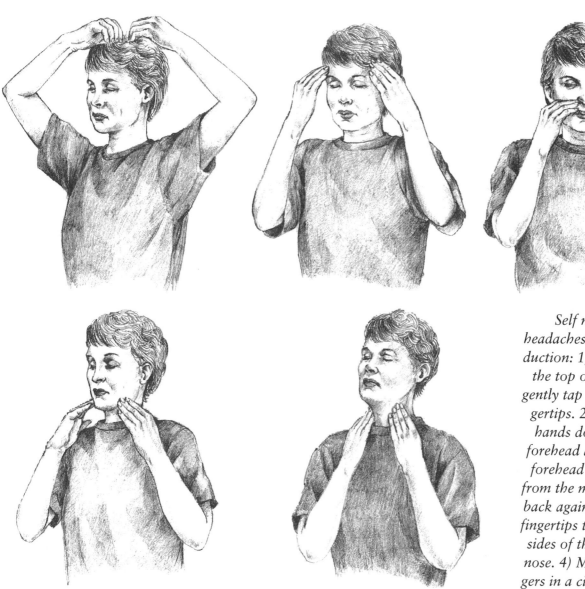

use their hands, but may also use their forearms, elbows, or feet. The basic goal of massage therapy is to help the body heal itself and to increase health and well-being.

Touch is the core ingredient of massage therapy and also combines science and art. Practitioners learn specific techniques for massage and use their sense of touch to determine the right amount of pressure to apply to each person and locate areas of ten-

sion and other soft-tissue problems. Touch also conveys a sense of caring, an important component in the healing relationship.

There are some 80 types of massage, many of which use a combination of techniques. About 60 of these are less than 20 years old, due in part to greater interest in massage in the 1970s as well as the introduction of other traditional forms of massage from other cultures.

Self massage for headaches and stress reduction: 1) Beginning at the top of your head, gently tap with your fingertips. 2) Move your hands down to your forehead and pull your forehead horizontally from the middle out and back again. 3) Use your fingertips to massage the sides of the tip of your nose. 4) Move your fingers in a circular motion along your jaw, slowly moving from your ears to your chin. 5) When you come to the tip of your chin, stroke gently down the front of your throat.

Swedish Massage—The most common massage therapy method used in the West is Swedish massage. This form of massage uses a system of long gliding strokes, kneading, and friction techniques. Swedish massage works on superficial layers of muscles, and sometimes includes active and passive movement of the joints. Swedish massage is used to promote general relaxation, improve circulation, increase range of motion, and relieve muscle tension.

Deep Tissue Massage—This form of massage uses greater pressure and works on deeper layers of muscle than Swedish massage does. Deep tissue massage is used to relieve chronic patterns of muscular tension by using slow strokes, direct pressure, or friction directed across the grain of the muscles.

Manual Lymph Drainage—This form of massage is used to improve the flow of lymphatic fluid (the fluid that runs through a system of ducts outside the bloodstream and is filtered by nodes found in the groin, armpits, neck, and other areas). Through light, rhythmic strokes, this method is used to treat conditions such as edema (or fluid buildup) in the extremities.

CAUTION

Don't Massage:
- Areas that are bruised, infected, inflamed, or swollen
- If you suspect a broken bone
- A person with a fever
- A person with phlebitis or thrombosis—massage can loosen blood clots
- Tumors
- Varicose veins

Neuromuscular Massage—Neuromuscular massage is a form of deep massage applied to specific individual muscles. Often used to reduce pain, it increases blood flow, releases trigger points, and relieves pressure on nerves caused by soft tissues.

Sports Massage—Sports massage uses techniques similar to those of Swedish and deep tissue massage. These methods are specially adapted to athletes' needs, such as preparing for a competition or helping restore the body after a rigorous workout.

Self Massage—Many massage therapies and other alternative practices, such as sports massage and qigong, teach techniques for self massage. (For a self-massage routine for headaches, see page 201.)

TRADITIONAL MASSAGE METHODS

Several alternative therapies incorporate massage into their overall treatment regimens. Here are a few of the systems that rely on massage therapy:

Ayurvedic Medicine—The ancient Hindu medicine of Ayurveda emphasizes the importance of regular massage as a method of increasing circulation to aid in the removal of waste from the tissues. Ayurvedic massage traditionally involves the use of oils, which may differ from season to season. (For more on Ayurvedic medicine, see pages 182–187.)

Traditional Chinese Medicine—Dating back to at least 200 B.C., traditional Chinese massage uses both tonification (energizing or stimulating) and sedation (relaxation) techniques to treat and relieve many conditions, including abdominal pain, the common cold, headache, lumbago, leg cramps, and sleeplessness. Techniques are generally used in combination, and include

- ma—rubbing with palm or fingertips
- pai—tapping with palm or fingertips
- ta—strong pinching with thumb and fingertip
- an—rapid and rhythmic pressing with thumb, palm, or back of the clenched hand
- nie—twisting with both thumbs and tips of the index finger grasping on the area being treated
- ning—pinching and lifting
- na—moving while performing *ning*
- tui—pushing, sometimes with slight vibratory effect

A wide variety of other methods of massage are also used in the United States, including techniques for movement reeducation (see pages 204–209), polarity therapy (see pages 209–210), pressure point techniques such as shiatsu and reflexology (see pages 211–212), and Therapeutic Touch (see page 197).

USES

Massage therapy has been shown to be effective for problems ranging from reducing anxiety and depression, to reducing pain and promoting weight gain in low-birth-weight infants.

Anxiety—A pilot study of five patients with symptoms of tension and anxiety found a significant improvement in one or more psychophysiologic parameters: heart rate, muscle response time on forearm extensor muscle electromyograms, and electrical skin resistance [5].

Depression—In a study of children and adolescents hospitalized with depression and adjustment disorder, those who were treated with massage were found to be less anxious and depressed than those who viewed relaxing videotapes [6].

Pain—Massage has been shown to be a cost-effective means of decreasing pain in patients with spinal trauma. The combination of shiatsu (a Japanese form of acupressure, see pages 169–172), Swedish muscle massage, and trigger point sedation in 52 patients with spinal injuries led to a significant decrease in pain and increase in muscle flexibility and tone [7].

A study of the use of massage in patients with pain from cancer found that those who received massage had a 60 percent lower level of pain perception and a 24 percent decrease in anxiety. More than half reported feeling more relaxed as well [8].

Premature Babies—Massage is a good way to help low-birth-weight babies born prematurely. Premature infants treated with daily massage gain more weight and have shorter hospital stays than infants who are not massaged. A Miami study of 40 low-birth-weight babies found that 20 massaged babies had a 47 percent greater weight gain per day and stayed in the hospital an average six days less than 20 similar infants who did not receive massage. In addition to more healthy babies, massage resulted in a cost savings of approximately $3,000 per infant [9].

Another study of 30 cocaine-exposed premature infants found that those who received massage for a 10-day period had a 28 percent greater weight gain than those who did not. They also had significantly fewer complications and displayed fewer stress behaviors and more mature motor behaviors [10].

Psychological Problems—Studies indicate that massage is beneficial for autistic children, abused and neglected children in shelters, and depressed and drug-exposed adolescents.

Relaxation—Researchers believe that massage may be an effective way to promote relaxation and improve communication with patients, such as elderly people who are in nursing homes. Such patients reported less anxiety, more relaxation, and had lower blood pressure and heart rates than patients who did not receive massage. Lavender oil can enhance the sense of relaxation from massage. The use of several types of essential oils can also enhance the effects of massage (see Aromatherapy, pages 178–181).

A very gentle touch or light stroking may be OK on unaffected areas, but check with your physician first. Massage can be very useful for pregnant women but should only be done by a therapist familiar with the situation's specific dangers. It is especially important to avoid pressure around the ankles and deep or percussive massage to the lower back or abdomen.

WHO DOES IT

There are approximately 50,000 qualified massage therapists in the United States. The number of massage therapists is increasing rapidly, with a corresponding increase in use by the public. There is a national certification exam for therapeutic massage, and currently 58 school programs are recognized by the Commission for Massage Therapy Accreditation/Approval. Associations include the 15,000-member American Massage Therapy Association and the National Association of Nurse Massage Therapists, a 300-member specialty organization.

RESOURCES

- American Massage Therapy Association
  820 Davis St., Ste. 100
  Evanston, IL 60201
  847-864-0123

- National Association of Nurse Massage Therapists
  1710 East Linden St.
  Tucson, AZ 85719
  602-325-0853

- National Certification Board for Therapeutic Massage and Bodywork
  1735 North Lynn St., Ste. 950
  Arlington, VA 22209
  703-524-9563
  800-296-0664

There are a number of good books on massage—check with your local library or bookstore.

MOVEMENT REEDUCATION THERAPIES

Movement reeducation therapies involve retraining your body to come into proper alignment. The new alignments can solve postural problems, improve balance and coordination, and relieve stress. All who have participated in these therapies agree that this body awareness has to be experienced and sensed rather than taught verbally. The increased awareness of using the body correctly can lead to more effective use of one's whole self.

THE ALEXANDER TECHNIQUE

Late in the 19th century, the Shakespearean actor F. Matthias Alexander

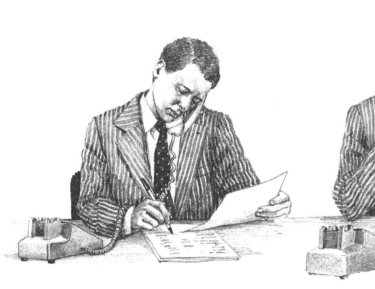

Posture and body attitude are crucial parts of many movement reeducation therapies such as the Alexander technique. Proper posture can make a difference in both mental and physical well-being.

developed vocal problems that threatened his career. The discovery that bad posture was responsible for his chronic voice loss led to his development of the Alexander technique for movement reeducation. The Alexander technique teaches simple, efficient movements designed to improve balance, posture, and coordination and to relieve pain. This practice has become especially popular with actors and musicians, and is taught in many drama programs throughout the United States.

WHO USES THE ALEXANDER TECHNIQUE?

According to the North American Society of Teachers of the Alexander technique, students of the technique have included well-known actors and writers. Here are just a few:
- John Cleese
- Kevin Kline
- Paul Newman
- Aldous Huxley
- George Bernard Shaw

Alexander discovered that a pattern of tension was interfering with the correct relationship between his head, neck, and back. The Alexander technique centers on reeducating people about everyday movements that are in actuality harmful. For example, actors who try to project their voices on stage by tilting back their heads actually wind up compressing their vocal chords.

The Alexander technique is taught in private half-hour to one-hour lessons. Students are guided through a series of simple movements and learn to observe and change habits that interfere with optimum functioning. The teacher may apply light pressure to points of contraction in the body. This awakens awareness of the position and movement of muscles and retrains the body to move more efficiently.

By working with a trained teacher, students learn to identify and stop destructive patterns of movement. Mastery of the technique leads to increased sensory awareness and more effective use of the whole self.

Practitioners of the Alexander technique say it is helpful in alleviating a variety of conditions, including
- anxiety
- breathing problems
- hypertension
- myalgia
- neck and back pain
- postural disorders
- repetitive strain injury
- rheumatica
- stress
- whiplash

Teachers approved by the North American Society of Teachers of the Alexander technique have undergone at least 1,600 hours of class instruction over a minimum of three years.

FELDENKRAIS METHOD

The Feldenkrais method combines movement training, gentle touch, and verbal dialogue to help people create freer, more efficient movement. Developed by the Russian-born Israeli physicist Moshe Feldenkrais, it is based on modern ideas and basic research about perception, motor learning, neural plasticity, and sensory integration.

Feldenkrais began studying human functioning in the 1940s. Integrating the physics of body movement with how people move, behave, and interact, he developed a system to improve movement and functioning.

There are two forms of Feldenkrais therapy: 1) awareness through movement and 2) functional integration. Both seek to help people relearn the proper way their body should move.

Awareness Through Movement—This approach uses gentle exploratory movement sequences focused on a specific function, such as bending, reaching, or walking. The teacher provides verbal directions to students to increase their awareness of the many possibilities of action. Thinking, sensory perception, and imagery are also used to examine each function.

Practitioners verbally guide students through a sequence of movements—sitting or lying on the floor, standing, or sitting in a chair—enabling the student to discover how they move and how to relax. The program helps students abandon habitual patterns so they can develop awareness, flexibility, and coordination.

Functional integration—This approach combines verbal instruction with gentle touch to help students become aware of existing and alternative movement patterns. The teacher tells students how they are organizing their movements and suggests other choices for movement patterns. This is done lying or sitting on a low padded table, or standing, walking, or sitting in a chair. The one-on-one sessions guide students through a series of precise movements that alter habitual patterns and provide new patterns directly to the neuromuscular system.

Feldenkrais practitioners believe that functional integration is especially helpful for people who need to overcome limitations brought on by accident, illness, misuse, or stress. It is also helpful with various postural and functional disorders. The method is frequently used to alleviate chronic pain and to help athletes and others improve their balance and coordination.

Possible uses include
- pain management
- physical therapy
- sports performance enhancement

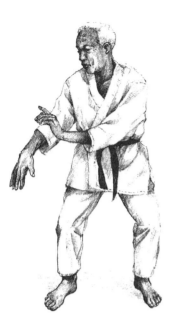
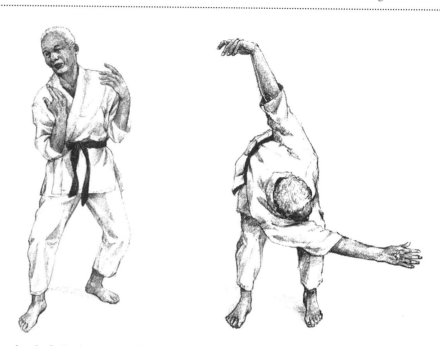

Although the Feldenkrais method combines ideas from many modern scientific disciplines, clinical studies of its effectiveness have been limited. Some reviews and studies suggest that movement reeducation is an important component in physical therapy and recovery for persons with lower-back pain and neurologic disorders such as Parkinson disease and stroke. Other studies suggest it is useful in pain management and as an exercise method for the elderly and people recovering from spinal injury [11, 12].

Unpublished research suggests that after semiweekly classes for six weeks, rheumatoid arthritis patients had decreased pain, improved walking performance, and improved ability to stand up from a sitting position, but the technique brought about no improvement in grip.

Case studies of patients suffering from acute and chronic back pain show that the Feldenkrais method helped even when a variety of other conventional and alternative methods had failed to produce results. Researchers believe it may have wide applications in the management of pain, stiffness, and restriction syndromes.

TRAGER APPROACH

A former boxer, acrobat, dancer, and physician specializing in neuromuscular disorders, Milton Trager began the foundations of his movement reeducation method more than 60 years ago. Dr. Trager's work focuses on the effects of gentle movement on the nervous system, which he associates with the unconscious mind.

The Trager approach seeks to increase relaxation and mobility through touch, movement, and an open meditative state. Practitioners use light, rhythmic rocking and shaking movements to loosen joints, ease movement, and release chronic patterns of tension. Sessions normally last 60 to 90 minutes. During a session, the practitioner cradles and moves the client's stiff limbs to retrain the body's old patterns of movement and prevent problems

All movement reeducation therapies use exercise to reinforce newly learned postures and movements. The exercises in the Trager approach, called mentastics *(examples of which are shown above), are designed to to maintain and enhance a sense of lightness, freedom, and flexibility.*

from recurring. Whereas some bodywork practitioners work more deeply when they encounter a tight muscle, Trager practitioners work more lightly to help patients recall the feeling of what it was like before it was tight. Practitioners work in a "hook up," a relaxed meditative state that allows them to connect with the client.

After the bodywork session, patients are given instruction in what Trager practitioners call *mentastics*. Developed by Dr. Trager to help maintain the sense achieved during the bodywork session, mentastics is a system of simple mentally directed physical movements designed to maintain and enhance a sense of lightness, freedom, and flexibility.

The Trager approach is used by athletes for performance enhancement and by persons with musculoskeletal problems, back problems, and more.

Reports on the effectiveness of Trager work tend to be case histories of people who have been helped by the technique. These suggest that it can provide long-term improvements in movement function in people with multiple sclerosis, cerebral palsy, chronic pain, muscle spasms, and stroke or spinal cord injuries.

One study of 12 people with chronic obstructive pulmonary (lung) disease found that Trager therapy seemed to produce better chest mobility and that persons treated with the technique had increased lung capacity and expiratory capacity [13].

Trager practitioners are certified by the Trager Institute, which offers a professional certification program in Trager work that takes a minimum of six months to complete.

ASTON-PATTERNING

Aston-Patterning, also called *Aston movement*, combines bodywork, ergonomics, fitness training, and movement coaching. The system is used to improve physical performance and to help the elderly and people in pain or with disabilities to minimize restriction and maximize movement capabilities.

Founder Judith Aston is a former professor of dance and movement who trained with Dr. Ida Rolf. Aston developed a movement maintenance program to help patients sustain the changes produced by Rolfing (see pages 212–213). In 1977, she formed her own organization to teach her integrated system of bodywork, movement education, and environmental education.

Aston-Patterning uses massage to help release the functional and structural holding patterns that create chronic stress. Therapy attempts to release unnecessary tension from all areas of the body, from the skin surface to the bone and address restrictions in the joints as well.

The technique also uses movement reeducation. Practitioners observe an individual's movements, posture, and tension-holding patterns. Movement lessons assist individuals in choosing alternatives to stressful patterns and movement habits.

Practitioners also offer consultation on how to modify physical surroundings, such as chairs and beds, to suit the body's needs better. Aston has developed a line of products such as cushions for chairs and car seats that are designed to support and adjust the position of the body to reduce unnecessary stress and promote ease of movement.

RESOURCES

- North American Society of Teachers of the Alexander Technique
P.O. Box 517
Urbana, IL 61801-0517
800-367-6956
NASAT offers general information on the Alexander technique and a directory of certified teachers.

- Feldenkrais Guild
P.O. Box 489
Albany, OR 97321
503-926-0981
The Feldenkrais Guild offers general information on Feldenkrais, books and videos, listings of practitioners, and training and certification for practitioners.

- The Trager Institute
21 Locust Ave.
Mill Valley, CA 94941-2091
415-388-2688
The Institute offers general information on the Trager approach and a directory of practitioners.

- Aston-Patterning
P.O. Box 3568
Incline Village, NV 89450-3568
702-831-8228
General information on Aston-Patterning, as well as training in the field, is provided by the group's Nevada headquarters.

POLARITY THERAPY

Polarity therapists believe that well-being and health are determined by the nature of the flow of the human energy field in the body and that this field can be affected by a variety of natural methods.

WHAT IT IS

Dr. Stone used the word *polarity* to describe energy's qualities of attraction and repulsion—a fundamental characteristic of all energy movement. Polarity therapists believe that the body, mind, emotions, and spirit are interdependent, that each person shares in the responsibility for his or her own health, and that simple steps can be taken to improve wellness.

Polarity therapy is designed to balance the body's subtle electromagnetic energy not only through touch or polarity contacts, but also through cleansing and building diets (with foods classified according to the five elements of Ayurveda [see page 182]), simple stretching exercises (called *polarity yoga,* or *polar energetics*), and self-awareness through changes in attitudinal and emotional habit patterns. These natural, self-guided techniques are combined to provide a simple, comprehensive method for health maintenance.

Polarity theory describes energy's qualities of attraction and repulsion through the concepts of charge: Every-

HISTORY

Polarity therapy was developed in the 1950s by Dr. Randolph Stone, a chiropractor, osteopath, and naturopath. Based on the idea of a human energy field, it draws from Oriental and Indian sources.

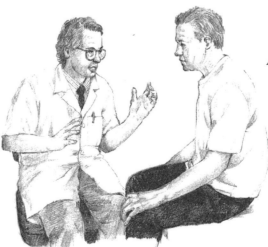

Polarity therapy often goes beyond bodywork. A typical polarity session involves the practitioner and client working together to address physical, mental, and emotional energy blockages.

thing has a positive, negative, or neutral charge. In the elaborate system of polarity therapy, the interactions of these three types of energy create the five elements of ether, air, fire, water, and earth, which further relate to ancient concepts from Chinese medicine and Ayurvedic medicine. It is the movement of these energies in the nervous system and musculoskeletal system of the physical body that is the focus of polarity theory's therapeutic efforts.

A typical polarity session involves the practitioner and client working together to address physical, mental, and emotional energy blockages. Polarity bodywork uses a variety of contacts and manipulations to stimulate and balance the body's electromagnetic fields. In somewhat of a counseling role, practitioners may help to process feelings and develop strategies for resolving issues causing tension. Physical techniques, such as primal therapy, may also be employed to this end.

Balancing polarity energy calms nerves, relaxes muscles, and opens up natural flow in the body's energy currents so that the body can heal itself.

USES

Commonly reported benefits of polarity therapy include
- relaxation
- pain reduction
- reduction of nervous conditions
- heightened self-awareness
- improvement in range of motion

Polarity therapy does not attempt to diagnose illnesses; rather it is a holistic approach to supplement and support medical treatment.

Polarity therapy, like many other forms of bodywork, has not been subject to rigorous scientific evaluation, such as controlled studies published in peer-reviewed scientific journals. It relies on reports of improvements observed by individual practitioners and experienced by those who undergo it and on scientific studies published in related fields.

WHO DOES IT

Polarity therapists are trained and certified by the American Polarity Therapy Association, established in 1983. A number of alternative practitioners from fields such as chiropractic, massage, and naturopathy are also registered polarity practitioners.

RESOURCES

- American Polarity Therapy Association
2888 Bluff St., Ste. 149
Boulder, CO 80301
303-545-2080
General information on polarity therapy and a directory of polarity practitioners across the country.

PRESSURE POINT TECHNIQUES

Pressure point therapies use finger pressure on specific points to reduce pain and treat various disorders. These points are usually related to traditional meridians, or pathways for vital energy, which are used in traditional Chinese medicine, acupuncture, and acupressure, but may also include other neurologic release points.

Writings dating back to the 1500s describe the use of pressure points to relieve pain. Westerners learned of Chinese pressure point therapy in the late 1700s through the writings of the Jesuit Amiat, which influenced the development of Swedish massage and traditional Japanese folk massage that would result in the form of therapy called *Shiatsu*. Pressure points are used under several systems of bodywork.

SHIATSU

Shiatsu involves applying pressure to meridian points to stimulate or sedate them (see Acupuncture, pages 173–177, and Acupressure, pages 169–172). Practitioners generally treat the meridians of the entire body in an attempt to bring relaxation, harmony, and balance. Based on traditional oriental medicine theory, shiatsu was developed in Japan and has been used extensively in the United States for the past 20 years.

Shiatsu literally means finger or thumb pressure. Shiatsu practitioners apply pressure to specific points, called *tsubos*, on the meridians, to rebalance the body's *ki* (the Japanese word for vital energy). It is traditionally used to promote health and well-being and relieve pain.

Shiatsu uses sequenced applications of pressure applied from one end of each meridian to the other. Clients recline, usually lying on their back, then front, as the practitioner uses thumb pressure to stimulate the acupressure point. Points are stimulated through a combination of thumb pressure and transfer of ki from the practitioner. Another form—barefoot shiatsu—uses foot pressure to stimulate the meridian points.

Therapy sessions focus on long-term health improvement. Shiatsu is also used for a variety of disorders, including emotional and stress-related problems and postural problems (see pages 199–204). Conditions that may be

helped by Shiatsu include

- circulatory problems
- depression
- headache
- pain

JIN SHIN JYUTSU AND JIN SHIN DO

"The art of circulation awakening," jin shin jyutsu was developed in Japan by Jiro Murai in the early 1900s and brought to the United States in the 1960s. Jin shin do was developed in America in the 1980s by Mary Iino Burmeister.

Both jin shin jyutsu and jin shin do involve sequences of meridian pressure-point applications that are specific to the ailment being treated. Like acupuncture and acupressure, jin shin uses meridian connections to organs. Pressure is applied to the meridian points and held in specific patterns to energize or enervate the meridian ki. The pressure applied is often no more than a light touch. Because sessions are primarily for the treatment of specific problems, rather than general well-being, jin shin is used more often than Shiatsu as an alternative treatment approach.

REFLEXOLOGY

Reflexology uses specific points on the hands and feet to relieve pain. These "zones" on the hands and feet are related to specific organs. Reflexology is used to treat a variety of disorders.

Scientific studies have shown that reflexology can reduce symptoms of premenstrual syndrome. One study of 38 women with a history of premenstrual syndrome found that women who received reflexology had a significantly greater decrease in symptoms than women who received "fake" reflexology. Researchers used reflex points on the ear, hand, and feet that related to the ovary, uterus, pituitary gland, adrenal gland, kidney, celiac or solar plexus, and sympathetic nervous system. The women had eight weekly sessions of 30 minutes each. Among women who received true reflexology, 83 percent showed a significant decrease in physical and psychological symptoms [14].

ROLFING

Most manual healing methods focus on muscles, the skeletal system, or both. Rolfing, also called *structural integration,* centers on fascia—sheets of connective tissue that support and hold the muscles and bones in place. Rolfers believe that fascia is shortened and thickened when the body is injured and attempt to bring the body back into realignment through manipulation of the fascia.

Dr. Ida P. Rolf pioneered the principles of Rolfing and founded the first school to teach these principles and techniques as part of the Rolf Institute in 1960. Although Dr. Rolf called her technique structural integration, the public referred to it as "Rolfing," and the name stuck.

Dr. Rolf believed that the body's attempt to distribute the stress of an injury leads to shortened fascia, and may, in turn, lead to symptoms no longer at the site of the original trauma. Rolfing attempts to unwind and stretch the fascia back to normal, thereby realigning the body. Rolfers believe that the alignment of the body in the field of gravity is extremely important to well-being. This alignment or misalignment is a function of fascia.

Practitioners stretch the fascia by applying sliding pressure to the affected area with their fingers, thumbs, and elbows. In its early days, Rolfing acquired a reputation of being uncomfortable. In recent years, however, refinements in technique have led to considerably less discomfort.

Rolfing is used to relieve pain, such as lower-back pain and whiplash, to relieve stress, and to improve performance. In addition to therapy, Rolfing attempts to reeducate people about how they move. (For more on movement reeducation, see pages 204–209.)

Studies suggest that Rolfing may be beneficial in reducing the stress and symptoms of lower-back pain and whiplash, and lead to more efficient use of the body. A California study measuring levels of anxiety in 48 people found that those who received Rolfing had significantly decreased anxiety after therapy than those who did not receive the therapy [15].

Graduates of The Rolf Institute call themselves *Rolfers.* The postbachelors degree training program requires 28 full weeks of classroom work.

RESOURCES

- The International Institute of Reflexology
  P.O. Box 12642
  St. Petersburg, FL 33733
  813-343-4811
  fax 813-381-2807

- The Rolf Institute
  P.O. Box 1868
  Boulder, CO 80306
  800-530-8875

The Rolf Institute provides general information on Rolfing, a list of certified practitioners, and training.

REIKI

The word reiki is a combination of the Japanese words *rei* (free passage) and *ki* (universal life energy). This form of therapy involves the transfer of energy from practitioner to patient to enhance the body's natural ability to heal itself through the balancing of energy.

WHAT IT IS

Reiki practitioners channel energy in a particular pattern to heal and harmonize. Like other healing therapies based on the premise of a human energy field, reiki seeks to restore order to the body whose vital energy has become unbalanced.

Although there are a few positions in which the practitioner is in contact with the patient (such as cradling the head), most reiki treatments do not involve actual touching. The practitioner holds his or her hands a few inches or farther away from the patient's body and manipulates the energy field from there.

WHO DOES IT

Practitioners study with reiki masters to learn how to access ki and become a channel for its transmission. Students learn basic healing patterns and the "laying on of hands" for themselves and others. More advanced practitioners may use absentee healing—which involves practicing reiki on someone from a long distance, such as a different part of the country—or goal-oriented healing to address specific problems.

USES

The vast majority of reports on the effectiveness of reiki appear in popular rather than scientific literature. Proponents of reiki cite the growing body of research in the field of Therapeutic Touch as evidence of the therapeutic transfer of energy through touch.

One California study showed that reiki can increase hemoglobin and hematocrit levels. The study compared 47 people participating in reiki training and a small control group of 9 healthy medical professionals. The study found a significant increase in hemoglobin and hematocrit levels among the reiki group and no significant change in the control group [16].

RESOURCES

- The Reiki Alliance
  P.O. Box 41
  Cataldo, ID 83810
  208-682-3535

Provides general information on reiki and reiki training, sponsors an annual conference for reiki practitioners, and provides referrals to reiki masters in your area.

HISTORY

Reiki was introduced to the Western world in the 1800s by Mikau Usui, head of a Christian seminary in Japan. Asked by his students why they had not been taught to heal, Usui undertook a ten-year worldwide search of the healing arts, during which he discovered the ancient Tibetan sutras containing the keys to healing that he would later identify as *reiki*.

Chelation Therapy

CHELATION THERAPY IS THE MOST COMMONLY USED CONVENTIONAL TREATMENT FOR LEAD AND OTHER TOXIC METAL POISONING. IT IS AN INCREASINGLY POPULAR ALTERNATIVE THERAPY FOR THE TREATMENT OF CARDIOVASCULAR DISEASE, PARTICULARLY ATHEROSCLEROSIS, AND OTHER CHRONIC DEGENERATIVE CONDITIONS.

HISTORY

EDTA was first used in the 1940s to treat heavy-metal poisoning. When elderly patients being treated for chronic lead poisoning showed dramatic improvement after EDTA chelation therapy, scientists became interested in its broader use.

The use of EDTA to treat cardiovascular disease has generated scientific interest since the 1950s. Researchers in those days, however, lacked the noninvasive tools available today, such as ultrasound, to evaluate changes in the arteries. Interest in the compound's use waned in the 1960s when new surgical techniques were developed to unclog blocked arteries. Furthermore the patent on EDTA expired, making it unprofitable for a drug company to sponsor research.

WHAT IT IS

Chelation therapy involves the intravenous infusion of EDTA (ethylenediaminetetraacetic acid) to remove heavy metals from the body and to reverse atherosclerosis. EDTA is usually given as a slow intravenous solution over a period of four hours.

EDTA binds to metals and minerals, thereby helping the body get rid of these compounds. Practitioners believe its ability to adhere to calcium helps decrease atherosclerotic deposits (or plaque) that clog the arteries and lead to heart disease.

EDTA may also function as a calcium channel blocker—a category of conventional drugs called vasodilators that cause blood vessels to relax and widen. EDTA has also been shown to increase the concentration of other vasodilators.

EDTA's ability to remove ions that cause harmful oxidation of fatty materials may also help maintain cellular health.

Chelation therapy generally requires 20 to 30 treatments at a cost of up to $120 per visit, or about $3,000 per patient for the whole course. While this represents a substantial amount of money when paid out of pocket, it is a tiny fraction of the cost of conventional therapies, such as bypass surgery, used to reduce cardiovascular disease, and carries none of the risks a procedure such as that entails.

CARDIOVASCULAR DISEASE

Chelation therapy is widely used for the treatment of atherosclerosis and other chronic degenerative diseases involving the circulatory system. An estimated 500,000 people undergo chelation therapy in the United States each year.

RESEARCH PROBLEMS

Although a number of studies have been published on the use of chelation therapy, critics say that most have been poorly designed, particularly because many did not compare patients who received the treatment with those who did not receive treatment. A large placebo-controlled study that began at three military hospitals in the 1980s was dropped before an answer was found because of the beginning of the Persian Gulf War.

Nonetheless, the possibilities of chelation therapy for cardiovascular disease have led to a recommendation for further research in a 1995 report by advisors to the Office of Alternative Medicine at the National Institutes of Health. The report suggests that one way to assess the effectiveness of chelation therapy would be to collect research information from physicians who are already using the procedure.

RESULTS FROM AROUND THE WORLD

A review of treatment results from 2,870 patients in Brazil found significant

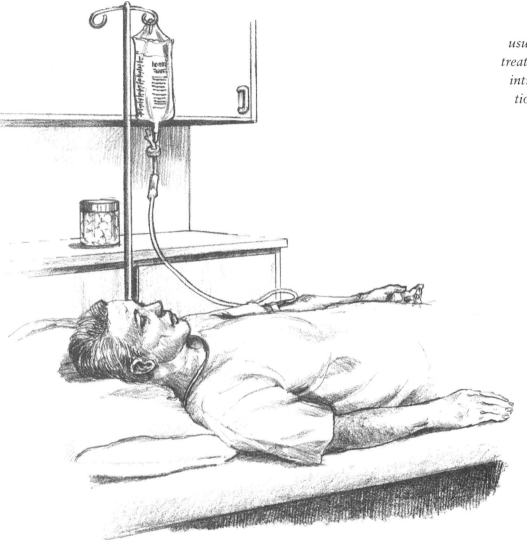

improvement in patients with heart disease or peripheral vascular disease who were treated with chelation therapy. Patients with heart disease were rated as showing "marked" improvement in 76.9 percent of cases and "good" improvement in 16.6 percent. Those with peripheral vascular disease showed a "marked" improvement in 91 percent of cases and "good" improvement in 7.6 percent [1].

In another study, the same researchers looked at patients with cerebrovascular disease and found 24 percent of the subjects showed "marked" improvement, and 30 percent showed "good" improvement [2].

WHO DOES IT

The American College of Advancement in Medicine (ACAM) has been granted approval by the Food and Drug Administration to study chelation therapy to treat peripheral vascular disease. The college provides a protocol for the use of chelation ther-

> ## CAUTION: SIDE EFFECTS
>
> Proponents of chelation therapy say its risks are similar to that of normal doses of aspirin and that early reports of side effects such as kidney toxicity were the result of doses that were too high. The American College of Advancement in Medicine provides recommendations for dose and rates of administration, as well as guidelines for dietary supplements with multivitamins and trace elements that should be taken during therapy.
>
> Others, however, are not so confident that the procedure is 100 percent safe. The therapy removes important substances such as calcium and magnesium from the blood and should always be performed in a setting with emergency cardiac equipment (a crash cart) ready.

apy and offers education and training in chelation therapy.

Chelation therapy may be legally practiced by a licensed medical or osteopathic physician. Look for a physician who has additional training and certification in the procedure. Approximately 160 physicians in the United States are certified by the American Board of Chelation Therapy, which requires physicians to undergo special training, pass a written exam, and give 1,000 administrations of chelation therapy before becoming a Diplomate (DIPL). Physicians who are in the process of completing their requirements for certification are called Diplomate Candidates, or D/C. Another ACAM designation is Fellow, which means that the physician has some training in chelation therapy but does not fulfill all the requirements to be a candidate for certification.

RESOURCES

- American Board of Chelation Therapy
  1407-B North Wells St.
  Chicago, IL 60610
  800-356-2228
  The ABCT provides certification for physicians in chelation therapy. Call or send a self-addressed stamped envelope for the names of board certified physicians.

- American College of Advancement in Medicine
  23121 Verdugo Dr., Ste. 204
  Laguna Hills, CA 92653
  714-583-7666
  800-532-3688
  fax 714-455-9679
  The ACAM offers education on chelation therapy for physicians and provides a treatment protocol with recommendations for dosage and rates of administration and dietary supplementation during treatment. The college provides a list of recommended readings and a directory of practitioners.

Chiropractic Medicine

CHIROPRACTIC MEDICINE OPERATES ON THE THEORY THAT THE IMPROPER ALIGNMENT OF THE VERTEBRAE (THE BONES THAT MAKE UP THE SPINAL COLUMN) AND THE SPINAL CORD THEY PROTECT IS THE CAUSE OF DISEASES AND DISORDERS. CHIROPRACTORS APPLY PRESSURE IN A SPECIFIC MANNER TO ALLOW THE BODY TO REALIGN THE VERTEBRAE IN THE SPINAL COLUMN.

Within two years of performing the first chiropractic "adjustment," Daniel David Palmer started his Chiropractic School and Cure. Palmer's son Bartlett Joshua (B.J.) graduated from and then took over control of the school in 1904. Two years later, there was a split amongst faculty members who did not agree with B.J.'s assertion that subluxation (misalignment of the vertebrae of the spinal column) is the cause of all disease. This led to the development of other schools of chiropractic, most notably John Howard's National School of Chiropractic, as well as the development of a variety of manual therapies.

THE JOURNEY TO THE MAINSTREAM

Chiropractors have faced a long, hard road in gaining acceptance from mainstream medicine. In fact, allopathic physicians were so opposed to chiropractic medicine that the American Medical Association (AMA) labeled chiropractors as "quacks" and forbade its member physicians to even associate with them.

In the 1960s, the AMA established a "Committee on Quackery," which worked aggressively to cut off chiropractors from their patients. It declared that it was unethical for medical physicians to associate with them and it even passed a resolution calling chiropractic an "unscientific cult."

This all-out campaign to destroy the credibility of chiropractors led to a restraint of trade complaint against the AMA by Illinois chiropractor Chester Wilk and four other doctors of chiropractic. In 1987, a federal judge ruled that the AMA, the American College of Radiology, and the American College of Surgeons had conspired to intentionally harm the chiropractic profession and were guilty of violating the Sherman Antitrust Act by conducting an illegal boycott of chiropractors. The AMA was ordered to cease and desist its hampering of chiropractors and to send a copy of the injunction to each of its members. The ruling was upheld through a series of appeals, and when an effort to appeal the case to the Supreme Court failed, the AMA lifted its ban and notified its members that they were free to refer patients to, and accept referrals from, chiropractors.

HOW IT WORKS

Nerve impulses travel from the brain to the rest of the body through the spinal cord, which is encased in a tunnel of interlocking bones called the spinal column. The spinal column is made up of 24 vertebrae separated by disks. Sometimes one or more vertebrae or disks can be displaced, resulting in pressure on the nerve, pain or

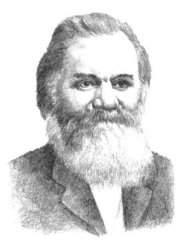

Daniel David Palmer

weakness, or other health problems.

Subluxation of the vertebrae refers to a misalignment of one or more of the vertebrae in the spinal column. Chiropractors perform "adjustments" to unlock subluxated vertebrae from their improperly aligned positions and restore normal nerve supply.

According to the World Chiropractic Alliance, chiropractors do not force misaligned vertebrae back into place, but work with the body's own inborn or innate intelligence, which knows how it should be aligned. Chiropractors believe that all living things have an innate intelligence that directs autonomic, or involuntary, functions, fights disease and infection, and heals damaged tissues. Chiropractic medicine attempts to help the body do its job to heal and to maintain the highest level of well-being possible.

The philosophy of chiropractic places strong emphasis on the body's ability to heal itself. Chiropractic seeks to help restore or maintain balance in the body, with the active participation of the patient. Chiropractors also believe that the nervous system is highly developed in humans and influences all other systems in the body. Therefore, the nervous system plays a significant role in health and disease. Chiropractors believe the presence of joint dysfunction and subluxation may interfere with the ability of the neuro-musculoskeletal system to act efficiently and may lead to disease.

WHAT IT IS

Chiropractors focus on dysfunctions that can result from irregularities of spinal structure or movement. They rely heavily on hands-on procedures to determine structural and functional problems, and they use manipulation to promote normal bodily function by correcting or preventing these structural deviations. Chiropractic "adjustment" refers to a variety of manual and mechanical interventions.

- *Manipulation* is movement of short amplitude and high velocity that moves the joint beyond where the patient's muscles could move the joint by themselves but short of ligament rupture.
- *Mobilization* is movements administered by the clinician within the physiologic joint space in order to increase overall range of motion.

Chiropractors have developed and refined a variety of manual therapies, particularly those known as high velocity and short amplitude. A number of systems have been developed and refined and may be used in a chiropractic session. These include

- activator technique
- applied kinesiology (see page 194)
- diversified technique
- flexion-distraction technique
- Gonstead technique
- Sacro-Occipital Technique, or SOT (see page 223)
- Thompson terminal technique

USES

Chiropractic is used both to maintain and to promote health, as well as to treat a variety of conditions. Adjustment of the spine normalizes the body's blood flow and allows the nervous system to balance itself—factors that affect every bodily organ and function. Many chiropractors assert that the method can optimize general health and help in the treatment of nonmusculoskeletal conditions, including

- headaches
- asthma
- digestive ailments

Skeptics in mainstream medicine, however, continue to question its use for these conditions. Although some promising results have been reported for other uses of chiropractic, these are often small studies or show mixed results.

RESEARCH PROBLEMS

The chiropractic profession has a long history of scientific research, but much of this early work was essentially lost because of difficulties in obtaining an appropriate forum for publishing. Even today, a visit to the Reading Room of the National Library of Medicine (the largest medical library in the world) will not yield a single journal devoted to chiropractic. In addition, chiropractic has been shut out from government funding for research studies, forcing the profession to rely on the limited resources of chiropractic colleges and the Foundation for Chiropractic Education and Research.

Conclusive scientific proof of the effectiveness of a treatment is based on large-scale studies involving hundreds of patients. These studies are very expensive to conduct. Whether the recent establishment of the Office of Alternative Medicine at the National Institutes of Health will help provide support for the studies needed in chiropractic and other areas of alternative medicine re-

mains to be seen. Current funding levels remain extremely low.

Despite these many difficulties, there are scientific studies that show that chiropractic medicine can positively affect health and is an effective treatment for a variety of conditions.

BACK PAIN

A London study of 741 men and women with lower-back pain found that patients treated by chiropractors reported 29 percent more improvement than those treated by standard medical practice in hospitals. The three-year study also found that patients treated by chiropractors reported more long-term satisfaction [1].

A Los Angeles study of 103 chiropractic patients and 187 medical patients with lower-back pain found that chiropractic care was at least as effective as medical care in reducing lower-back pain and functional disability and that patients who received chiropractic care were more satisfied with their treatment than medical patients. Three months after their initial visit, a greater proportion of chiropractic than medical patients perceived their treatment to be successful. More chiropractic patients reported they had no days with back pain in the preceding week and no functional impairment due to lower-back pain than did patients who received medical treatment [2].

A "meta-analysis" by the RAND Corporation looking at all published literature on the use of chiropractic manipulation for lower-back pain concluded that there is enough evidence to show chiropractic to be an effective treatment for a number of conditions that cause lower-back pain.

OTHER CONDITIONS

Recent studies suggest that spinal adjustment may be effective in many other conditions:

- painful menstrual periods
- migraine headaches
- infant colic
- carpal tunnel syndrome
- cervical disk herniation
- multiple sclerosis

Animal studies show that spinal manipulation can produce a number of physical responses, such as decreased blood pressure and renal and adrenal nerve activity. It may also enhance immune function by increasing metabolic rates of certain white blood cells and increasing other substances that play a role in immune regulation and inflammation. These studies also show that spinal adjustment can reduce levels of inflammatory prostaglandins and possibly increase levels of beta-endorphins, the natural painkillers in the body [3].

COST-EFFECTIVENESS AND PATIENT SATISFACTION

Perhaps more startling than its success stories in the scientific field is chiropractic's consistently high marks with individual patients. Chiropractic medicine continues to have a fiercely loyal following. It has also shown itself to be very cost-effective when compared with conventional medicine.

LOWER COSTS

An analysis of workers' compensation claims for back injuries in Australia found that the cost of chiropractic treatment was less than half that of standard medical treatment [4].

A Minnesota study compared the health care costs of patients who received chiropractic treatment in insurance plans that do not restrict chiropractic or medical benefits with those of patients treated solely by medical and osteopathic physicians. Researchers analyzed two years of claims data on total insurance payments and total outpatient payments and found that patients receiving reimbursed chiropractic care had significantly lower total health care costs and lower hospitalization rates than those who received only medical and osteopathic care [5].

A comparison of health care costs of patients who received chiropractic treatment for common neuro-musculo-skeletal disorders with costs of those treated solely by medical and osteopathic physicians found significantly lower health care costs among patients who received chiropractic care. The analysis of 395,641 patients found that nearly one-fourth were treated by chiropractors. Those patients who received chiropractic care experienced significantly lower health care costs, largely due to lower hospitalization rates than patients treated by medical physicians. The study's author suggests that insurance practices and programs that restrict chiropractic coverage should be reexamined [6].

THE FIRST TIME'S THE CHARM

The first patient to receive a chiropractic adjustment was Harvey Lillard in 1895. After having suffered from nerve deafness for 17 years, he is reported to have had his hearing restored.

BETTER CARE

A number of studies have also found that patients who visit chiropractors report more satisfaction with their care than those who visit conventional physicians for the same complaint. Whether this is a result of better effectiveness of chiropractic treatment for certain complaints or stems from the doctor–patient relationship is unclear.

A Minnesota survey of 541 chiropractic patients found high levels of satisfaction with their doctors and the care they received. Patients were most satisfied with the accessibility of their doctors and least satisfied with the financial aspects of treatment, particularly those with lower incomes and no insurance for chiropractic care [7].

PATIENT EDUCATION

Effective communication between practitioner and patient can be an important component in chiropractic care. An Indiana survey looked at 61 patients with lower-back pain and/or leg pain who attended a three-part lower-back wellness school conducted to teach them how to control their back pain in daily living. Almost all (95 percent) of the patients surveyed after the class responded that they felt it was worth their time to attend and that they felt they had learned something to prevent reinjury in daily living [8].

WHO DOES IT

There are more than 50,000 licensed practitioners in every state in the United States. Chiropractors see more than 15 million patients each year. Chiropractors are trained and licensed to use manual procedures and interventions, not surgical or drug therapies.

Modern chiropractic education consists of five years of training in chiropractic philosophy, basic and clinical science, and clinical care in outpatient settings. Degrees for the Doctor of Chiropractic are granted by 18 colleges in the United States that are accredited by the Council for Chiropractic Education, which has been recognized by the Department of Education since 1974 and by the Council on Postsecondary Accreditation since 1976. The extent of chiropractic practices varies from state to state.

A survey of state licensing authorities found that more than half allow chiropractors to order or perform clinical lab procedures, conduct components of a routine physical exam, and conduct electromyographic, electrocardiographic, and nerve-conduction studies. Most (more than 80 percent) allow chiropractors to perform and order a variety of X-ray procedures, as well as computed tomography and magnetic resonance imaging.

RESOURCES

- American Chiropractic Association
1701 Clarendon Blvd.
Arlington, VA 22209
703-276-8800
fax 703-243-2593
The Association offers an Information Resource Center (800-IRC-8448) as well as suggested readings and other materials on chiropractic.

- The World Chiropractic Alliance
2950 North Dobson, Ste. 1
Chandler, AZ 85224
800-347-1011
The Alliance offers fact sheets and general information on chiropractic.

Craniosacral Therapy

Just as the heartbeat signals the body's cardiac rhythm and breathing indicates respiratory rhythm, the craniosacral rhythm is created by the functioning of the craniosacral system—the head and spine. Craniosacral therapy monitors this rhythm and uses gentle, hands-on manipulations to correct abnormalities and enhance well-being.

HISTORY

The origins of craniosacral therapy can be traced back to the early 1900s, when William Sutherland, a Missouri osteopathic student, experimented with ways to manipulate the cranial bones. He called his technique craniosacral osteopathy. At Michigan State University in the 1970s, osteopath John Upledger did further research on the entire craniosacral system, resulting in the therapy now known as craniosacral therapy.

The word *cranio* is a Latin word referring to the head; *sacral* relates to the spine and tailbone. Thus, the craniosacral system comprises

- the brain and spinal cord
- the cerebrospinal fluid that envelops the brain and spinal cord
- the membranes (or meninges) that surround the brain, spinal cord, and cerebrospinal fluid
- the bones of the spine and skull that surround the meninges

Proper functioning of the craniosacral system is key to the health of the body's nervous system, which in turn is vital to overall well-being. During the normal workings of the craniosacral system, the pressure of the cerebrospinal fluid rises and falls. This produces a slight but perceptible wave-like motion known as the craniosacral rhythm.

DIAGNOSIS

A craniosacral therapist is trained to read the craniosacral rhythmic motion in the body by lightly touching with the hands. The locations at which it's easiest to detect this rhythm include the skull, the sacrum (the triangular bone at the base of the spine that forms the back of the pelvis), and the coccyx (tailbone)—the three sites that are attached to the membranes that encase the cerebrospinal fluid. By feeling the craniosacral rhythm, the therapist can diagnose any problems that may exist in the craniosacral system, and detect where there may be restrictions or dysfunctions. Then by using gentle, hands-on manipulations, the therapist makes adjustments to restore the craniosacral system's proper balance and healthy functioning.

TYPES

Today, different craniosacral therapists practice different methods. Three key approaches that have evolved over the years include sutural, meningeal, and reflex. Another system called Sacro-Occipital Technique blends aspects of all of the other three.

SUTURAL METHOD

Missouri osteopathic physician William Sutherland developed this technique in the early 1900s. It involves manipulating the bones of the skull at the places where they meet (called sutures). The idea is to relieve any pressures that may have built up, thus enhancing the functioning of the entire craniosacral system. Sutherland's technique came to be known as cranial osteopathy.

MENINGEAL METHOD

This method was the creation of John Upledger, a Michigan osteopathic physician who worked with a multidisciplinary team of health professionals and scientists at Michigan State University in the late 1970s. Upledger's technique focuses on manipulating the meninges, or the membrane that encases the brain, spinal cord, and cerebrospinal fluid.

REFLEX METHOD

This approach stimulates nerve endings in the scalp and between cranial sutures to relieve stress in the craniosacral system and elsewhere in the body. Applied kinesiology, developed by chiropractor George Goodheart, utilizes the reflex approach, along with specific cranial adjustments, to treat craniosacral problems. (For more on applied kinesiology, see page 194.)

SACRO-OCCIPITAL TECHNIQUE (SOT)

Created by Major DeJarnette, a chiropractor who studied under Sutherland in the 1920s, this method blends the three above methodologies. It's also known as craniopathy and aims to remove restrictions in the craniosacral system and between the cranial bones.

UNWINDING TO RELEASE TRAUMA

Unwinding is an advanced craniosacral therapy technique that helps the body to release previous trauma that manifests later as pain or dysfunction in the body. With this technique, the person undergoing treatment assumes the same position the body was in when the trauma happened. Unwinding releases the tension and serves as a self-correcting mechanism for the body.

This technique requires special training for the practitioner, who must be able to follow the client's movements during the procedure, while also staying attuned to the client's craniosacral rhythm. Some observers have likened these movements and countermovements in craniosacral therapy to dancing or the Chinese technique Tai Chi Chuan (see Traditional Chinese Medicine, pages 346–353).

USES

Abnormalities in the craniosacral system can result from injuries, spinal and cranial joint inflexibilities, and other dysfunctions in the body. Although the therapy can have application for many illnesses, conditions that craniosacral therapy often treats successfully include

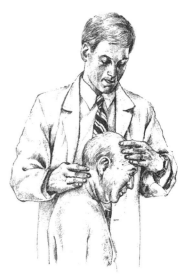

- trauma to the head and spine (resulting from car accidents, sports injuries, falls, and so on)
- chronic pain
- headache
- temporomandibular disorder (TMD)
- dizziness
- cerebral palsy
- neck and spine stiffness
- ear problems
- eye problems
- dyslexia
- hyperactivity
- learning difficulties
- balance problems
- autism
- mood disorders
- ringing in the ear (tinnitus)
- high or low blood pressure
- edema (swelling)
- recurrent infections
- stroke
- epilepsy
- some types of musculoskeletal conditions

SACRO-OCCIPITAL TECHNIQUE

Therapists who use SOT claim it has been found useful in treating additional conditions related to the central nervous system, as well as other disorders including diabetes, constipation, anxiety, impotence, asthma, cataracts, and inflammation.

TREATMENT IN CHILDREN

Craniosacral therapists say their techniques can be highly effective for children, especially for infants whose cranial bones and membranes are still in early stages of development. In fact, therapists point out that the birth process may be a trigger for craniosacral imbalances. These may result from a difficult delivery, the extreme backward extension of the head during delivery, improper use of forceps, suction procedures, and so on.

Also, improper nutrition before birth can cause facial and jaw bones to develop inadequately, which can lead to craniosacral problems later in life. For these reasons, craniosacral therapists suggest that infants receive treatment soon after birth. Craniosacral therapy also can be used to alleviate various problems during infancy, including

- earaches and ear infections
- sinus congestion
- vomiting
- irritability
- hyperactivity

WHO DOES IT

If you are interested in trying craniosacral therapy, first find a qualified practitioner. Ask where the therapist received training and which of the craniosacral therapy methodologies he or she uses.

Health care professionals from many disciplines have received training at the three centers mentioned below. Counted among these professionals are

- medical doctors
- osteopaths
- chiropractors
- naturopathic physicians
- physical therapists
- occupational therapists
- massage therapists
- dentists
- acupuncturists

RESOURCES

- Cranial Academy
  8606 Allisonville Rd., Ste. 130
  Indianapolis, IN 46250
  317-594-0411
  The academy teaches Sutherland's method of cranial osteopathy and provides referrals to its members.

- SORSI (SOT)
  P.O. Box 8245
  Prairie Village, KS 66208
  913-649-3475
  Teaches postgraduate courses and certifies chiropractors in DeJarnette's method, Sacro-Occipital Technique. Provides referrals to SOT practitioners.

- Upledger Institute
  11211 Prosperity Farms Rd.
  Palm Beach Gardens, FL 33410
  407-622-4706
  Teaches courses in Upledger's technique to health care professionals from many disciplines. It also has a clinic and provides general information to the public. A directory listing craniosacral therapists nationwide is available for $5 plus $2 shipping and handling.

Detoxification, Fasting & Colon Therapy

WE LIVE IN AN INCREASINGLY POLLUTED WORLD. OUR BODIES HAVE BECOME STOREHOUSES FOR PESTICIDE RESIDUES, HEAVY METALS, FOOD ADDITIVES, CHEMICAL CONTAMINANTS, PHARMACEUTICALS, INDUSTRIAL POLLUTANTS, AND OTHER TOXIC SUBSTANCES. DETOXIFICATION THERAPY HELPS US TO CLEANSE OUR BODIES, THUS IMPROVING VITALITY AND BOOSTING OUR ABILITY TO FIGHT MANY TYPES OF ILLNESS.

The air we breathe, the food we eat, and the water we drink all bear multiple toxic pollutants—many of which we can't taste or see or smell. Our bodies' own metabolism produces toxic by-products, too. Plus, we may take in additional toxic substances by choice, such as tobacco, alcohol, pharmaceuticals, illegal drugs, caffeine, and others.

The body has a natural ability to neutralize and eliminate these toxins. The liver, the kidneys, the respiratory system, and bodily processes such as perspiration and elimination do their part to filter out and cleanse the body of toxins. But occasionally, the contaminants may be more than our bodies can handle, resulting in heightened vulnerability to various health disorders. Detoxification therapy is a way to help the body cope with the overload of toxins it's subjected to by life in the modern world.

TYPES OF TOXINS

Various types of toxins can accumulate in the body. Some are external pollutants; others are substances the body itself produces. The body's capacity to rid itself of these contaminants is crucial to optimum health.

Heavy Metals—These include aluminum, nickel, cadmium, arsenic, mercury, and lead. Industrial pollution and automobile exhaust are major sources of heavy-metal contaminants. Exposure to mercury can come from contaminated fish or dental fillings; aluminum is found in cookware and antacids; and cadmium and lead are components of cigarette smoke. Effects on the body are diverse. Headache, indigestion, tremors, anemia, dizziness, coordination problems, fatigue, and constipation have all been linked to exposure to heavy metals. Several studies over the years have cited exposure to heavy metals as a possible cause of childhood learning disorders and even criminal behaviors.

Chemicals—Today these come in an astounding number of forms: pesticides, herbicides, solvents (such as cleaning materials, formaldehyde, and benzene), food additives, and dry-cleaning fluids, to name only a few. Adverse effects on the body can include nervous system impairment, allergies, cancers, headaches, depression, and mental confusion.

Microbial Compounds—These are toxins produced by bacteria and yeast in the gut. These substances can be absorbed into the bloodstream and have been linked to various disorders, such as liver diseases, ulcerative colitis, thyroid disease, allergies, immune disorders, and other health problems.

HISTORY

Detoxification practices go way back in history. A few examples: Ancient Greeks and Romans used enemas as a sort of internal bath. Native Americans have long used sweat lodges and fasting to purify the body and mind. And among the world's major religions, Hinduism, Christianity, Islam, and Judaism all include fasting traditions.

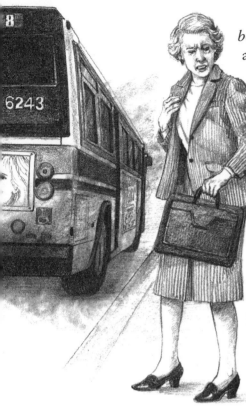

Waste Products of Metabolism—Waste products, such as ammonia and urea, are produced by the body when proteins are broken down. The kidneys do most of the work of eliminating these substances. Drinking plenty of water and eating a balanced diet with primarily easy-to-digest proteins are keys to helping the kidneys perform this purification function adequately.

BENEFITS OF DETOXIFICATION

Detoxification proponents point to several benefits:
- greater resistance to health disorders, including serious conditions such as cancer, heart diseases, obesity, and arthritis
- reduced blood pressure
- reduced cholesterol and triglycerides (culprits in heart conditions)
- better digestion and assimilation of nutrients
- increased mental alertness
- clearing up skin problems
- help in quitting smoking
- better resistance to allergies
- enhanced physical energy

FINDING TOXINS

One way to find out whether detoxification therapy can benefit a given condition is to have your stool, urine, blood, liver function, or hair analyzed. Stool, urine, blood, and hair can be examined for specific toxins or the byproducts of the body's attempt to eliminate toxins. Examination of hair can be very telling, as toxins are often stored in hair as it grows, giving a timeline of environmental exposure. Liver function tests reveal how hard the body's main toxin filter is working. An overtaxed liver can indicate significant toxin buildup.

Another way to determine if you need detoxification is to look for cues from your body, including
- headaches
- joint pain
- allergies
- ulcers
- skin conditions
- constipation
- back pain
- insomnia
- sinus congestion
- mood swings
- hemorrhoids
- recurrent respiratory problems
- fatigue
- lack of mental clarity

FASTING

Say the word *fasting* and most people think of starving saints and people on hunger strikes. But fasting advocates claim that it's a technique for renewal and rejuvenation, not harsh deprivation, and that it comes naturally: When, for instance, an illness

---

WHILE YOU'RE FASTING ...

- Avoid strenuous exercise, so as to conserve your energy for healing.
- Give yourself plenty of rest; take naps, and relax.
- Wash or brush your skin to aid elimination through the skin, but don't use harsh soaps, shampoos, deodorants, and so on. These just add to the detoxification load.

causes you to avoid food for a day or two, it may be your body's way of communicating what it needs for healing. Among the detoxification methods, fasting is the easiest and least expensive.

Length—Fasting periods can range from a day or two to a month or longer. Short fasts are a good technique for tuning up your body's well-being and energy or for fending off mild diseases such as flu or colds. Some people regularly fast one day every week, for example. Longer fasts are suited for combating more serious conditions, such as arthritis or chronic headaches.

Supervision—Short fasts (three days or less) can usually be done without supervision, but health care professionals stress that any fast of more than a couple days should be done under professional guidance. Obviously, the longer you fast, the more critical it is that you have someone monitoring how you're doing. Even for a short fast, however, you might want to talk it over with your health care professional first. Whatever fasting duration you choose, select a time for fasting when there are few demands in your life. You'll be able to rest more and conserve your energy for healing.

Fluids—During a fast, you need to take in fluids, but experts disagree on whether you should include fruit and vegetable juices or just water. Some therapists recommend either juices or water; others argue that if you're drinking juices you're not really fasting because you're taking in some sustenance. (Unsweetened herbal teas usually count as just water.) Both types of fasts can be effective, and it is usually a matter of individual choice.

AVOID FASTING IF ...

- You have a debilitating disease that is leaving you weak and causing you to lose weight.
- You are on certain medications, such as steroids and anti-inflammatory agents.
- You have insulin-dependent diabetes.
- You are scared or turned off by the whole idea of fasting.

Special Limited Diets—A variation on the fasting approach is to not avoid food entirely, but to eat only certain foods during a given period of time. For instance, the monodiet approach calls for eating only one food, such as apples or rice. Special limited diets are not simply fad diets; any kind of special diet detoxification regime should be discussed with a health care practitioner experienced in detoxification.

Breaking the Fast—How you come off a fast is just as important as the fast itself. Flipping from fasting to feasting will quickly undo any healing benefits gained. Experts advise starting out with juices, fruits, and vegetables and then working back to a wholesome, varied diet. The longer the fast period, the more gradual the reintroduction to foods will need to be. The same is also true for the beginning of a fast; start preparing for a fast by eating only rice and vegetables for a few days before the fast begins, and don't forget to drink plenty of water.

COLON THERAPY

Colon therapy (also called colon hydrotherapy) cleanses and detoxifies the large intestine by irrigating it with purified water. Vitamins, herbs, helpful bacteria, or oxygen also may be added to the water.

This procedure dates back to the 1890s, when Dr. Elmer Lee designed an irrigating apparatus to use for cholera patients. In fact, the origins of colon therapy can be traced much further back to the Ancient Egyptians who performed enemas (which are only partial colonic irrigation) by using reeds to introduce water into the body through the rectum. As recently as the 1940s, colon therapy was still being used to treat various diseases, but fell into disuse with the advent of antibiotics and other drugs. Today, however, many natural health practitioners, as well as some mainstream doctors, view colon therapy as an effective detoxification therapy.

The colon is a roughly five-foot section of the large intestine. It's the last part of the digestive system where nutrients and water can be extracted from food before it is eliminated. Stagnant waste products and toxic substances can accumulate along the colon walls over time if the colon is not functioning as it should. Some of the key causes for this malfunctioning might include

- emotional stress
- physical stress or defects, such as genetic problems or a neurological impairment
- bad diet and health habits, such as not eating enough fiber, eating too much fatty food, or eating too fast
- not drinking enough water (However, drinking too much water with meals can dilute digestive enzymes, contributing to waste buildup problems.)
- drinking caffeinated beverages (such as coffee, tea, colas) that dehydrate the stool, making it harder to move along through elimination
- having been bedridden for a while, so that your colonic functions have become sluggish

When wastes collect and stagnate, toxins can be released into the bloodstream and can then be distributed throughout the body. This, colon therapists believe, is a major reason for disease and poor health. Flushing the colon with a gentle flow of water dislodges the wastes and other toxins and pushes them out of the body. It may also exercise and tone the colon, allowing it to function more efficiently. The colon therapist might massage the colon through the abdomen during the therapy to help break up collected materials.

Colonic irrigation is one way to cleanse the colon. Another is to ingest certain herbs or other substances, such as psyllium seed husks, which loosen and break up stagnated materials in the colon. (If you use the psyllium, it is very important to increase your intake of water to ensure that it doesn't block the colon and actually worsen the con-

---

COLON THERAPY CAUTIONS

Be sure the colon therapist takes all necessary precautions to avoid spread of communicable diseases from one patient to another via the colonic equipment. Sterilization or use of disposable parts is crucial in preventing the spread of any kind of infection.

dition.) You might also use this type of colonic therapy as a follow-up to colonic irrigation.

CHOOSING A COLON THERAPIST

Finding a therapist you feel comfortable with is the first crucial step in getting effective colon therapy. You may want to do a preinterview before setting up an appointment. Ask about the training and certification the therapist has received. Some states have certification programs. Qualified colon therapists should be informed about all aspects of this therapy: colonic anatomy and physiology, colonic disorders, contraindications to therapy, coping with aftereffects, ethics, safety, and sanitation.

WHAT TO EXPECT

Many patients describe coming out of a therapy session feeling light and calm. Some people feel very tired after a colonic, and it is not uncommon for patients to sleep for hours after the procedure. Colon therapy can stimulate a general overall body cleansing; in the aftermath of a colonic, other organs may also eliminate wastes and toxins. Therefore, some people experience diarrhea, flu, or vomiting. Some people also experience emotional releases as part of the cleansing.

You should drink plenty of room-temperature (not cold) water after a colonic treatment. Your therapist might also advise you to take nutritional supplements to replace lost potassium, cell salts, and acidophilus (a helpful bacteria for digestion) and may suggest you also do other detoxification routines, such as fasting or a sauna.

OTHER DETOXIFICATION THERAPIES

CHELATION THERAPY

Chelation is a medical process used to remove toxic metals, such as lead and cadmium, from the bloodstream. The chelating agent, which is a synthetic amino acid, binds with the metals and exits with them through the kidneys. Many United States medical doctors offer chelation therapy. (Chelation therapy is discussed in its own chapter, pages 214–216.)

VITAMIN C THERAPY

Vitamin C has become widely recognized in recent years for its role in healing. It also enhances the body's ability to detoxify naturally. Some researchers believe vitamin C bolsters our ability to fend off environmental pollutants and that it neutralizes toxins in the body. (See also Nutritional Therapy, pages 303–333.)

HYPERTHERMIA

Hyperthermia takes the form of saunas, hot baths, steam baths, sweat lodges, and high-tech medical procedures. By raising the body's temperature above normal, invading organisms susceptible to heat can be eradicated from the body. Hyperthermia also purifies by facilitating elimination of body wastes through sweating. Toxins such as pesticides, chemicals, or drug residues also can be expelled. Negative responses might occur when certain toxins are released, so medical supervision is essential. (Hyperthermia is discussed on pages 269–271.)

USES

The detoxification process of one kind or another has been used for al-

---

WHO SHOULD AVOID DETOXIFICATION?

If your health is fragile, proceed extremely cautiously with detoxification. Do it only with the advice and guidance of a health professional who is experienced in detoxification processes. Among those who need to be extra careful are people who

- are recovering drug users or alcoholics
- have been taking many medications
- have eating disorders
- have diabetes
- are recuperating from surgery
- are underweight
- have a serious illness that has left them physically weak
- have hypothyroidism
- are hyperglycemic

Some of the most common therapeutic uses, though, include

- headaches
- allergies
- constipation
- chronic fatigue

RESOURCES

- International Association of Hygienic Physicians
  Regency Health Resource and Spa
  204 Stambaugh Bldg.
  Youngstown, OH 44503
  330-746-5000

  Members are doctors who specialize in fasting supervision. Referral list of physicians available.

- International Association of Colon Therapy
  2204 Northwest Loop, #410
  San Antonio, TX 78230-5352
  210-366-2888

  Provides referrals to colon therapists nationwide. Presents seminars and training for the general public and health professionals. Certifies teachers. Publishes pamphlets for general information and a quarterly newsletter for therapists.

most every conceivable condition and health objective—from general health promotion and prevention to psychological problems and serious diseases. Different people find detoxification useful for different problems, and almost everyone's experience is different.

Environmental Medicine

IN ENVIRONMENTAL MEDICINE, THE CAUSES OF ILLNESSES ARE SOUGHT IN THE SUBSTANCES THAT ARE FOUND IN THE INDIVIDUAL'S SURROUNDINGS. INDEED, RESPONSES TO FOODS, CHEMICALS IN THE HOME AND WORKPLACE, AND COMMON ALLERGENS, SUCH AS DANDER, DUST AND DUST MITES, MOLDS, AND POLLENS, ARE IMPLICATED IN MANY AILMENTS. INDIVIDUAL RESPONSES TO THESE EXPOSURES VARY AND ARE SPECIFIC TO EACH PERSON'S LEVEL OF SUSCEPTIBILITY. ILLNESS CAN BE THE RESULT OF A LARGE ONE-TIME EXPOSURE, OR LOW LEVEL, GRADUAL EXPOSURES.

Humans are wonderfully adaptable in their efforts to deal with hostile environments, but they are not infinitely adaptable. The nature of a person's interactions with different foods and environmental exposures changes dynamically over time and is individually specific. Every person's immune system is different and reacts in various ways and with various intensity to different environmental substances. The way an individual's immune system reacts may play a big role in many illnesses, and this is precisely what environmental medicine explores.

WHAT IT IS

Strictly speaking, practitioners of environmental medicine assess the impact of environmental factors on health. They study the relationship between chemicals, foods, inhalants, and other stressors in the environment and the functioning of the individual.

Environmental medicine began with the identification of many different symptoms caused by allergies to common foods, such as corn, wheat, milk, and eggs. Using Herbert Rinkel's method of unmasking food allergies by avoiding suspect foods for four days, Dr. Randolph identified food-related triggers for conditions such as

- anxiety
- arthritis
- asthma
- colitis
- depression
- fatigue
- hyperactivity

Researchers soon began to look at the effects of chemicals, such as car emissions, formaldehyde, industrial solvents, natural gas, and pesticides. Dr. Randolph found that some people are more sensitive to exposure of even small amounts of these compounds and that illness could be triggered in these people by the amounts of chemicals that others could tolerate without any evident symptoms.

Illness may be caused by a broad range of substances, such as chemicals found in the home and workplace; chemicals in the air, water, and food; and inhalants such as dust, dust mites, molds, and pollen. Specific responses to these exposures vary from individual to individual. Practitioners of environmental medicine seek to learn why a particular patient has a particular symptom at a particular time.

HISTORY

In the 1940s, Theron Randolph, the father of environmental medicine, identified a wide range of medical problems he believed were caused by food allergies. His work developed methods still used today to test for the role of food allergies in a number of conditions. In the 1950s, Dr. Randolph's work expanded to focus on health problems caused by sensitivity to small amounts of chemicals, such as car exhaust, pesticides, and solvents.

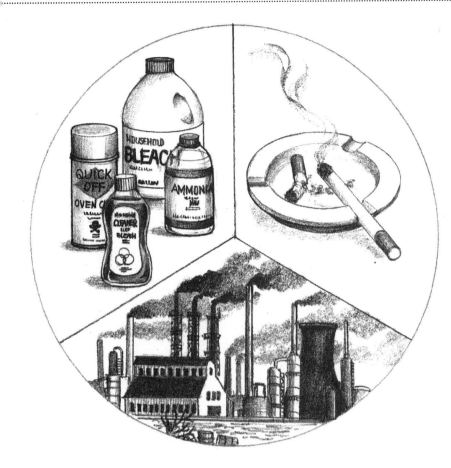

Although environmental medicine practitioners believe that toxic substances affect everyone exposed, they acknowledge that small amounts may affect only persons who are unusually susceptible to the material. For example, 10 percent of people are highly sensitive to small amounts of formaldehyde, whereas 90 percent are not. This may lead to patients being misdiagnosed or labeled as hypochondriacs. An estimated 4 million to 5 million Americans are believed to have illnesses related to chemical sensitivities, but only about 5 percent of these have been identified and treated.

In addition to conditions that are considered traditional allergic reactions, such as asthma and hay fever, environmental medicine physicians treat other conditions for which the immunologic basis is not yet fully understood, including

- arthritis (and other autoimmune diseases)
- attention deficit disorder
- cardiovascular disease
- colitis
- depression
- fatigue
- migraines

PRINCIPLES OF ENVIRONMENTAL MEDICINE

Susceptibility is the possibility of a person falling ill because of some abnormal interaction between a patient and his or her diet or environment. This could be due to an allergy, hypersensitivity, or intolerance. Factors that can affect a person's susceptibility include genetics, nutritional status, stress, the body's ability to detoxify, and the total allergic and chemical load the person is enduring at the time.

Environmental medicine is based on five governing principles:
- total load
- adaptation
- bipolarity of responses
- spreading phenomenon
- switch phenomenon

TOTAL LOAD

Total load is the sum total, at any one time, of all the stressors to which an individual is susceptible. Because a person's total load is always changing (depending on what foods a person has eaten, what substances they may have been in contact with, and what kind of emotional stresses they have encountered), reactions and symptoms can vary considerably over time and even from hour to hour and day to day.

ADAPTATION

Adaptation is when the body attempts to maintain balance by adjusting to the changing environmental conditions. This adaptation takes place in the following stages that may change from time to time:

- Preadapted and nonadapted alarm stage—when initial symptoms occur in response to an environmental stressor encountered for the first time.
- Adapted, or masked, stage—when the body adjusts to the stressor and the initial symptoms fade.
- Maladapted stage—when the accommodations the body has made in response to a stressor cause other health problems.
- Nonadapted exhaustion stage—the final stage when more serious symptoms occur that may damage and scar chronically inflamed tissues.

For example, a wheat allergy may initially cause a symptom such as fatigue. Then there is a period with no symptoms until, after more exposures, other symptoms, such as migraine headaches, may occur. The final stage—nonadapted exhaustion stage—occurs when the body is so overloaded that serious and sometimes irreversible health problems crop up.

BIPOLARITY OF RESPONSES

Bipolarity refers to the changing nature of environmental illnesses. Initial responses often have a clear environmental trigger, but later symptoms may persist even in the absence of a trigger. This puzzling phenomenon may be caused by tissue changes brought on by the long-term (chronic) allergic condition.

SPREADING PHENOMENON

The spreading phenomenon is the new onset of acute or chronic sensitivity to substances that were previously tolerated, or the spread of susceptibility to organs not previously affected. This spreading phenomenon is frequently seen when people who have had a single large exposure to a pesticide or solvent begin to react to many other chemicals.

SWITCH PHENOMENON

This means that symptoms can change and affect different organ systems from one time to another.

DIAGNOSIS

Environmental medicine practitioners use conventional diagnostic procedures, physical exams, and laboratory tests (such as blood and skin) to detect allergies. A key component in diagnosis by an environmental medicine physician (sometimes called a clinical ecologist), however, is a detailed chronological history that looks at the patient's environment and stressors over time. Environmental medicine practitioners require a detailed history that can provide important clues to a patient's illness. Careful listening and detailed medical histories allow physicians to learn from patients. Therefore, diagnosis and treatment is highly individualized in environmental medicine to take into account each patient's individual biochemistry and unique susceptibility.

Environmental physicians also look for special symptoms such as shiny dark circles and/or swelling below the eyes ("allergic shiners"), coated tongue, hair loss, spots on the nails, and a line across the bridge of the nose caused by frequent wiping (the "allergic salute"). Diagnostic techniques may also include tests to determine metabolic function, immune system function, endocrine system function, and nutritional status.

Sometimes patients with complex multiple sensitivities are evaluated in environmental control units that are free of all common exposures. Often the patients fast or go on hypoallergenic diets until all of their symptoms disappear. Then they are exposed to certain foods and chemicals to determine their response and the cause of their illness. (This process is called *challenging*.) Other methods of investigation include blood tests, electroacupuncture testing, and examination of the patient's environment by trained researchers with special equipment to test for common irritants.

TREATMENT

Education about what substances to avoid and how to avoid them successfully is a key part of treatment by an environmental medicine physician. Dietary management involves avoiding certain foods altogether and adopting a four-day rotation diet, which reduces sensitivity to foods by ensuring that the patient is not exposed to the same food or food group more frequently than once every four days.

Nutritional supplements are often prescribed to correct dysfunctions and to help improve detoxification pathways within the body. Patients are also advised to avoid emotional stressors.

Sometimes immunotherapy is used when it is not possible for a patient to avoid a stressor. This therapy attempts to neutralize the reaction by giving extremely small amounts of the substance to build up the body's tolerance for it. In the therapy called provocative neutralization, patients are tested using several dilutions of environmental extracts until symptoms occur; then, a weaker dilution of the same extract is used as therapy. (Sometimes, this desensitization can also be accomplished orally with homeopathics.)

DISEASES WITH ENVIRONMENTAL CAUSES

A number of studies have shown compelling evidence that a variety of conditions are, in fact, due to environmental causes. Studies have found that patients with chronic conditions often written off as "psychosomatic" share striking similarities to those with chemical sensitivities.

One study compared 90 persons with either chronic fatigue syndrome, fibromyalgia, or multiple chemical sensitivities. These conditions are all associated with fatigue and a variety of other symptoms. The investigators found that patients in the three groups were remarkably similar in demographic characteristics and in the specific symptoms that they noted [1].

FIBROMYALGIA

Between 2 and 4 percent of Americans are affected with fibromyalgia, a disabling disorder of the immune system that causes a variety of symptoms, such as pain, fatigue, and mood and sleep disorders. But patients with fibromyalgia—and other chronic conditions such as chronic fatigue syndrome—are often dismissed as being hypochondriacs, despite clear evidence of the autoimmune nature of their disease.

A recent controlled study of 51 patients with fibromyalgia found that just eliminating allergic substances in the diet and home and providing nutritional supplementation can significantly decrease pain and accompanying depression. The study compared 40 patients whose blood was first tested for food and environmental sensitivities then provided with individualized diets and nutritional supplementation, with 11 control subjects. The treated patients had 15 to 32 multiple food or environmental sensitivities, whereas the control group reacted to only a few of the items on the test. The most common sensitivities were to monosodium glutamate (MSG), yeast, caffeine, food coloring, chocolate, shrimp, and dairy products.

Patients were given detailed dietary guidelines to help them avoid substances they were sensitive to. By four months, most of the treatment group reported feeling markedly better than they had in the past years, despite prior failures with other treatments. At the end of six months, treated fibromyalgia patients had more than a 50 percent reduction in pain, whereas the control group reported an increase in pain. Treated patients also reported less depression, whereas those in the control group had higher depression scores than at the beginning. Treated patients rated their overall health as twice as good as it had been before the program [2].

MIGRAINE

Food allergies have long been implicated in migraine headaches. One study found that two-thirds of people with severe migraines have allergies to certain foods [3].

A study of children with severe, frequent migraines found that 93 percent recovered when placed on special diets to avoid substances to which they were sensitive. The study compared 40 children with a control group that did not undergo individualized dietary modification [4].

THROMBOPHLEBITIS

Thrombophlebitis is a condition in which veins (usually in the legs) become inflamed, allowing blood clots to form. The condition can be uncomfortable and very dangerous. A five-year study of 20 disabled patients with recurrent intractable phlebitis found that treatment focusing on the removal of environmental triggers results in significant improvement over conventional therapy.

The patients were divided into two groups: The control group received standard anticlotting medication, bed rest, and support hose. Patients in the treatment group were placed in a specially designed environmental control unit where air, food, and water could be controlled. They were taken off all medication and not fed until their leg swelling and pain had disappeared, which occurred in about four to seven days. When tested for specific sensitivities to foods and inhaled chemicals such as formaldehyde, eight of ten experienced phlebitis again. When symptom-free, the patients were able to ride an exercise bike for one mile daily, whereas none was able to walk across the room at the beginning of the study.

Five years later, patients in the environmental treatment group reported only two 48-hour episodes of phlebitis that cleared up upon bed rest and food abstinence. Those in the control group that received conventional therapy experienced more than 60 episodes of phlebitis at home and 41 episodes in the hospital [5].

WHO DOES IT

Environmental medicine practitioners are graduates of conventional medical and osteopathic schools and may be certified in a variety of conventional specialties. More than 3,000 physicians, most in the United States, Canada, and England, practice environmental medicine.

Although trained in conventional allopathic medicine, these physicians have an expanded view of health and illness that includes an emphasis on the role the environment plays in a variety of disorders. Environmental medicine practitioners describe their field as "comprehensive patient-oriented medicine," but their broader range of thinking about the cause of illness and

their comprehensive treatment approach has led them to be classified as "alternative" practitioners. Many naturopathic physicians also use environmental medicine as a major component in their practices.

RESOURCES

- American Academy of Environmental Medicine
4510 West 89th St., Ste. 110
Prairie Village, KS 66207
913-642-6062
fax 913-341-6912
Established in 1965, AAEM provides general information on environmental medicine and a list of providers. The Academy issues practice guidelines and makes available its detailed history questionnaire for patient assessment. AAEM offers seminars and courses for physicians in environmental medicine. Full members have undergone training and an examination in the field of environmental medicine.

Guided Imagery & Visualization

IMAGERY IS THE PROCESS OF IMAGINING THROUGH ANY SENSE—HEARING, SIGHT, SMELL, TASTE, OR TOUCH. SOMETIMES THE WORD IMAGERY IS USED IN THE SAME WAY AS VISUALIZATION, BUT VISUALIZATION REFERS ONLY TO SEEING SOMETHING IN THE MIND'S EYE.

WHAT IT IS

Imagery is commonly used as a technique to encourage changes in attitudes, behavior, or physiologic reactions. It is used in a wide variety of therapies and may also be used as a form of meditation. A number of therapies include imagery in their work, including

- autogenic training
- biofeedback
- desensitization and counterconditioning
- Gestalt therapy
- hypnosis
- Jungian active imagination
- neurolinguistic programming
- rational emotive therapy
- relaxation techniques
- Transcendental Meditation

Imagery can be taught individually or in groups and is often used for specific purposes, such as bolstering the immune system to attack cancer cells. It has been shown to affect a number of functions, such as the following:

- brain-wave activity
- blood glucose levels
- cardiovascular function
- gastrointestinal activity
- oxygen supply in tissues

MENTAL REHEARSAL

Imagery can be used to help relieve anxiety, pain, and side effects from medical techniques. An integral part of natural childbirth training, imagery can be helpful in a variety of other situations, such as burn debridement.

"Rehearsing" a surgery or difficult procedure before it happens helps patients to be prepared and to get rid of unrealistic fantasies. Patients are taught coping techniques such as abdominal breathing, distraction, mental dissociation, and muscle relaxation.

These mental rehearsals, also known as sensory education, can have dramatic results, including

- reduced pain and anxiety
- shorter hospital stays
- use of less medication

IMAGERY AS THERAPY

Imagery may be best known as a way to help patients mobilize their immune system. It has also shown results in alleviating nausea and vomiting from cancer chemotherapy and in reducing pain. Patients are shown how to use their own flow of images about the healing process or are guided through a series of images intended to soothe and focus attention elsewhere.

Imagery has been used in a number of therapeutic settings to

- enhance immunity
- relieve stress
- treat aspects of heart disease, diabetes, and chronic pain

TYPES OF IMAGERY

Components of imagery are used in a variety of therapeutic approaches.

HISTORY

Imagery has been used to promote healing and happiness since ancient times. Shamanism is one kind of healing that employs the use of the mind or imagination, but there are many forms.

The following are some of the terms you may come across:

Creative Visualization—Popularized by Shakti Gawain in her 1979 book, *Creative Visualization*, this term refers to the use of mental energy to improve health and life situations through affirmations, exercises, and meditations to make positive ideas and concepts become a reality.

Guided Imagery—Guided imagery frequently employs audiotapes and other methods to help people imagine specific images, such as calming situations, or to imagine that their body's immune system is attacking cancer cells.

Interactive Guided Imagery—Interactive guided imagery seeks to enhance awareness of the unconscious imagery patients already have and help them learn tools to mobilize their innate healing abilities. For example, patients

may be asked to close their eyes and imagine a picture that represents their problem. They may then be guided in an imaginary dialogue with the image to explore and reveal its meaning. Such images can provide information about the problem, as well as the person's beliefs, hopes, fears, and resources.

USES

Imagery is used in a variety of ways, from evaluation and diagnosis to mental rehearsal and therapy.

DIAGNOSIS AND EVALUATION

Imagery can be used for diagnosis and evaluation by asking patients to describe their condition in sensory terms. In psychotherapy, for example, patients may be asked about their dreams to gain insight into a situation. From this imagery information a practitioner can provide the basis for mental rehearsal and therapy strategies.

ANXIETY

A study of 51 patients undergoing abdominal surgery found that those who were taught guided imagery before surgery had less postoperative pain than those who did not. They were also less distressed by the surgery, felt as if they coped with it better, and requested less pain medication than patients who did not practice imagery [1].

Magnetic resonance imaging is a diagnostic test in which patients must lie still inside a cylindrical tube. The procedure can be anxiety producing because of concerns about what it may find and the claustrophobic feelings from being inside the cramped machine.

A study of 41 patients found that those who listened to a guided im-

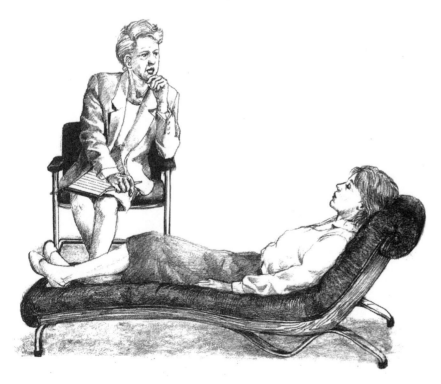

agery/relaxation tape before their magnetic resonance scan and used guided imagery during their scan had less anxiety and moved less frequently during the procedure than those who did not use the techniques [2].

The use of imagery is not limited to adults. A study of 24 children undergoing cardiac catheterization found that those who were taught imagery displayed fewer distress behaviors during the procedure [3].

BREAST-FEEDING

Mothers of babies who are born prematurely and are hospitalized in neonatal intensive care units often want to express breast milk to feed their babies. However, their milk production can frequently be inhibited by anxiety, fatigue, and stress.

A study of 55 mothers found that those who listened to a 20-minute audiocassette tape of relaxation and guided imagery training produced 63 percent more breast milk than those who did not receive any relaxation training [4].

CANCER

A study of 38 cancer patients compared those who practiced imagery in combination with chemotherapy with those who did not. The patients in the imagery group learned mental imagery techniques and were given two imagery audiotapes to listen to daily. After four months, those who practiced imagery were found to have significantly better function of cancer-attacking cells than those patients who did not practice imagery. Six months later, patients in both groups had significant increases in disease state. However, after one year, fewer patients in the imagery group had died (14 percent) than in the control group (36 percent) [5].

Another study of 154 women with early breast cancer compared those using relaxation therapy or relaxation plus imagery with a control group undergoing neither therapy. At six weeks, women in the relaxation plus imagery group were more relaxed than those who received relaxation training only, whereas the mood of women in the control group worsened [6].

Guided imagery has also been found to be effective in reducing symptoms associated with cancer chemotherapy. A study of 28 cancer patients undergoing chemotherapy found that those who used chemotherapy-specific guided imagery reported a significantly more positive experience with therapy than those who did not [7].

IMMUNE ENHANCEMENT

A study of 45 college students found that guided imagery can increase antibody production. The study compared students who were taught to focus on the immune system and who were given a tape with guided imagery instructions with students who were not. Antibodies to fight infection were significantly higher in the therapy group than in the other subjects [8].

MOTOR SKILLS ENHANCEMENT

A study of 32 adolescents with mild mental retardation found that those who used both physical practice plus imagery practice before carrying out a task performed the task with significantly greater accuracy than those who used physical practice alone [9].

Imagery is widely used by athletes and coaches alike to enhance athletic performance. Although a number of studies have suggested that guided imagery can enhance sports performance, others have found no evidence that imagery is successful in improving physical performance. Further research will undoubtedly address the technique's usefulness in this area.

POSTPARTUM DEPRESSION

Postpartum depression can be alleviated by imagery, recent studies have found. A study of 60 first-time mothers found that those who practiced guided imagery during the first four weeks after delivery had less anxiety and depression and greater self-esteem than women who did not [10].

SMOKING CESSATION

As any former or current smoker can tell you, quitting cigarettes can be an arduous task. In fact, many ex-smokers fail to stay off cigarettes even after completing smoking cessation programs. Relapse rates of 60 to 80 percent are common even for people who make it through such programs.

People who start smoking again identify stress as a major factor in their picking up another pack. Studies confirm that staying off cigarettes is closely related to the coping skills of the ex-smoker in dealing with stress.

An Ohio study of 76 people who had successfully completed a smoking cessation program found that training in relaxation imagery results in significantly reduced stress and lower relapse rates. The study compared ex-smokers who were trained in imagery techniques to those who attended support groups with no imagery training. Imagery techniques used included positive images of improved health, thoughts to delay a return to smoking and to distract, and deep breathing and relaxation methods. After three months, 72 percent of the imagery group had stayed off cigarettes and only 28 percent had relapsed, whereas 49 percent of the control group relapsed [11].

WHO DOES IT

Imagery is practiced and taught by a wide variety of conventional and alternative health care professionals. Nurses, who have traditionally focused on the whole person, are among practitioners in the forefront of imagery as a therapeutic intervention. Much of the recent research on the use of imagery in healing has been conducted by doctorally trained nurses, but many different types of practitioners use the technique.

RESOURCES

- The Academy for Guided Imagery
  P.O. Box 2070
  Mill Valley, CA 94942
  800-726-2070
  fax 415-389-9342

The Academy for Guided Imagery has provided training and certification in Interactive Guided Imagery to more than 10,000 health professionals such as clinical social workers, counselors, physicians, and nurses. The Academy publishes a directory of imagery practitioners and sponsors conferences on mind/body issues in cancer treatment, heart disease, and emotional and spiritual healing.

HERBAL MEDICINE IS OFTEN THE FIRST THING YOU THINK OF WHEN SOMEONE MENTIONS ALTERNATIVE THERAPIES. INDEED, HERBS ARE THE BASIS OF MANY DIFFERENT MEDICINAL SYSTEMS AROUND THE WORLD. ESPECIALLY POPULAR IN ASIA, INDIA, AND EUROPE, HERBAL MEDICINE IS USED BY AN ESTIMATED 80 PERCENT OF THE WORLD'S POPULATION. MODERN CONVENTIONAL MEDICINE OWES MUCH TO ITS HERBAL PAST. DRUG COMPANIES STILL USE THE NATURAL PLANT WORLD AS A SOURCE OF MANY OF ITS PHARMACEUTICAL INSPIRATIONS. IN FACT, 77 PERCENT OF THE 150 MOST COMMONLY PRESCRIBED DRUGS ARE OF PLANT ORIGIN. MORE AND MORE CONVENTIONAL PHYSICIANS HAVE BEGUN TO RECOGNIZE THE POWER OF PLANTS TO HEAL.

DIVERSE TRADITIONS

Every culture has a long history of using plants as medicine (also known as phytomedicine or botanical medicine). Well into the 20th century, many of the agents used in scientific medicine were derived from herbal lore. Even today, about three-fourths of the drugs commonly used in the United States are of plant origin. These include such drugs as aspirin, digitalis, and the anticancer agents vincristine and taxol.

CHINA

Medical texts that may date as far back as the third century B.C. have been found in a burial site in the Hunan province of China. Written on silk, they include a pharmacologic volume that lists more than 250 medicinal substances. Most are derived from herbs and wood.

The first Chinese book to focus on individual herbs was the *Classic of the Materia Medica*. Written around the first century A.D., it includes more than 250 botanical substances.

Today, herbal remedies remain the backbone of traditional Chinese medi-cine. Practitioners in China and abroad continue to use a variety of herbs, often in combinations, to treat a variety of conditions (see page 349).

MIDDLE EAST

Ancient Mesopotamian clay tablet writings and Egyptian papyrus contain some of the first written records of herbs for the treatment of illness. The first known pharmacopeia—a compilation of drugs, formulas, and uses—was written around 2000 B.C. Ordered by the Sumerian King Assurbanipal, it contains some 250 herbs. The Ebers Papyrus, written around 1500 B.C., contains 876 prescriptions.

ANCIENT GREECE AND ROME

A pupil of Aristotle known as Diocles of Caryotos is reported to have written an early materia medicus, which has since been lost. One of the most influential compilations of drug and herbal usage, however, was written by Dioscorides in the first century A.D. Entitled *De Materia Medica*, it contains 950 curative substances of which some 600 are plant products.

HISTORY

The history of herbal medicine can be traced back some 60,000 years. When the body of a Neanderthal man was discovered in a cave in northern Iraq in the 1960s, scientists found that his body was surrounded by eight species of plants, seven of which are still widely used as herbal medicines today. Although the medicinal use of herbs predates written language, the first written records of herbs as medicine were found in China and the Middle East and go back thousands of years.

MUSLIM WORLD

The text of Jami of Ibn Bair (who died in 1248 A.D.) lists more than 2,000 substances, including many plant products.

INDIA

Herbs play an important role in India's traditional Ayurvedic medicine. The major writings date back more than 2,000 years and include the *Characka Samhita,* an Ayurvedic book on internal medicine that includes 582 herbs, and the *Sushruta Samhita,* an ancient book on surgery that includes 600 herbal remedies. Ayurvedic physicians continue to use a number of herbs, many in combinations (see pages 182–187).

UNITED STATES

Much of North America's herbal history is based on traditions and uses established by Native Americans. European immigrants to this country exchanged knowledge with Native Americans and learned how to use herbs for a variety of purposes.

Until the beginning of this century, physicians commonly used herbal preparations to treat a wide range of illnesses, but such treatments were gradually replaced with more sophisticated remedies, including many over-the-counter products that are based on time-honored herbal cures. In the United Sates today, herbal products are marketed and sold as food supplements.

FORMS OF HERBS

The goal of the herbalist is to release the volatile oils, antibiotics, aromatics, and other healing chemicals an herb contains. Dried, powdered herbs can be made into pills or capsules. Others can be brewed with water to make teas. Herbs can be soaked in alcohol, vinegar, or glycerine to produce long-lasting tinctures. Herbs can be mashed for poultices and plasters, or they can be heated in oil to make salves, balms, liniments, and creams.

TEAS

One of the easiest and most popular ways of preparing an herbal medicine is to brew a tea. There are two types of teas: infusions and decoctions. An infusion is simply herbs steeped in hot water. A decoction is herbs boiled in water.

In general, delicate leaves and flowers are best infused; boiling may cause them to lose the volatile essential oils. To prepare an infusion, use one tablespoon of herbs per one cup of hot water. Pour the hot water over the herbs in a pan or teapot, cover with a lid, and allow to steep. You can make your own herbal tea bags, too. Tie up a teaspoon of herbs in a small muslin bag (sold in most natural food stores) or a piece of cheesecloth, and drop it in a cup of hot water. Let the tea steep for 15 minutes. You can also steep a teaspoon of loose herbs in a cup of hot water; then strain and drink. To make larger quantities of hot infusions, use one ounce of herb per one pint of water.

Roots, barks, and seeds, on the other hand, are best made into decoctions because these hard woody materials need a bit of boiling to get the constituents out of the fiber. Fresh roots should be sliced thin. To prepare a medicinal decoction, use one teaspoon of herbs per one cup of water, cover, and gently boil for 15 to 30 minutes. Strain the decoction. Use glass, ceramic, or earthenware pots to make your decoction: Aluminum tends to taint herbal teas and impart a bitter taste to them. A tea will remain fresh for several days in the refrigerator.

TINCTURES

Another popular way of making herbal medicines is to produce a tincture, an herb extracted in water mixed with alcohol, glycerine, or vinegar. These solvents are strong enough to release the herbs' chemical constituents without heat. A combination of the solvent and water is used because some constituents in herbs are more soluble in the water, whereas others are more soluble in the alcohol. Tinctures can be added to hot or cold water to make an instant tea or mixed with water for external use in compresses and foot baths. The advantage of tinctures is that they have a long shelf life, they're available for use in a pinch, and you can add tinctures to oils or salves to create instant healing ointments.

PILLS AND CAPSULES

We have come to rely on pharmaceutical pills to cure many of our ailments. There is nothing inherently wrong with taking pills, but if you're uncomfortable with the notion of ingesting synthetic chemicals, you can turn to herbal capsules, tablets, or lozenges. Capsules and tablets provide a convenient method of ingesting herbs that have strong, harsh flavors. They're also an alternative for people who do not enjoy drinking herbal teas or using alcohol-based tinctures.

SYRUPS

Syrups can make even the most bitter herbs taste good. They're ideal for coating and soothing sore throats and for respiratory ailments. You can make herbal syrups by combining sugar, honey, or glycerine with infusions, decoctions, tinctures, herbal juices, or medicinal liquors.

HERBAL OILS

Oils provide a versatile medium for extracting herbal constituents. You can consume herbal oils in recipes or salads or massage sore body parts with medicinal oils. Oils are usually made with a common base oil, such as olive, almond, grape seed, or sesame oils, but any vegetable oil will do. Select an oil with a light fragrance that won't overpower the herbs. Avoid mineral oil. Add herbs to an oil of your choice, allow it to sit for a week; then strain and bottle. Refrigerate the oils you plan to use in cooking to avoid rancidity.

SALVES

Salves, also called ointments, are fat-based preparations used to soothe abrasions, heal wounds and lacerations, protect babies' skin from diaper rash, and soften dry, rough skin and chapped lips. Salves are made by heating an herb with fat or vegetable oil until the fat absorbs the plant's healing properties. Beeswax is then added to the strained mixture to give it a thicker consistency.

LINIMENTS

A liniment is a topical preparation that contains alcohol or oil and stimulating, warming herbs such as cayenne. Since a liniment is for external use only, sometimes isopropyl, or rubbing, alcohol is used instead of grain alcohol. *Do not take products made with rubbing alcohol internally.* Liniments warm the skin and turn it red temporarily. It is best to test your tolerance to liniments by rubbing a small amount on your wrist to make sure it does not burn.

BUYING HERBAL PREPARATIONS

Commercial herbal remedies are a little different from the kind that you might prepare in your own home. Here are some basics you need to know about shopping for herbal remedies.

Increasingly, herb suppliers are standardizing the botanical extracts they sell to consumers. This means these herbal preparations have been tested to determine the type and amount of at least one chemical constituent contained in the plant. Standardization sounds like a good idea. But the practice has its pros and cons. Standardization ensures the correct potency of an herbal product. Many of the healing properties of ginkgo biloba, for example, are thought to reside in chemi-

Buying herbs may be confusing at first, but it's often safer than gathering them (see page 256).

cals called heterosides. Thus, if you buy a standardized ginkgo preparation, you can be fairly certain that you're getting a sufficient amount of heterosides. The problem is ginkgo also contains other compounds that are not standardized.

Another problem with standardization is that as we study the medicinal effects of herbs, we're learning that healing may result not from a single element contained in a plant, but from a complex combination of constituents. Standardization implies that an herb is good only for the standardized constituent. But herbs contain many nourishing substances; unlike drugs, herbs are not administered to produce a single chemical effect. If we begin to value plants for their standardized chemicals only, it won't be long before pharmaceutical companies are isolating extracts and packaging them as drugs. And that's not what herbal medicine is about.

USEFUL HERBS

The long and rich history of herbal medicine is worthy of a book in itself, and there are many that can provide a good overview of medicinal herbs. This chapter will provide a brief introduction to the use of herbs, focusing on some of the most popular and most widely available herbs in use in the United States today, as well as some of the more controversial ones.

ALOE (ALOE VERA)

The most popular medicinal variety of aloe is aloe vera, also known as *Aloe barbadensis* and *Aloe vulgari*. A perennial plant with yellow flowers and tough triangular or spearlike leaves, aloe vera is a common houseplant in

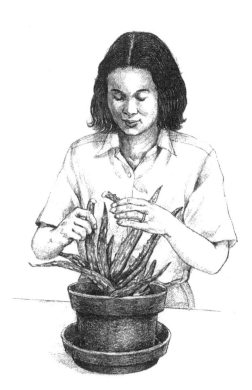

the United States and is easily grown. In many households, it is as much appreciated for the beauty of its tough triangular or spearlike leaves as for its usefulness in treating burns and abrasions.

The ancient Egyptians and Greeks wrote thousands of years ago of aloe's ability to treat wounds and heal skin infections. Although it may have originated in Egypt or the Middle East, aloe is also grown today in many areas, including the southern United States, Mexico, the Caribbean, Latin America, India, and Asia.

Burns, Cuts, and Abrasions—Aloe vera gel promotes wound healing and has been shown to have anti-inflammatory, antimicrobial, emollient, and moisturizing effects. Aloe vera contains a number of compounds that promote wound healing, such as vitamins C and E and zinc. Laboratory studies suggest that aloe vera has antibacterial effects

against a number of organisms, as well as antiviral effects against some viruses.

Pure aloe vera gel can be used to treat minor burns and abrasions. Aloe vera gel can be purchased at the store, or you can simply break off a leaf from your aloe vera plant and use the gel contained inside the fleshy leaf.

Aloe Vera Juice—Some consumers drink oral preparations of aloe vera juice as a tonic. Several studies point to its effectiveness in treating asthma, non–insulin-dependent diabetes, and wounds [1]. One study seems to indicate that one of its constituents may be beneficial in the treatment of AIDS, increasing the activity of white blood cells and reducing the dose of the drug zidovudine that patients need. The juice may also have some antiviral properties [2].

Cautions and Side Effects—Be careful with which wounds you treat with aloe. Although it promotes the healing of minor wounds, it may delay healing of deep surgical wounds and should not be used to treat such deep wounds. Also, although rare, some people have developed skin reactions such as dermatitis to topical aloe vera. When taken internally, it can have potent laxative effects.

CAPSICUM (CAYENNE, HOT PEPPER)

Capsicum annum is a woody perennial native to Central and South America, but commonly cultivated in North America. It is an important source of cayenne pepper, chilies, and red pepper. Capsaicin is the active principle in capsicum.

A number of scientific studies have shown that topical creams containing capsaicin are a safe and effective way to relieve pain from arthritis and a variety of painful nerve disorders. Capsicum is available as a tincture, capsule, or topical ointment.

Arthritis—A study of 21 patients with osteoarthritis or rheumatoid arthritis of the hand found that a topical capsaicin solution applied to each painful joint reduced tenderness and pain in those with osteoarthritis but not rheumatoid arthritis. The only adverse effect noted was a local burning sensation [3].

Fibromyalgia—Capsaicin may also benefit persons who suffer from fibromyalgia—a chronic musculoskeletal condition characterized by chronic, widespread, aching pain and stiffness and tenderness of soft tissues. A study of 45 patients found that those who received a capsaicin topical cream reported significantly less tenderness in the tender points and had a significant increase in grip strength. The most common adverse effect was a temporary burning or stinging at the application site [4].

Neuralgia and Neuropathy—Capsaicin cream has also been found to be effective in reducing nerve pain after outbreaks of herpes and may benefit persons who suffer from diabetic neuropathy—a disease of the peripheral nerves in the hands and feet that causes pain, numbness, and tingling.

Capsaicin cream has been shown to be safe and effective in reducing pain from diabetic neuropathy. A study involving 252 patients

found that, compared with an inactive cream, capsicum cream applied four times a day resulted in a statistically significant improvement in pain relief and a decrease in pain intensity. The only side effects were temporary burning at the application site and some sneezing and coughing [5].

About 10 percent of patients experience severe pain a month after an outbreak of herpes zoster infection (or shingles). This delayed pain is known as postherpetic neuralgia. A study of 33 such patients treated with topical capsaicin found that 39 percent achieved at least a good result and 55 percent were improved or better. Of those who completed the study, 56 percent had good or excellent pain relief after four weeks, and 78 percent noted at least some improvement in pain. Burning was a common side effect and was so severe in one-third of the original group that they withdrew from the trial early [6].

Another study in 33 elderly patients with chronic postherpetic neuralgia comparing capsaicin cream with an inactive cream found significantly greater relief in the treated group than the placebo group. Almost 80 percent of the treated group experienced some relief from their pain [7].

Postmastectomy Pain—A study of 23 patients with persistent pain after a mastectomy (removal of part or all of the breast) believed to be due to nerve injury compared capsaicin cream with an inactive cream. Among the group receiving capsaicin cream, 62 percent had a 50 percent or greater improvement in pain compared with only one person in the group that didn't receive capsaicin treatment [8].

ECHINACEA (PURPLE CONEFLOWER)

Echinacea, also known as purple coneflower, is a perennial herb found in the Midwest and was the most widely used medicinal plant of the Central Plains Indians. The leaf and root of echinacea are reputed to have mild antibacterial and antiviral effects and to aid in wound healing. Echinacea is available as tincture, tea, or capsule.

Topical preparations made from echinacea are used to treat eczema, burns, herpes, psoriasis, and wounds. Preparations designed for internal use can prevent the onset of cold and flu symptoms and may hold promise for arthritis and other ailments. Anecdotal reports (that is, reports by, or observations in, people who take a compound outside of a scientific study) suggest that taking echinacea extract at the first sign of a cold can ward off its symptoms.

Most scientific studies of echinacea have been conducted in Europe, particularly in Germany. These have shown that echinacea both stimulates the immune system and inhibits an enzyme needed by bacteria to enter tissues and cause infection. Laboratory studies have found that echinacea can stimulate the activity of phagocytes, important immune system cells that fight infection, and increase their ability to kill harmful bacteria, such as staphylococci. Echinacea also stimulates monocytes to secrete tumor necrosis factor-alpha and interleukins 1 and 6—important immune system components in fighting infection and tumors. Other laboratory studies suggest that echinacea may have an antiviral effect against influenza, herpes, and other viruses.

CRANBERRIES

Cranberries, particularly cranberry juice, have long been used as a folk remedy to prevent and cure urinary tract infections. Although many conventional doctors have recommended its usage, it is only in recent years that scientists have sought to determine how and why it works. Cranberry is available as juice (the unsweetened is best) or as capsules.

Scientists have shown that cranberry juice inhibits bacteria that may cause urinary tract infections. Many urinary tract infections are caused by *Escherichia coli,* a bacteria normally found in the digestive tract. A study of 77 different types of *E. coli* found that cranberry juice inhibited the adherence to the bladder wall (the ability of the bacteria to anchor themselves and build a colony) of more than 60 percent of the isolates. The same study found that when mice were given cranberry juice, their urine inhibited the adherence of *E. coli* by 89 percent. In humans, 15 of 22 subjects showed antiadherence activity in their urine one to three hours after drinking 15 ounces of cranberry cocktail [9].

A study of 153 elderly women found that those who drank ten ounces of cranberry juice per day were significantly less likely to have bacteria in their urine than women who drank a similar drink that contained no cranberry juice. The study found that the beneficial effects of cranberry juice occurred after four to eight weeks. The researchers speculate that cranberry juice given with antibiotics for urinary tract infections may turn out to be more helpful than antibiotic treatment alone [10].

FEVERFEW (*TANACETUM PARTHENIUM* OR *CHRYSANTHEMUM PARTHENIUM*)

Grown throughout Europe and the United States, feverfew is a composite plant with small daisylike flowers. Feverfew has been used for centuries to treat fever, arthritis, menstrual cramps, and migraines. It is available as tea, capsules, and tincture.

Arthritis—Although feverfew has been used in folk medicine as a treatment for arthritis, no modern clinical trials have been conducted of its use for arthritis. Studies that examine the pharmaceutical properties of the plant show that feverfew does have anti-inflammatory properties similar to those found in nonsteroidal anti-inflammatory drugs, such as ibuprofen, commonly used to treat rheumatoid arthritis.

Migraines—Feverfew is used widely as a home remedy for migraine prevention. In recent years, clinical trials have supported this use. A British study of 59 migraine sufferers found that those who took capsules containing dried feverfew leaves had a significant reduction in the frequency of migraines and a reduction in vomiting associated with migraines compared with a group receiving a placebo. Patients taking feverfew also tended to have reduced severity of their migraines [11].

While not a controlled scientific study, a survey by a group of British scientists found that 70 percent of 270 migraine sufferers who ate feverfew leaves each day reported a decrease in the frequency or severity of attacks, or both.

While the cause of migraines remains unknown, studies show that platelets (components of blood) release serotonin during an attack. Laboratory studies show that feverfew extract inhibits serotonin release from platelets. This action may explain how it helps migraine sufferers. Commonly used drugs to prevent migraines, such as pizotifen and methysergide, are also serotonin antagonists, as is ergotamine, which is used to treat acute attacks.

Cautions and Side Effects—Feverfew use has been associated with mouth ulcers and inflammation of the lips, mouth, and tongue, but these side effects were in cases in which the subjects chewed the leaves (not the preferred method of ingestion). Although the studies cited above found no side effects associated with feverfew treatment, they were conducted for brief periods, such as four months. No serious side effects have been reported from people who have taken feverfew regularly. Because it has historically been used to induce abortion, feverfew should not be taken by pregnant women.

GARLIC (*ALLIUM SATIVUM*)

Garlic is a member of the lily family and is found throughout the world. Its principal active ingredient is alliin, a sulphur-containing compound that converts to allicin, which gives garlic its well-known pungent odor. Garlic has been used as a folk medicine as well as a food and spice since ancient times. It is available as food, as a condiment or tincture, and as deodorized capsules. While garlic has long been thought to have antimicrobial and antitumor properties, its protective effects against heart disease have received the most widespread attention in recent years.

Coronary Heart Disease—In Germany, where the government approves health claims for garlic's cardiovascular benefits, garlic supplements are the best-selling nonprescription medicine. Garlic's effectiveness in protecting against heart disease is due to its activity in reducing a number of risk factors for conditions such as atherosclerosis. Often referred to as "hardening of the arteries," atherosclerosis is the leading cause of heart disease and stroke. It is caused by deposits of fats and other substances on the insides of arteries that can reduce or even block blood flow.

Scientific studies suggest that garlic protects the heart and cardiovascular system through a variety of ways [12]. Garlic has been shown to

- inhibit the aggregation, or clumping, of blood platelets that leads to the formation of blood clots
- disperse blood clots
- decrease blood levels of lipids (fats) and cholesterol
- reduce blood pressure
- enhance antioxidant activity

High Blood Cholesterol Levels— More than half of all Americans are estimated to have hypercholesterolemia (high blood cholesterol levels; that is, greater than 200 mg/dL) and are, thus, at risk for coronary artery disease. Scientific studies show that garlic can be useful in reducing cholesterol levels in people with increased levels of blood cholesterol.

A study of 42 people with total blood cholesterol levels of 220 mg/dL or greater found that daily garlic supplementation produced a significant reduction in total blood cholesterol levels and low-density lipoprotein cholesterol (the most dangerous kind of blood cholesterol). The subjects were given 300 mg of garlic powder in capsule form three times a day [13].

Another study of 40 people with high cholesterol levels found that those who received 900 mg of garlic powder per day had significantly lower levels of total blood cholesterol, blood triglycerides, and blood pressure than those who received placebo capsules. Patients who received garlic also reported a greater feeling of well-being [14].

Another study looked at the effects of garlic on 20 healthy volunteers and 62 patients with coronary heart disease and elevated cholesterol. Among healthy patients who were fed garlic for six months, blood cholesterol and triglyceride levels were significantly lowered, and blood levels of "good" high-density lipoprotein cholesterol were raised. The 62 patients with coronary heart disease and high blood cholesterol levels were given either garlic for ten months or no treatment. Those who took garlic had significant decreases in blood levels of total cholesterol, triglycerides, and low-density lipoprotein cholesterol [15].

A study that analyzed many controlled scientific trials of therapeutic garlic use found that garlic significantly reduced total cholesterol levels. The analysis of five studies involving 410 persons estimates that garlic, in an amount equivalent to one-half to one clove per day, decreases total cholesterol levels by at least 9 percent [16].

Blood clots can have devastating effects if they lodge in an artery carrying blood to the heart, brain, or lungs. Clots are of particular concern to people with atherosclerosis, as these people have already narrowed blood vessels. Laboratory studies have shown that garlic inhibits the aggregation, or clumping together, of blood platelets that leads to the formation of blood clots [17].

High Blood Pressure—Garlic has also been shown to help patients with mild hypertension, or high blood pressure. A study of 47 patients with mild hypertension found that those who received doses of garlic powder daily for 12 weeks had significant reductions in blood pressure compared with those who received a placebo. Patients receiving garlic also had significant reductions in blood cholesterol and triglyceride levels [18].

Antifungal and Antimicrobial Properties—Garlic has long been used as a folk remedy for conditions such as ear infections and vaginal yeast infections. Although its antibiotic effects were noted by Louis Pasteur in the 1800s and many laboratory test have confirmed it, its use as an antibacterial has not been widely studied in controlled clinical trials in humans.

Garlic has been shown to have activity against the fungus *Candida albicans,* the cause of common vaginal yeast infections and other infectious conditions such as oral thrush. Animal studies have shown that it is effective in protecting against infections in experimental conditions [19].

Laboratory studies have shown that garlic has measurable antibacterial activity against a variety of bacteria, including *Salmonella typhimurium* and *Escherichia coli* [20].

Antitumor Properties—Scientists have observed that people who report eating large amounts of allium vegetables, such as garlic, have as much as a 60 percent lower incidence of stomach cancer. Studies in mice have shown that garlic inhibits experimentally induced colon cancer, skin cancer, and mammary cancer. These studies suggest that garlic acts to inhibit very early steps in tumor development [21, 22, 23].

GINGER (*ZINGIBER OFFICINALE*)

A tropical perennial, ginger grows as tall as three or four feet. While the root, or rhizome, is used as a spice and medicine, ginger stems are sometimes crystallized for candy. Ginger is commonly used as a spice, particularly in Asian and Indian foods, as well as in many baked goods, drinks (such as ginger ale), and other products. It is available as food, tincture, capsules, or tea.

Used in China since at least the fourth century B.C., ginger has been used in traditional Chinese medicine, Ayurvedic medicine, and other traditional medicine systems for a wide variety of conditions. Ginger promotes gastric secretion and aids in digestion, stimulates the circulatory system, and has anti-inflammatory activities.

Arthritis—Ginger's usefulness in treating inflammation and rheumatism has long been described in Ayurvedic and other traditional systems of medicine. Although there are a wide variety of drugs used to treat rheumatoid arthritis, all have at least some side effects, making ginger and other plant-based remedies more attractive.

A Danish report suggests that gingerroot capsules may help reduce pain and swelling in persons suffering from arthritis and musculoskeletal disorders. Among 46 patients with rheumatoid or osteoarthritis, more than 75 percent reported some degree of relief from pain and swelling. All 10 patients with muscular discomfort reported relief from pain [24].

Morning Sickness—A Danish study of 30 women with morning sickness so severe that it required hospitalization found that gingerroot worked better than a placebo in reducing or eliminating nausea and vomiting. Patients were given either powdered gingerroot capsules or placebo capsules for four days, then were switched to the other treatment. When asked which treatment period they preferred, 70 percent of women identified the period that was later disclosed to be the one during which they had received the real ginger capsules [25].

Motion Sickness—Although there are effective drugs to treat motion sickness, they may cause side effects, such as sedation or visual disturbances.

HOME CURE FOR NAUSEA

Finely chop ¼ inch of gingerroot. Bring it to a boil in a cup or two of water. Let it steep for five to ten minutes, then add honey or brown sugar to taste.

Therefore, the use of ginger and other alternative therapies with no reported side effects is of special interest for use by people who must remain alert on the job. A Danish study of 80 naval cadets embarking on their first sea cruise found that those who received capsules containing one gram of powdered gingerroot had significantly less vomiting and cold sweats than those who received a placebo capsule [26].

Another study of 36 college students with very high susceptibility to motion sickness found that gingerroot was more effective than dimenhydrinate (Dramamine) in reducing motion sickness induced by blindfolding the students and placing them in a tilted rotating chair [27].

Nausea—A British study of 60 women undergoing major gynecologic surgery found that gingerroot significantly reduced nausea and vomiting after surgery when compared with a placebo and that gingerroot was as effective as the antinausea drug metoclopramide [28].

GINKGO BILOBA

Gingko, the world's oldest living tree species, can be traced back more than 200 million years. Almost destroyed by the Ice Age, the ginkgo survived in China. It was brought to the United States in the late 1700s and can now be found throughout the country. Ginkgo trees have distinctive fanlike leaves that turn a bright gold in the autumn. Aside from being appreciated for their beauty, the leaves of ginkgo, when dried, are used for a variety of medicinal purposes. It is most often found in the form of a standardized extract or capsules.

Ginkgo has long been used in traditional Chinese medicine to treat asthma and bronchitis. In Europe and the West, ginkgo is mainly used to counteract symptoms of aging and increase circulation, especially to the brain.

Cerebral Insufficiency—Decreased blood flow to the brain can cause a variety of symptoms, including difficulties in concentration and memory, absent-mindedness, confusion, lack of energy, fatigue, decreased physical performance, depression, anxiety, dizziness, tinnitus (ringing of the ears), and headache. This collection of problems is known as cerebral insufficiency—sometimes referred to as dementia or senility. A number of clinical studies have shown that ginkgo extract can help alleviate many of these symptoms. No significant side effects have been reported from the use of ginkgo extract.

A German study of 99 people suffering from cerebral insufficiency found that those who received 150 mg of ginkgo per day had significant improvement in most of their symptoms compared with those who received a placebo. Almost 70 percent of the patients who received ginkgo reported that they felt improved compared with only 14 percent in the placebo group.

A study of 70 patients with vertigo and associated symptoms such as ringing in the ears, hearing loss, headaches, and nausea found that symptoms disappeared after three months of treatment in 47 percent of patients who received ginkgo compared to only 18 percent of those who received a placebo.

Ginkgo also appears to be effective in enhancing memory and concentration. A study compared ginkgo with a placebo in 100 elderly patients with at least four of the following symptoms: difficulties of concentration and memory, anxiety, dizziness, tinnitus (ringing of the ears), and headaches. After 12 weeks of treatment, improvement was significantly more noticeable in every category [29].

Alzheimer Disease—Alzheimer disease shares many symptoms with cerebral insufficiency, and treatment with ginkgo has been found to have a similarly beneficial effect. A German study of 40 patients with early stage Alzheimer disease found a significant improvement in memory and attention and in psychomotor performance compared with the group receiving a placebo [30].

GINSENG

A perennial plant cultivated in the Far East, panax ginseng (not Siberian ginseng) has been used in Chinese medicine for thousands of years. Ginseng has traditionally been used as a tonic alone or in combination with other herbs to restore yang. Ginseng has been used in folk medicine to treat virtually every condition imaginable. Recent studies suggest it may help reduce stress, increase performance, and protect against cancer. Usually sold in capsules, it can be made into teas and tinctures, too.

Cancer Prevention—Scientific studies lend support to ginseng's protective effects against cancer. A Korean study found that ginseng intake appeared to reduce a person's odds of developing cancer. The researchers found that ginseng extract and powder seemed to be more effective than fresh sliced ginseng, juice, or tea in reducing the odds ratio for cancer [31].

Performance—Studies suggest that ginseng may improve certain psychomotor functions. A study showed that 100 mg of ginseng twice a day for 12 weeks produced significantly superior performance in mental arithmetic and showed a favorable, although not statistically significant, effect on other functions such as attention and reaction time compared with matched control subjects [32].

Stress and Fatigue—Animal studies suggest that ginseng can enhance the ability to cope with both mental and physical stress.

Caution—Ginseng has been shown to have an estrogenlike effect, and vaginal bleeding has been reported in postmenopausal women taking ginseng formulas and using ginseng face cream. Ginseng may also increase blood pressure. Prolonged use of the herb can lead to ginseng abuse syndrome, which causes sleeplessness, irritability, and headaches.

Some scientists believe there is not enough information to support the long-term ingestion of large quantities of ginseng as the risks may outweigh the benefits. In addition, there is a great deal of variability in the amount of ginseng in products on the market. Seek the advice of a trained herbalist before taking large amounts of ginseng.

GOLDENSEAL
(*HYDRASTIS CANADENSIS*)

A perennial herb native to eastern North America, goldenseal's dried rhizome and roots have long been used as a medicinal herb. Its active ingredient, berberine, has been shown to have an-

tibiotic, antiviral, and immune stimulating effects.

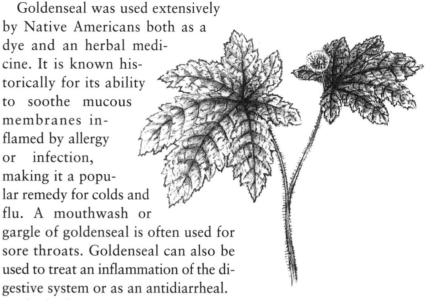

Goldenseal

Goldenseal was used extensively by Native Americans both as a dye and an herbal medicine. It is known historically for its ability to soothe mucous membranes inflamed by allergy or infection, making it a popular remedy for colds and flu. A mouthwash or gargle of goldenseal is often used for sore throats. Goldenseal can also be used to treat an inflammation of the digestive system or as an antidiarrheal.

The herb has a bitter taste, so it is often given in capsules, but powder for teas and a tincture form are also available. Preparations for topical use are also prominent.

Eye Infections—Extracts of goldenseal have also been used for a variety of eye problems. In recent years, berberine—one of goldenseal's components—has been shown to be an effective treatment for trachoma, an infectious eye disease caused by *Chlamydia trachomatis* and a major cause of blindness in developing nations.

Standard drug therapy for trachoma is sulfacetamide, but a study of 32 people with trachoma found that berberine was more effective than the drug sulfacetamide in the clinical course of trachoma. It was also able to reduce antibodies against *Chlamydia* [33].

Infectious Diarrhea—Berberine has also been shown to be effective against diarrhea caused by a variety of organisms—sometimes called traveler's diarrhea. One study of 165 patients with acute diarrhea due to a disease-causing strain of the usually benign *Escherichia coli* found that patients who received a single oral dose of 400 mg of berberine sulfate had significantly less diarrhea in the hours after treatment than those who received no treatment. Patients treated with berberine also were more likely to stop having diarrhea 24 hours after treatment than those who received no medication [34].

Herbalists recommend that persons planning to travel to developing countries or areas with poor water quality take berberine-containing herbs before and during their visit to prevent diarrhea.

Caution—Because one of its active ingredients, berberine, stimulates the uterus, pregnant women should not use goldenseal.

LICORICE (*GLYCYRRHIZA GLABRA*)

One of the most popular herbs used in traditional Chinese medicine, licorice has long been used to treat a variety of conditions, including ulcers, asthma, malaria, and infections. Licorice is a perennial herb that grows three to seven feet high. Its dried roots and runners are collected in the fall and used for herbal remedies. One of the major active ingredients in licorice is glycyrrhizic acid. Licorice is available as a tea, a tincture, capsules, and a solid extract.

Ulcers—The use of licorice to treat gastric ulcers has been extensively studied. It has been compared favorably with antacids and the successful antiulcer medication cimetidine. In the treatment of gastric conditions, the herb is usually deglycyrrhizinated—has the glycyrrhizic acid removed—because this component can cause elevated blood pressure and water retention.

A study of 100 patients with gastric ulcers found that licorice is as effective as cimetidine. Once the ulcers were healed, patients were placed on lower doses for maintenance therapy. After one year of maintenance therapy, there was no difference in the rate of ulcer recurrence [35].

Many people on aspirin therapy for cardiovascular reasons have difficulty with aspirin's tendency to cause stomach bleeding. Research has shown that deglycyrrhizinated licorice can reduce blood loss induced by aspirin in humans and reduce gastric mucosal damage caused by aspirin in rats [36].

Licorice has also been used historically to treat a variety of other conditions. Laboratory studies show that it has anti-inflammatory and antiallergic effects and that it may help stimulate the immune system and inhibit the growth of certain viruses. Treatment of menstrual problems, menopausal complaints, gastritis, and several lung conditions are among its common uses.

Cautions—Excessive use of licorice, either as a medication or as a food, can lower the amount of potassium and other minerals in the blood to dangerous levels. Large amounts of licorice also can affect blood pressure–regulating hormones and contribute to high blood pressure. It may also cause water and sodium retention.

MILK THISTLE (*SILYBUM MARIANUM*)

An annual or biennial plant found in dry rocky areas in Europe and the United States, milk thistle has reddish-purple flower heads. One of its active ingredients is silymarin, which is found in the fruit, leaves, and seeds of the plant. Milk thistle is usually sold in capsules and tinctures.

Milk thistle has been used as a liver remedy for 2,000 years. Silymarin has a long history of folk use against poisoning from the toxic *Amanita phalloides* mushroom, which kills as many as 30 percent of its victims. Studies in mice show that it can prevent liver toxicity from phalloidin (the mushroom's toxin). European hospitals routinely use intravenous milk thistle extracts to counteract liver poisoning from toxins. This observed protective effect has led researchers to examine how the compound might be used in other disorders that affect the liver.

A study of 106 patients with liver disease accompanied by increased levels of liver enzymes known as transaminases compared silymarin with placebo treatment. Patients receiving silymarin for four weeks had significant decreases in the level of enzymes, indicating an overall improvement in their condition [37].

A study of 170 patients with cirrhosis of the liver found that those who received silymarin lived significantly longer than those who received placebo therapy [38].

ST.-JOHN'S-WORT (*HYPERICUM PERFORATUM*)

St.-John's-wort is a perennial plant with bright yellow flowers that is native to many parts of the world, including Europe and the United States. St.-John's-wort has been used since ancient times for a variety of conditions. The herb is generally available as a tea or a tincture.

One active ingredient in St.-John's-wort appears to be hypericin, a photosensitive compound that has chemical and pharmacologic similarities to medications known as tricyclic antidepressants. The herb *is* widely used for the treatment of depression; in fact, it is the most commonly used antidepressant in Germany.

Depression—The scientific literature on the use of hypericin reveals that hypericin is a safe and effective treatment for depression. A review of recent stud-

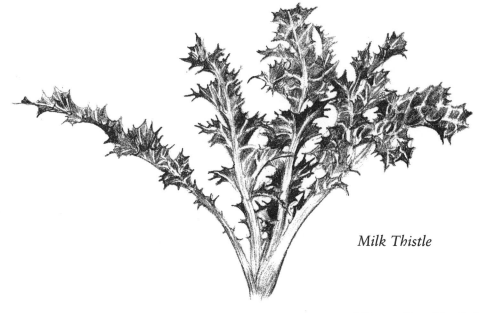

Milk Thistle

ies found that hypericin was superior to a placebo in alleviating symptoms of depression. It also appears to be as effective as standard medication, such as maprotiline and imipramine, but without the side effects [39].

Researchers believe St.-John's-wort may have an advantage over standard antidepressant medications because it seems to be effective in treating many different kinds of depression. St.-John's-wort also lacks the side effects and dangers associated with synthetic antidepressants. For example, suicide through overdose can be a problem with antidepressants. While there is an estimated death rate following overdose of synthetic antidepressants of 30 deaths per 1 million prescriptions, there have been no reports of overdoses or intoxication from ingestion of hypericin.

CAUTION

Although everyone needs to exercise caution when using herbal preparations, the following groups need to be especially careful:

- Pregnant women and nursing mothers should always consult with their physician before taking any herbal or other over-the-counter remedies.
- People with hay fever and allergies to foods and drugs should be aware that certain herbs may cause dangerous allergic reactions.
- People taking prescription medication need to check with their physicians before taking herbs. Some herbs may interact with the medications.

Side Effects—Photosensitivity (sensitivity to sunlight) has been observed in animals that eat large quantities of St.-John's-wort. While reports of photosensitivity in humans are rare and have only been in people taking excessive amounts, some herbalists advise that people taking the herb, particularly those with fair skin, avoid strong sunlight. Hypericin requires the same precautions as the class of drugs called monoamine oxidase inhibitors, or MAO inhibitors: Avoid foods that contain tyramine, such as cheeses, beer, wine, and yeast, and avoid drugs that interact with MAO inhibitors, such as levodopa.

SAFETY CONCERNS

Just because something is "natural" does not mean that it is safe. There are plenty of plants out there that can harm you. And others that, while helpful in small amounts, can be harmful and even fatal when taken in large amounts. Just as not all mushrooms are safe to eat, not all herbs are safe to use on your own. It takes an expert to identify which mushrooms are safe to eat, and likewise, expert identification is crucial for collecting herbs, many of which are grown in the wild. Misidentification of one herb for another, more toxic one does occur sometimes even in commercial preparations.

The potency of an herb can vary dramatically from plant to plant, location to location, and season to season. This depends on a variety of factors, such as variations in climate and soil. How and when the herb is collected and how it is processed can also affect its potency. Sometimes this variability can be extremely dangerous. For example, the flower foxglove was long noted to have beneficial effects on the heart, but in too small doses it did not work, and in too large doses it could kill. Modern medicine uses the prescription drug digitalis, which is carefully controlled to contain just the right amount of the active ingredient for therapeutic use.

Because there is no standardization of herbal products in the United States, different brands of a product may vary considerably in strength. Responsible manufacturers employ measures to ensure that their products are equivalent from batch to batch. Look for the words *standard* or *standardized extract* on the label.

Many herbs have been used safely for thousands of years. Try using small doses of those herbs that have a long track record of safety.

Information on herbs is available from a wide variety of sources including books, associations (several of which are listed at the end of this chapter), and even on the Internet. Read up on the herb you plan to use, and seek the advice of a naturopathic physician or other holistic practitioner for how best to use herbs to treat serious conditions.

The bottom line: Educate yourself about the herbs you are interested in, and seek the advice of a competent herbalist. Some herbalists suggest that when trying an herbal remedy, you choose one brand and experiment within that one because herbal products may not be equivalent from one brand to another. Start slowly with small doses and amounts. Only buy herbal remedies that list the plants used and their relative amounts.

HERBS TO LOOK OUT FOR

A number of herbs are considered controversial, even by members of the herbal industry. While this list is not exhaustive, these are a few herbal products that are causing concern and, in some cases, creating headlines.

Comfrey—Reports of liver disease and toxicity have led to concerns about the safety of comfrey, which is sold as tea, capsules, and other formulations. Comfrey roots and leaves contain pyrrolizidine alkaloids, which are known liver toxins and cause cancer in rats. The sale of comfrey is banned in Canada and Germany. External use of this herb may still be safe.

Chaparral—Reports of liver toxicity have led to concerns about the safety of this herb, which has been linked to serious liver injury in case reports to medical journals. The American Herbal Products Association recently voted to end the voluntary suspension of chaparral sales, though, after determining that the herb was probably not to blame in the four cases of liver failure studied. You may want to consult with a practitioner to discuss the risks and benefits of this herb.

Other herbs that are suspected to cause liver toxicity include

- germander
- mistletoe
- skullcap
- margosa oil
- mate tea
- gordoloba yerba tea
- pennyroyal oil
- Jin Bu Huan (a Chinese product)

Ephedra—Also known as Ma huang, this is a key component in products sold as "natural stimulants" and diet aids. Ephedra's major active ingredient is ephedrine, which can cause heart palpitations, raise blood pressure, and result in heart attack, seizures, stroke, psychosis, and death.

Although ephedra has been used for thousands of years, in recent years it has generated alarm because it is included in strong concentrations in diet and stimulant products. Ephedra presents special risks to people with high blood pressure, heart disease, and diabetes. However, there have been a number of deaths reported from its use among healthy people who have taken high doses of "natural stimulants." Some manufacturers have taken voluntary action to post warnings and limit the maximum dose that should be taken.

Herbal Diet Products—In addition to the concerns about ephedra, which is found in many of these products, other herbal ingredients in these diet products present other dangers. Many of these products are based on laxatives and diuretics, which cause weight loss through dehydration. This water loss can drain electrolytes from the body and cause cardiovascular problems, such as increased blood pressure.

Herbal Laxatives—Although many herbal products act as laxatives, they should not be used on a regular basis. For example, senna and cascara laxatives can be habit-forming and cause serious side effects, such as severe electrolyte imbalances leading to cardiac arrhythmia and death.

Teas—There have been a variety of reports of liver disease and other adverse effects from persons who drink herbal teas, especially ones that are homemade or contain herbs that have not been extensively studied. Many of

these reports involve herbal tea preparations purchased in other countries, but others, such as comfrey, are sold in the United States. Remember that in some cases, herbal tea is not just a beverage; it is also a medicine. Check to see what ingredients are used.

SOME GENERAL ADVICE

Many herbs have not been extensively studied and their potential risks, especially at high doses, are not known. For example, only after hundreds of years of use was tobacco discovered to cause cancer.

Toxicity from herbs is most likely to occur in people who take large amounts or use a wide variety of herbs. The very young, the elderly, the sick, and the undernourished are at special risk for toxicity. Pregnant and nursing women should not use herbs or consume herbal teas without consulting their physician.

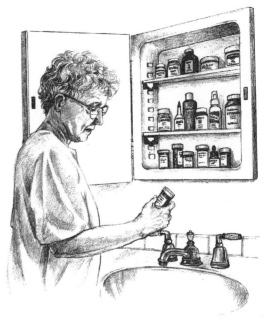

RESOURCES

- American Botanical Council
  P.O. Box 201660
  Austin, TX 78720
  512-331-8868
  fax 512-331-1924

  A good resource for information on herbs for consumers and professionals alike. Publishes a magazine and many other valuable publications on herbal medicine.

- Herb Research Foundation
  1007 Pearl St., Ste. 200
  Boulder, CO 80302
  303-449-2265
  fax 303-449-7849
  http://sunsite.unc.edu/herbs/

  Provides data and information resources on botanicals worldwide. The Web site provides timely and valuable information on medicinal herb usage and safety.

- American Herbal Pharmacopeia
  P.O. Box 5159
  Santa Cruz, CA 95063
  408-461-6317
  fax 408-438-7410

  This nonprofit corporation is devoted to creating a meaningful, contemporary series of monographs on medicinal herbs.

- American Herbal Products
  Association
  P.O. Box 2410
  Austin, TX 78768
  512-320-8555
  fax 512-320-8908

  The trade association for manufacturers of herbal products.

Homeopathy

Derived from the Greek words homeo *(similar) and* pathos *(suffering from disease), homeopathy is based on the principle of similars. That is, an infinitesimal dose of a substance can heal the symptoms caused by a larger amount of the same substance.*

HISTORY

Homeopathy was founded in 1796 by German chemist and physician Samuel Hahnemann. Known as the father of homeopathy, he is reported to have been curious about why quinine could cure malaria. Hahnemann found that when he ingested quinine bark, he experienced the classic symptoms of malaria—chills, fever, and weakness. Hence, he made the connection that lead to homeopathic medicine: the principle of similars.

WHAT IT IS

The principle of similars, "like cures like," holds that a substance that causes certain symptoms when given in large doses to a healthy person can cure an ill person with the same symptoms when given in very small doses. This idea that the same substance that can cause symptoms can also be used to heal is often met with skepticism. However, conventional medicine uses some analogous approaches:

- Allergy shots involve a tiny bit of a substance given to neutralize the immune response against it.
- Radiation therapy for cancer involves small doses of radiation that can be used to cure cancer, whereas large doses are well known to cause cancer.
- Vaccines involve a small number of, or part of, an organism given to stimulate protection against it.

Dr. Samuel Hahnemann's observation that the same compound (quinine) that cures the symptoms in a person with malaria can cause the symptoms of the disease in a healthy person and his development of the principle of similars led to an extensive series of tests of other agents and how they might be used to treat a variety of conditions and illnesses. Common herbal and medicinal substances were tested in healthy persons to see what symptoms they produced. The results of these tests, or provings, led Hahnemann to

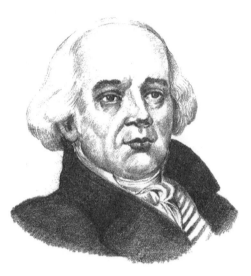

Dr. Samuel Hahnemann

try using these substances to treat persons who were ill with the symptoms the agents caused in healthy persons.

The results of these provings were carefully recorded and resulted in the homeopathic materia medica. The *Homeopathic Pharmacopoeia of the United States* includes thousands of homeopathic medicines made from naturally occurring plant, animal, and mineral substances.

HOMEOPATHY IN THE UNITED STATES AND ABROAD

At the turn of the century, homeopathic medicine was in widespread use in the United States. More than 100 homeopathic hospitals were located around the country, 22 homeopathic medical schools taught its use, and an estimated 15 percent of physicians in the United States practiced homeopathy. Homeopathy was widely used to treat the infectious epidemics of the day, including cholera, yellow fever, scarlet fever, and typhoid. Homeopathic hospitals are reported to have had death rates of one-half to one-eighth of those in allopathic institutions at the time.

Like other types of alternative medicine in the United States, however, the use (and especially the teaching) of homeopathy dramatically declined after the publication in 1910 of the Flexner Report on medical education and its crippling effects on any alternatives to allopathic institutions approved by the American Medical Association. The advent of "miracle" drugs such as antibiotics also led to homeopathy's decline in the United States. Even Hahnemann Medical College in Philadelphia, named after the founder of homeopathy, taught its last class in 1950.

Throughout much of the rest of the world, however, homeopathic medicine has remained a popular traditional treatment approach, particularly in Europe. An estimated 42 percent of British physicians refer patients to homeopathic doctors. In France, 39 percent of physicians and 40 percent of the public use homeopathic medicine. In Germany, where some training in homeopathic and natural medicine is now required for all medical students, an estimated 20 percent of physicians use homeopathic medicine. India has 120 five-year homeopathic medical colleges and more than 100,000 homeopathic physicians.

Despite the tremendous setbacks experienced by homeopathy and other types of alternative therapies in the United States, homeopathy is making a remarkable comeback. Sales of homeopathic remedies in the United States have grown from $100 million in 1988 to $250 million in 1992. And while usage estimates are difficult, at least 3,000 physicians are reported to use homeopathic remedies.

HOW IT WORKS

One of the least understood and, therefore, most controversial aspects of homeopathy is its use of doses so small that modern Western pharmacology considers them to be pharmacologically inactive or to lack completely an "active" ingredient.

Homeopathic remedies are prepared by a process called *potentization*. Dr. Hahnemann discovered that even toxic substances could be given safely without side effects if they were diluted in water, then shaken, then diluted again, shaken again, and the process repeated. For example, a substance would be diluted in a solution of 1 part to 9 parts water, then shaken vigorously; this would be repeated two more times. When a solution is diluted 1 to 9 over three times, it is known as *3x*. If diluted 1 part to 99 parts water, and the process is done a total of three times, it is known as a *3c* solution.

In his early work, Dr. Hahnemann rarely used remedies diluted more than 6x. But later work by him and by others in the field found that even more diluted solutions could have a therapeutic effect. Nowadays, homeopathic solutions may be diluted to as low as 1 in $10^{20,000}$.

The use of such dilute concentrations is perhaps the most perplexing as-

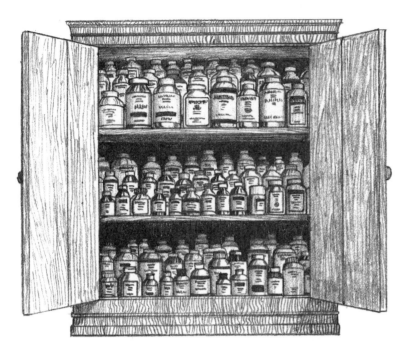

Homeopathy uses thousands of medicines made from naturally occurring plant, animal, and mineral substances.

pect of homeopathy to modern Western scientists who believe that if a solution is so diluted that no molecules of the original substance can be found, it is not logical that it can work. If there are no molecules of the substance, the solution cannot carry any of the substance's properties.

Homeopaths have a number of theories as to why homeopathy works. And while these theories challenge the thinking of scientists who think in terms of molecules and active ingredients, advances and new understanding in other areas of science are providing new insights.

MEMORY OF WATER

One of the more popular theories of how homeopathy works is that the water used to dilute the substance retains a memory of the original substance. Some physical chemists have speculated that the structure of the water solution is altered by the medicine during the dilution process and retains this structure even after none of the original substance can be detected. For example, water may have a magnetic property that allows it to "remember" a substance, much like the way a computer diskette can "remember" and retain information even though a chemical analysis of the diskette would not reveal the information contained within.

CHAOS THEORY

Chaos theory states that many simple, nonlinear interdependent systems can behave in a seemingly unpredictable or chaotic manner. It is based on the French mathematician Jules-Henri Poincaré's observation that "small differences in the initial condition produce very great ones in the final phenomena." In recent years, the availability of advanced computers has led to new understanding of phenomena in many fields, including physics and medicine. Many homeopaths believe such research may be able to help explain how homeopathy works.

HOLOGRAM THEORY

Holograms (those colorful little images that appear on many credit cards) are photographs that look three-dimensional. They are made by illuminating an object with a laser to create a true three-dimensional image of the subject. When a hologram is broken into pieces, each piece retains the same image in its entirety, although in a smaller size. A similar phenomenon could occur as a result of the serial dilutions used to prepare homeopathic medicines.

Other possible explanations for how homeopathy works may lie in the areas of quantum physics or biological phenomena such as field effects that are not molecular.

USES

Homeopathy is used to treat both acute and chronic health problems and to promote health and prevent illness in healthy people. Classical homeopathic treatment is highly individualized, with a single remedy prescribed to treat a sick person's specific illness and symptoms. Over-the-counter homeopathic remedies generally include a formula of several or a few remedies that are known to be effective in treating similar illnesses.

Homeopaths believe symptoms are the body's way of defending and healing itself and that specific symptoms are the guide to choosing the correct remedy. Sometimes a homeopathic remedy may cause a temporary exacerbation of symptoms, known as a healing crisis. Persons with a chronic ailment may have a temporary increase in symptoms before noticing a significant improvement in health.

Homeopathy has the ability to address almost any health problem. Since the therapy really treats the whole person and not the disease, it is difficult to enumerate the specific conditions for which homeopathy is effective. However, the following are just a few of the conditions for which it is frequently used:

- arthritis
- asthma
- colic
- flu
- hay fever
- insomnia
- migraine headaches
- respiratory conditions
- rheumatic conditions
- teething

ASTHMA

Asthma, a disease that is known to be caused in some circumstances by minute quantities of allergens, has long been of interest to homeopathic medicine. Homeopathy has had great success in the treatment of asthma. A study of 28 patients with allergic asthma compared those who received homeopathic immunotherapy to their principal allergen (mostly the dust mite) with patients who did not receive active homeopathic therapy. All patients continued to receive conventional treatment. Patients who also received homeopathic treatment reported a significant decrease in symptoms after one week of treatment and had improved respiratory function and bronchial reactivity tests as well [1].

DIARRHEA

A trial comparing homeopathic medicine with a placebo in 81 children with acute childhood diarrhea found that those who received homeopathic treatment had a statistically significant decrease in the duration of diarrhea compared with the children receiving the placebo [2].

HAY FEVER

A trial of 144 patients with hay fever compared a homeopathic remedy made of mixed grass pollens with a placebo. Patients who received the homeopathic treatment had a significant reduction in symptoms and needed half the antihistamines as those who received the placebo. As can be expected with homeopathic treatments, patients in the homeopathy group were more likely to have an initial aggravation of symptoms after starting therapy before improving [3].

WHO DOES IT

State licensing of health care professionals varies from state to state. Practitioners who practice homeopathy may include: acupuncturists, chiropractors, dentists, medical doctors, naturopathic physicians, doctors of osteopathy, nurse practitioners, physician's assistants, and veterinarians.

Many physicians study homeopathy as a postgraduate specialty; those who have board certification in homeopathy are known as Diplomates. Other health care professionals may receive a CCH designation, which means Certified in Classical Homeopathy.

Check with the National Center for Homeopathy (listed below) for a list of homeopathic practitioners. Questions to ask when seeking a homeopathic practitioner include whether they are certified in homeopathy, what their training is, and what their experience is in homeopathy (and specifically in treating your condition).

Homeopathic remedies are recognized and regulated by the Food and Drug Administration and are manufactured under strict guidelines established by the *Homeopathic Pharmacopoeia of the United States*. Although products in high potencies are limited to licensed practitioners, many over-the-counter preparations (30c and less) are available for the treatment of conditions such as colds and hay fever.

RESOURCES

- Homeopathy Online
  http://www.wolfenet.com/~enos/ho_web/index.html
  A noncommercial magazine about homeopathy, this World Wide Web site has discussions of remedies, uses, history, and education on homeopathy from around the world.

- Homeopathic Academy of Naturopathic Physicians
  P.O. Box 69565
  Portland, OR 97201
  503-795-0579
  fax 503-829-8541
  The Academy provides services for professionals and consumers. Promotes continuing education, provides referrals, and sponsors an annual conference.

- National Center for Homeopathy
  801 North Fairfax St., Ste. 306
  Alexandria, VA 22314
  703-548-7790
  fax 703-548-7792
  e-mail nchinfo@igc.apc.org
  http://www.healthy.net/nch
  The NCH provides self-help as well as professional training courses in homeopathy. Publishes a *Directory of Homeopathic Practitioners*—a listing of licensed health care providers who dedicate anywhere from 25 to 100 percent of their practice to homeopathic treatment.

AS THE NAME IMPLIES, HYDROTHERAPY IS THERAPY WITH WATER IN ANY OF ITS FORMS—ICE, COLD WATER, HOT WATER, STEAM, FRESHWATER, OR WATER IMBUED WITH SPECIAL MINERALS. WATER CAN BE USED ON OR IN THE BODY TO ENHANCE HEALTH AND TREAT A VARIETY OF HEALTH PROBLEMS.

WHAT IT IS

People are increasingly leery of the rising use of medications to treat all sorts of health problems, minor or major. One of the key appeals of hydrotherapy is its simplicity. It uses the most common substance in our environment and one that we know to be essential to us.

The different ways in which water is used therapeutically are almost too numerous to mention. For instance, while fasting, it's important to drink enough water to help cleanse the body of wastes and toxins. Swimming in water exercises muscles and relieves tensions. Taking a steam bath or sauna invigorates the body and induces sweating to flush out impurities. Taking a hot bath can help us combat a flu or cold. And the list could go on and on. Some forms of hydrotherapy are found only in clinic settings, such as whirlpools for rehabilitating injuries, and colon therapy, which uses special equipment to flush water through the colon (see chapter on Detoxification, Fasting & Colon Therapy, pages 225–230). Hydrotherapy also is offered by special spas that provide access to the healing effects of hot springs or mineral waters. Still other hydrotherapies are easily and inexpensively available right at home.

HYDROTHERAPY AT HOME

Water—whether in frozen, liquid, or vaporized form—can be used at home in various therapies to treat many common health conditions.

BATHS AND SHOWERS

Although they may seem routine, baths and showers are healing and health-promoting activities. A hot bath or shower can encourage relaxation and invigorate the immune system. Soaking in a hot bath causes one to work up a sweat, flushing out impurities built up in the body and inducing a fever (see also Hyperthermia, pages 269–271).

Cold baths and showers, on the other hand, can be energizing and stimulating and can combat fatigue. Cold water also reduces inflammation. Alternating hot and cold showers (or going from a hot sauna to a cold snow drift—a Scandinavian tradition) can have invigorating effects. The hot-cold contrast enhances circulation and organ functioning.

BATH ADDITIVES

Adding certain natural ingredients to bathwater can boost its detoxifying power and relaxation potential. Essential oils used in aromatherapy are one option (see pages 178–181). A blend of four drops of juniper (to enhance blood flow), two drops of grapefruit, two drops of rosemary (for calming), and one teaspoon of vegetable oil added to a tubful of water is one suggestion.

HISTORY

As water is the most prevalent substance on earth, it's no surprise that humans have long used water therapeutically. The oldest records describing hydrotherapy methods can be found in 6,000-year-old Sanskrit writings. Today's Jacuzzis are but one of the latest in a long line of hydrotherapy methods developed over the centuries.

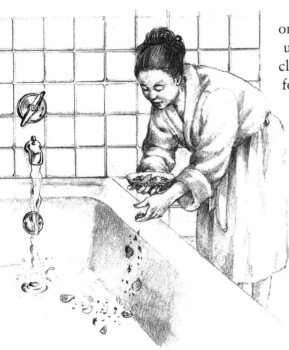

Another bath recipe—one that can restore natural body salts and cleanse the body—calls for combining a half-cup each of sea salt and Epsom salts, plus one-third cup of dried kelp or dulse seaweed in a blender to form a powder, and then adding this mixture to your bathwater. As an alternative, you can use it as a skin scrub. Put some of the powdered mix on a washcloth or a loofah, dampen slightly, and work it into your skin with a massaging motion. Follow with a bath or shower.

SITZ BATH

A European tradition, the sitz bath calls for immersing the pelvis and lower abdomen in hot or cold water or alternating hot and cold. The upper torso and the feet should be out of the water.

A hot sitz bath is recommended for uterine cramps, painful ovaries or testicles, prostate infections, and hemorrhoids. A brief cold sitz bath is good for inflammation, constipation, vaginal discharge, and impotence. Alternating five minutes in hot water and one minute in cold water (alternating three times ending with cold) is used for relieving congestion in the pelvis.

FOOT BATH

Dizziness, nausea, insomnia, shivering, cold feet, foot and leg cramps, sore throats, colds, and flu respond to a hot foot bath, but be sure to wrap the upper body in a blanket to avoid chills and promote sweating. Alternating hot and cold foot baths can treat swollen ankles, foot infections, toothaches, and abdominal congestion. The latter is also a good technique for headaches, when a cold compress is also placed on the head.

HAND BATH

Dipping a hand into hot water relieves hand cramps. Immersing the hand in cold water is helpful for stopping nosebleeds and treating sunstroke.

HOT PACKS AND COMPRESSES

Hot packs are commercially available, but to make a hot compress, soak a towel in hot water and wring out. Hot packs or compresses applied to the body can relieve sciatica, intestinal colic, painful menstrual periods, gallstones, muscle spasms, and pain. Be careful not to use water hot enough to cause scalding.

ICE PACKS AND COLD COMPRESSES

Ice or gel packs are available on the market, but you can devise your own ice pack with a plastic bag of ice cubes. A bag of frozen peas works well, too. To make a cold compress, soak a cloth in ice water and wring out. Ice packs

CAUTION

Oils added to bathwater can make the tub slippery. Lay a rubber mat on the tub bottom and hold on to something stable as you enter and exit the bath.

help to reduce swelling, inflammation, pain, or congestion. Thus, they are useful for sprains, tendinitis, bursitis, crushing injuries, and injuries due to blows.

Cold compresses provide the benefits of forcing blood away from an area, removing the toxins with it and relieving heat. Cold compresses can relieve or prevent headaches accompanying a fever and can reduce minor inflammations. A cold compress on the back of the neck can relieve nosebleeds.

CONTRAST HYDROTHERAPY

This type of hydrotherapy involves alternating hot and cold compresses or hot and cold water immersions. The alternations increase blood flow through an area. In the case of injuries, ice should be applied during the first 24 to 36 hours. After that, alternate hot (five minutes) and cold (one-half to one minute). Always end with cold. Also use alternations for tendinitis, bursitis,

---

MORE BATH ADDITIONS

Herbs, oils, and other home ingredients can be added to bathwater for health benefits. Here are a few samples:
- Chamomile, lavender, and linden flowers create a calming bath.
- Essential oils such as lavender, rose, clary sage, ylang ylang, and patchouli relieve stress, headaches, muscle tension, and symptoms of premenstrual syndrome.
- Epsom salts contain magnesium sulfate, which relaxes muscles and calms the nervous system.

---

arthritis, and local infections.

STEAM

Steam cleansing in the form of a sauna, Turkish bath, or Russian bath is excellent for eliminating impurities and stimulating circulation throughout the body. Most people do not have these available at home, but one simple strategy for using steam as a health aid can easily be done in your kitchen. Boil a pot full of water, adding a little wintergreen oil or mint leaves if you like. Remove the pot from the burner. Then place a towel over your head to form a tent and lean over the steaming pot to breathe in the vapors. (Be careful not to get too close or to breathe too deeply because steam can cause scalding.) This procedure soothes the respiratory tract and helps to clear congestion.

PROFESSIONAL HYDROTHERAPY

Some hydrotherapies cannot be done at home. Special equipment, such as whirlpools and steam baths, or special expertise, such as certain wraps or manipulations, often require the treatment be performed at a treatment facility.

CONSTITUTIONAL HYDROTHERAPY

Naturopathic physicians use this method for promoting overall health and immune system strength. Many conditions respond to constitutional hydrotherapy, including
- asthma
- gastroenteritis
- arthritis
- upper respiratory infections
- bronchitis
- ulcerative colitis
- premenstrual syndrome

You can also do an adapted version of constitutional hydrotherapy at home, with a little help from a friend, by following these steps:

- Have the person lie faceup on top of a sheet and blanket. Cover his or her trunk from the neck to the waist with two hot wet towels that have been wrung out.
- Over this, wrap the person in the sheet and blanket and leave on for five minutes.
- Lift the blanket and sheet and place a fresh hot bath towel on top of the other two hot towels.
- Flip all three at once so the fresh towel is on the person's skin.
- Then remove the two old towels, leaving the new hot towel in place.
- Place a cold towel on top of the new hot towel and flip again so the cold one is against the person's skin.
- Remove the hot towel, leaving the cold one, and wrap the person in the sheet and blanket again. (Add an extra layer of blanket if the person is cold.) Leave on for ten minutes until the cold towel is nicely warmed.
- Lift the blanket and remove the now-warm towel.
- Have the person turn over to lie facedown.
- Repeat the process on the back side.

ENEMAS

The above hydrotherapy methods involve the external use of water. An enema is an internal therapy using water to irrigate the lower portion of the colon, thus encouraging elimination and aiding detoxification. Cool water can be used to stimulate, whereas warm water can be used to soothe spasmodic conditions.

An enema solution is made up of one tablespoon baking soda per quart of body-temperature water. Follow instructions that come with the enema bag. Consult a professional before using an enema for children or someone who is pregnant, elderly, or ill.

For a more complete intestinal cleansing, colon therapy can be used. It must be provided by a trained colon therapist (see pages 227–229).

RESOURCES

- American Association of Naturopathic Physicians
  2366 Eastlake Ave. East, Ste. 322
  Seattle, WA 98102
  206-323-7610
  fax 206-323-7612
  http://infinite.org/Naturopathi.Physician

The AANP is the professional association for naturopathic physicians. Publishes a listing of naturopathic physicians in the United States. The Web site provides consumer information and an extensive listing of self-care information on a wide variety of conditions and ailments.

CAUTION

Many hydrotherapy techniques must be used extremely cautiously by anyone with reduced sensations that would impair monitoring heat and cold. In such cases, have an assistant help you to assure safety. Also, if you have heart problems, diabetes, neurologic impairments, or other serious conditions, talk to a health professional before using hydrotherapy.

HYPERTHERMIA IS A THERAPY THAT USES ONE OF THE BODY'S OWN DEFENSE MECHANISMS: FEVER. FEVER HELPS TO DESTROY INVADING ORGANISMS AND SWEAT AWAY IMPURITIES. HYPERTHERMIA TREATMENTS RANGE FROM LOW-TECH, DO-IT-YOURSELF METHODS, SUCH AS HOT BATHS AND SAUNAS, TO HIGH-TECH APPROACHES THAT NEED TO BE ADMINISTERED AND SUPERVISED BY A TRAINED PROFESSIONAL.

WHAT IT IS

The principle behind hyperthermia is fairly simple: Pushing body temperature above 98.6°F (37°C) kills off viruses, bacteria, and other invading organisms that can't take the excess heat, while not inflicting any damage on the more heat-tolerant human body tissues.

Even if the invading organisms don't all succumb to the heat, the idea is that their number will be diminished enough so that the body's own immune system can handle the rest. In addition, the state of hyperthermia stimulates the immune system by boosting production of antibodies and interferon, a protein created by the body's virus-invaded cells that blocks reproduction of the virus.

METHODS

Hyperthermia can be applied to the entire body, such as for fighting a systemic viral infection, or to just a specific part or area, such as to treat a tumor. The techniques for inducing hyperthermia are many and varied, ranging from at-home methods, such as a hot bath, to strategies that need to be done in a medical setting.

Therapists may use any of the following methods:

- Radiant heating applies infrared heat to the body.
- Ultrasound applies high-energy sound waves that raise body temperature by creating molecular friction when they hit body tissue.
- Diathermy applies shortwave or microwave electromagnetic energy to the body to elevate temperature.
- Extracorporeal heating involves removing blood from the body, heating it, and putting the heated blood back in the body.

To help fight off common illnesses such as colds and flu, at-home hyperthermia can be very effective. Here are some ways to induce a fever response:

- Take a hot bath, drink a hot beverage, and wrap yourself up in blankets. Put a hot water bottle on your abdomen. You should start to sweat. Endure it as long as you can (it may take hours), and then cool off with a neutral (not cold) shower.
- Skip the bath and just wrap up in dry blankets. Sweat as long as you can and then cool off with a shower.
- Wrap up in a wet, cold sheet (this is more comfortable if you've just warmed up by exercising or bathing in hot water), and then wrap up in layers of dry blankets. The wet sheet against your skin prompts your body to produce heat, so you'll work up a sweat. Again, it may take one or two hours.

HISTORY

Hyperthermia has been a part of human health care traditions for millennia. Native American sweat lodges, Turkish hot baths, and Finnish saunas are all variations on the hyperthermia theme. Today hyperthermia has become accepted in mainstream medicine as a tool for combating serious illnesses, such as cancer.

GUIDELINES FOR HYPERTHERMIA AT HOME

- Wait for one hour after a meal.
- Drink plenty of neutral (not cold) water before and after the hyperthermia session.
- If you've just exercised, give your body a chance to cool down a bit first.
- Be sure you don't have a condition that might preclude hyperthermia (see Caution, page 271).

- Inhaling steam is an example of localized hyperthermia and is an excellent technique for treating colds and sinus congestion. Steam can cause scalding so be careful not to get too close.

USES

Simple hyperthermia techniques, such as hot baths, steam baths, or saunas, have been shown to be effective for many common illnesses. Among them are
- colds and flu
- bronchitis
- pneumonia
- sinusitis
- infected wounds
- bladder problems
- urinary tract infections
- chronic fatigue syndrome

DETOXIFICATION

Toxins such as pesticides, herbicides, chemical solvents, and prescription and recreational drugs build up in the body's fat and cells. Hyperthermia is often used as part of detoxification programs. Close monitoring is essential, however, as medical emergencies (such as breathing difficulties, heart problems, or flashbacks) can arise during detoxification. Never attempt detoxification without professional supervision.

HIV/AIDS

Hyperthermia techniques are being used by health professionals to combat HIV infections, although the therapy is still far from prevalent. A 1992 study conducted at the Natural Health Clinic of Bastyr College in Seattle found hyperthermia effective in giving clients a greater sense of well-being [1].

Other research, which was reported in 1988, showed that 30 minutes in a hot water bath (107.6°F; 42°C) resulted in 40 percent inactivation of HIV. Inactivation climbed to 100 percent at a temperature of 132.8°F (56°C) [2].

In Europe, extracorporeal heating (removing the blood from the body, heating it, and putting the hot blood back in the body) has been used successfully to treat full-blown AIDS. This is still a highly controversial procedure in the United States and has not received the Food and Drug Association's stamp of approval.

CANCER

Medical doctors have found hyperthermia useful as an adjunct therapy in treating cancer. A treatment regimen combining hyperthermia with conventional chemotherapy and radiation has proved to be more effective than chemotherapy or radiation alone. A survey of cancer experts reported that they viewed hyperthermia as a "promising technology" in treating chest wall recurrences in breast cancer [3].

Some research into the applications of hyperthermia techniques in the treatment of breast cancer showed complete response in combination with other treatment in roughly two-thirds of patients [4]. Another study reported that hyperthermia significantly improved tumor control in malignant melanoma (the deadliest form of skin cancer) when used with radiation treatment [5]. The use of hyperthermia for cancer treatment is still highly controversial in the United States.

RISKS

Hyperthermia is not a risk-free therapy. In the case of high-tech hyperthermia methods, medical studies have cited surface burns, blistering, ulceration, pain, and infection as the most common adverse effects.

Implanted hyperthermia devices (through which, for example, electromagnetic energy may be channeled) have been associated with scalp infection, swelling, increased intracranial pressure, dangerously elevated body temperature, nausea, hemorrhage, and neurologic problems.

Cataracts can be a problem if hyperthermia is applied in the area of the eyes. Male sterility has also been reported as an aftereffect. Even the at-home hyperthermia procedures can be risky for some people who are overly sensitive to heat.

RESOURCES

- American Association of Naturopathic Physicians
2366 Eastlake Ave. East, Ste. 322
Seattle, WA 98102
206-323-7610
fax 206-323-7612
http://infinite.org/Naturopathic.Physician

Many naturopathic physicians are trained in hyperthermia. To receive a national referral directory of naturopathic physicians and a general brochure about naturopathy, send $5 to AANP, or fax your request with all necessary credit card information.

CAUTION

Hyperthermia can be dangerous for people who are sensitive to heat. Check with your health professional first if you are pregnant or have any of the following conditions:
- heart problems
- seizure disorders
- diabetes
- anemia
- tuberculosis
- loss of sensation in an area of your body, which may put you at risk for burns
- high or low blood pressure
- temperature regulatory problems, common in the elderly or very young children

Hypnotherapy

Hypnotherapy is therapy using hypnosis—sometimes called the art of suggestion. Physical, psychological, and emotional disorders have been found to respond to hypnotherapy. Today, many medical doctors, dentists, psychologists, psychiatrists, and natural health practitioners are using hypnotherapy for conditions ranging from asthma and overeating to skin diseases.

THE HYPNOTIC STATE

Hypnotism may seem unfamiliar to most, but common experiences do give a glimpse of what the hypnotic state is like. On a long, boring drive when suddenly you realize you have no recollection of what you've seen for the last several miles, or when you are so engrossed in doing something that you shut out everything else—these can be thought of as slightly hypnotic states.

The hypnotic state is not sleep, but it's also not a state of full wakefulness in the usual sense either. It's somewhere in between. In fact, electroencephalography (EEG) shows that a hypnotized person's brain rhythm is in neither a waking nor a sleeping pattern. Still, no one can say for sure exactly how hypnosis works. During hypnosis, the normally "in-charge" conscious mind somehow takes a backseat to let the subconscious—and some would say also our higher consciousness—come to the fore.

HYPNOSIS VERSUS HYPNOTHERAPY

Hypnosis is the inducing of the altered state described above. Hypnotherapy, on the other hand, is using hypnosis for therapy—to deal with some psychological, physical, or emotional condition or conflict. This therapeutic process becomes possible because while under hypnosis, a person is open to suggestion. New ways of thinking about the body, feelings, or abilities are opened up during hypnotherapy that rational, intellectual logic might normally reject out of hand.

USES

Hypnotherapy experts are quick to point out that hypnotherapy cannot heal every condition, nor does it work for every person. Still, unlike the sideshow image that some people have of hypnosis, health professionals in diverse disciplines have found hypnotherapy useful. It's being used in psychiatry, psychotherapy, general

THE ROAD TO CREDIBILITY

Although healing by suggestion has roots in almost every human culture, hypnosis has been through ups and downs in recent centuries in gaining credibility. A key shift came in 1955, when the British Medical Association approved hypnotherapy as a valid medical treatment. Three years later, the American Medical Association also granted its stamp of approval.

medicine, and dentistry to treat conditions such as

- chronic pain
- pain during childbirth
- bed-wetting
- muscle spasms
- asthma
- high blood pressure
- skin disorders
- headaches
- migraines
- ulcerative colitis
- anorexia
- anxiety
- pain and discomfort during dental procedures
- addictions (to alcohol and other drugs, smoking, overeating)
- inflammation
- nausea (such as from morning sickness or chemotherapy)
- irritable bowel syndrome
- weight problems
- sexual dysfunction
- phobias
- stress
- depression
- menstrual discomforts
- impaired immunity

PAIN MANAGEMENT

One of the major clinical applications of hypnosis is in the management of pain. Chronic and episodic pain can often be ameliorated by hypnotherapy. In one case, a woman suffering from painful attacks of sickle-cell disease was unresponsive to pain medication and other conventional interventions. Using a technique called glove anesthesia, she was able to obtain immediate relief. In this technique, the subject under hypnosis imagines her hand becoming numb in an ice-cold bucket of

---

A MISNOMER

The word *hypnosis* comes from *hypnos*—the Greek word for sleep. Scottish physician James Braid so named the technique because he thought it was related to sleep. By the time he realized it wasn't accurate, he tried to change the name to *monoeidism*, which means "concentrating on one idea." It never caught on. The word *hypnosis* was here to stay.

---

water, and the suggestion is given that the numbness can be transferred to any part of the body to numb pain [1].

People with other conditions such as arthritis that cause chronic pain can also benefit from this and other forms of hypnotherapy. Perhaps one of the more astounding uses of hypnotherapy has been as a substitute for anesthesia during minor and major surgery—a practice first employed by the French physician Jules Cloquet in 1829. It has also been used to aid in pain management and recovery after surgery and during the treatment of serious burns.

PREGNANCY AND CHILDBIRTH

In addition to the pain-management benefits that hypnotherapy can bring to women in labor, certain suggestion techniques can also be useful in focusing the mother's breathing and relaxation during labor. Maternal anxiety is associated with an increase in childbirth complications, and hypnotherapy may be able to influence the expectant mother to produce a smoother labor [2]. One study even found that hypnotherapy conducted in the weeks before delivery

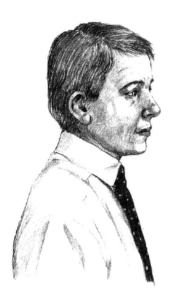
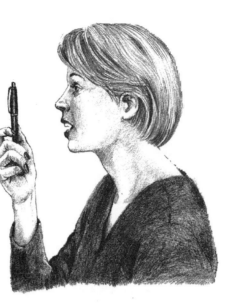

was able to turn fetuses in the breech position to the head-first position [3].

ADDICTION

Hypnosis is beginning to gain wide acceptance in the addiction-treatment community. In smoking-cessation programs, hypnotherapy has proved comparable to other treatment methods and is showing great promise as an adjunct to more conventional therapy [4].

PROFESSIONAL AND PERSONAL GROWTH

This has become a popular use of hypnosis and self-hypnosis. For instance, athletes and business people use these techniques to bolster performance levels on the playing field or in the corporate office. Hypnosis can also be used to enhance relaxation, concentration, and creativity.

MYTHS ABOUT HYPNOTHERAPY

Some people shy away from hypnotherapy because of unfounded fears.

The following is a rational look at some of the myths:

I'll lose control. It is only natural to be afraid to submit oneself to someone else's suggestions, but the fact is the patient remains in control at all times during hypnosis. That's why some hypnotherapy experts say that all hypnosis is really self-hypnosis. The patient actually chooses if and when to enter the hypnotic state and when to leave it. Furthermore, the power of suggestion only works with the patient's consent—if it's something that he or she truly wants to do. (You can't be made to do anything against your will.)

I might get stuck in the hypnotized state. This cannot happen, hypnotherapists say. The patient retains the ability at all times to come back to full consciousness instantly.

If I can't be hypnotized, it must be my fault. Some people, for whatever reason, just don't take to hypnotic suggestion. That doesn't mean you're in any way deficient or lacking. Not everyone is "hypnotizable." The World Health Organization estimates that 90 percent of the population can be hypnotized, while other sources put it at about 70 percent. If you decide to try it, a qualified hypnotherapist can test you for suggestibility.

WHO DOES IT
PROFESSIONAL HYPNOTISTS

Working with the right hypnotherapist for you is a crucial part of successful treatment. Many states have no certification process for hypnotherapists. Inquire about the therapist's training and experience. Ask around for referrals in your community, or call one of the organizations listed below.

Trust and a good rapport are key. Incompatibilities between the personalities of therapist and subject can quickly sabotage the chances for effective hypnotherapy. The hypnotherapist should be willing to take time to talk with you about any concerns you have about this form of treatment. If you feel the hypnotherapist is trying to foster dependency on him or her in your relationship, walk away.

SELF-HYPNOSIS

The other person qualified to perform hypnosis is you. In self-hypnosis, you act as your own hypnotherapist, after learning a few techniques. You might use self-hypnosis as an adjunct to working with a hypnotherapist, or you might decide to do it on your own. It's important that you feel comfortable with the latter idea, however, and not just pursue it to cut costs. Most hypnotherapists will teach their clients techniques to use. And there is a wide range of literature on the subject, too.

RESOURCES

- Academy of Scientific Hypnotherapy
  P.O. Box 12041
  San Diego, CA 92112
  619-427-6225
  Provides referrals nationwide and in some other countries to professionally trained hypnotherapists.

- American Academy of Medical Hypnoanalysts
  107½ West Jefferson
  Joliet, IL 60432
  800-344-9766
  Provides referrals nationwide and offers professional training.

- American Guild of Hypnotherapists
  2200 Veterans Blvd.
  New Orleans, LA 70062
  504-468-3223
  Offers professional training and also referrals to practitioners.

- American Board of Hypnotherapy
  16842 Von Karman Ave., Ste. 475
  Irvine, CA 92714
  714-261-6400
  800-872-9996
  Offers books and tapes on hypnotherapy; trains and certifies hypnotherapists. Provides referrals.

- American Society of Clinical Hypnosis
  2200 East Devon Ave., Ste. 291
  Des Plaines, IL 60018-4534
  847-297-3317
  Send a stamped, self-addressed envelope for referrals to medical doctors and dentists trained in hypnotherapy. Offers professional training.

- National Guild of Hypnotists
  P.O. Box 308
  Merrimack, NH 03054
  603-429-9438
  Offers training and certification programs; provides books and tapes on hypnotherapy. Referrals also available.

- Society for Clinical and Experimental Hypnosis
  3905 Vincennes Rd., Ste. 304
  Indianapolis, IN 46268
  fax 317-872-7133
  Send a stamped, self-addressed envelope to obtain a list of professional hypnotherapists in your area, or request the list by fax.

Meditation

MEDITATION COMES IN DIVERSE FORMS AND HAS BEEN SHOWN TO ENHANCE PHYSICAL, PSYCHOLOGICAL, AND EMOTIONAL WELL-BEING. HIGH BLOOD PRESSURE, PAIN, AND ANXIETY DISORDERS ARE BUT A FEW OF THE CONDITIONS THAT MEDITATION CAN AMELIORATE. THE KEY TO SUCCESSFUL MEDITATION PRACTICE IS TO FIND A TECHNIQUE SUITED TO YOU.

HISTORY

Human beings have long been fascinated with the power of the mind to help promote healing. Sacred traditions have included various types of meditation as spiritual practices. In the West, interest in meditation has spiraled since the 1960s, when people became aware of Eastern practices such as yoga and Zen Buddhism.

POTENTIAL BENEFITS

Meditation might be defined as a mental exercise aimed at training the mind to let go and become free. Others have described it as learning how to stay anchored in the present moment. Different motivations spur people to try meditation. They look to meditation as a means to enhance the mental, physical, or emotional aspects of their lives.

CONCENTRATION

Some turn to meditation to learn how to quiet the mind—to counteract the condition one old Buddhist saying describes as being "like a drunken monkey stung by a bee." The feeling is familiar to most: The mind seems overflowing with disjointed ramblings—worries about the mortgage payment, fuss about what to make for dinner, or the reliving of a tense moment over and over. Meditation is a way to get a grip on the endless, mostly useless, internal chatter.

PHYSICAL WELL-BEING

Another appeal of meditation is that it can help relieve tensions in the body, promote relaxation, and help recharge physical energy. Beyond helping to enhance physical vitality, meditation has been shown to play a role in treating various health problems.

EMOTIONAL FITNESS

Many who practice meditation regularly find they become more resilient to life's ups and downs. Frustrations, disappointments, and worries don't get to them as much. They feel on a more even keel, better able to deal with whatever the day may bring their way. In addition, meditation helps to relieve more serious emotional disorders, such as anxiety or mild depression. Meditation also appears to affect the physiologic responses that reflect emotional states, such as muscle tension, brainwave activity, and levels of brain chemicals called neurotransmitters.

THE FOURTH DIMENSION

While many people are originally drawn to meditation to learn to relax or to boost their energy, they might also discover that meditation is a window to self-exploration. Sometimes without intending it, people who practice meditation find themselves opening up to new ways of questioning and thinking about themselves and their lives. This is a more difficult benefit to describe, to be sure, but nonetheless, it's one that many meditators come to experience personally.

TYPES OF MEDITATION

Meditation can take many forms. It may be sitting quietly and freeing the mind, but it does not have to be a stationary practice. Walking meditation involves walking while focusing our attention completely on what our body is doing with every step. Even common daily activities such as knitting or washing the dishes can be meditative if we perform them attentively.

While meditation techniques are diverse, overall they can be grouped into two broad categories: concentration and insight. The concentration method focuses the attention on something, such as the breath, a candle flame, a sound, or a repeated word or thought. The insight technique (also called *mindfulness*) involves expanding the awareness by opening up one's attention to assorted passing feelings, thoughts, images, sounds, and so on without reacting to them. The idea is to stay calm, just noticing whatever is there, without judging or getting emotionally wrapped up in it.

Transcendental Meditation, or TM, is one particular type of concentration meditation practice—probably the one best known in the West. TM involves meditation focusing on a single object, a sound, a word, or short phrase; the sound, word, or phrase is called a mantra.

Maharishi Mahesh Yogi of India introduced TM to the United States in the 1960s. He was also the developer of a form of Ayurvedic medicine (see pages 182–187). With a well-funded institute behind it, the relatively simple, easy-to-learn TM technique has become quite popular in this country and has been the subject of numerous studies, many of which attest to TM's effectiveness. Still, while TM's benefits seem clear, it remains debatable in many experts' eyes whether it's more beneficial than other meditation forms.

USES

In addition to enhancing well-being and generally bolstering mental clarity and physical energy, meditation has been found effective in treating almost all health problems to some extent. Some of its greatest therapeutic successes have been in dealing with the following conditions:

- stress
- addictions to alcohol and other drugs
- anxiety
- mild depression
- chronic pain
- hypertension
- heart disease
- weakened immune systems
- epileptic seizures
- pain after surgery

Not all meditation involves sitting in the lotus position with your eyes shut. Mindfulness is a type of meditation practiced throughout your daily activities.

CHRONIC PAIN

People living with chronic pain face a daily challenge of coping. Pain in itself can be debilitating, but the depression and isolation that can accompany pain can also be extremely difficult for sufferers. These people often cope with a great deal of physical and emotional stress. Drug therapy for these patients is often limited in effectiveness, but certain meditation techniques are emerging that can offer help.

In a study of 51 chronic pain sufferers—ranging from back pain to chest pain (angina)—a form of mindfulness meditation was used for a ten-week outpatient treatment program. The technique involved "detached observation" of the pain, evaluating it as an observer, rather than experiencing it as a subject. After the ten-week program, 65 percent reported a significant reduction in their perceived pain; in fact, 50 percent said their pain was reduced by more than half. Significant reductions in mood disturbances and psychiatric symptoms accompanied the reduction in pain, as well [1].

ANXIETY DISORDERS

A study examined the effects of a mindfulness meditation–based stress-reduction program for treating anxiety disorders. The researchers at the University of Massachusetts Medical Center found "significant improvements" in anxiety and panic symptoms after an eight-week outpatient group stress-reduction program. Three years later, they found that these patients' gains were still evident. Also, the majority had stayed with the meditation practice over the years. The researchers concluded that mindfulness meditation can have long-term beneficial effects in the treatment of anxiety disorders [2].

HIGH BLOOD PRESSURE

Meditation can have significant effects on cardiovascular health. People with high blood pressure (hypertension), in particular, can experience dramatic improvement through several forms of meditation. In a study conducted at an inner-city health care center, older people with mild hypertension were divided into three groups: those who learned TM, those who participated in a progressive muscle-relaxation program, and those who were educated in lifestyle changes. After a three-month follow-up, the TM and muscle relaxation groups fared the best in lowering blood pressure, with TM proving to be twice as effective as muscle relaxation [3].

MOOD CHANGES

Meditation's effect on different mood states is just beginning to receive attention. It may have therapeutic value similar to regular exercise in improving actual physiologic changes in the brain related to mood. Researchers in the United States and Australia compared a group of runners with trained meditators to assess changes in levels of three hormones related to mood state. The research team found that hormone levels and moods were elevated in both groups, with no significant differences between runners and meditators [4].

MONITOR MEDICAL CONDITIONS

If you have conditions such as diabetes and high blood pressure, you may find that meditating causes changes in how much medication you need. Be sure to be monitored by a health professional who can advise you on medication adjustments. Also, some people with serious asthma may find it difficult to practice meditation that focuses on the breath. In such cases, use another technique.

FIBROMYALGIA

Fibromyalgia is a chronic illness characterized by widespread pain, fatigue, sleep disturbances, and resistance to treatment. However, meditation may hold promise for people with the disease. A study evaluated the effectiveness of a mindfulness meditation–based stress-reduction program for helping fibromyalgia patients cope with their disease. All program participants had at least some improvement, but 51 percent showed "marked to moderate improvement" in their symptoms [5].

SEIZURE DISORDERS

Drug therapy has helped millions with seizure disorders such as epilepsy, but often these drugs have significant side effects, and there are many people for whom medication is unable to control their condition. A small group of people with epilepsy, whose seizures were not adequately controlled by drugs, practiced meditation for 20 minutes a day for a year. Researchers found that the meditators had fewer and shorter seizures. Electroencephalography (EEG)—a measurement of brain-wave patterns—showed the meditation group had significant improvements when compared with a control group that had not practiced meditation [6].

THE ROUGH ROAD OF MEDITATION

For all of meditation's benefits, researchers also have found that meditation can bring on negative physical and emotional experiences. These aren't necessarily "bad" in and of themselves; troubled feelings may just be part of the process of opening up. However,

---

MEDITATION IN MOTION

Meditation doesn't have to be a sedentary practice. For instance, walking meditation involves purposeful walking, with total attention focused on the sensations and movements in your body as you walk. The phrase "meditation in motion" is often used to describe Tai Chi Chuan, a gentle, slow-moving Chinese exercise form. The phrase also appears quite often in the practice of a yoga technique called Kripalu Yoga.

---

people who undertake meditation should be aware of these possible reactions and get help if needed. Professional support during the learning process can be very helpful.

Some of the reported problems that people experience include anxiety, depression, and even physical discomforts such as headaches, sore throats, cramped muscles, sweating, shivering, trembling, racing heartbeat, and tingling or stinging sensations in parts of the body. Other side effects might include having certain smell or taste sensations or sudden laughing or crying outbursts. Some experts attribute these symptoms to tension release.

Usually, these symptoms are only experienced by new meditators, who soon see the problems vanish. Such side effects are not indicators to stop or reduce meditation time—unless the effects persist and make you really uncomfortable. The path to self-awareness can be a bumpy one, but almost without exception, those who travel it consider it worth the trip.

GETTING STARTED

If you decide meditation is appealing, you might want to take a class to learn some techniques. Private teachers, health care centers, fitness clubs, or community organizations in your area may teach classes in meditation. Books and tapes can also provide a good introduction to the subject.

A crucial first step is finding the meditation technique that's best suited to you. For instance, you may be someone who gets overanxious sitting still, in which case a meditation form based on movement may be more appropriate. Or if you're an analytical person, a more structured meditation might be the optimum fit, at least for starters, rather than a free-flowing form. With a little investigating and experimenting, you'll find a technique that feels comfortable for you.

Once you choose a technique, stick with it. Regular practice each day, even if you don't feel like it, is key to deriving full benefit from meditation. And as is the case with any sport or art form, don't expect to master it in a few weeks or months. Be patient. Practice faithfully. And you will begin to see benefits in time. Don't get discouraged if your initial meditation sessions don't turn out as you'd hoped. It's only natural for the mind to wander, for distractions to pop up that steer us off track. Just remember, even people who have been practicing meditation for a long time still have an unsatisfying session now and then. Be patient with yourself.

RESOURCES

- Insight Meditation Society
  1230 Pleasant St.
  Barre, MA 01005
  508-355-4378
  Publishes a newsletter and organizes retreats and seminars on meditation and mindfulness.

- Institute of Noetic Sciences
  475 Gate Five Rd., Ste. 300
  Sausalito, CA 94965
  415-331-5650
  Promotes human consciousness research and education, including meditation.

- The Maharishi University of Management
  1000 North 4th St.
  Fairfield, IA 52557
  515-472-5031
  800-888-5797
  School and research facility on Transcendental Meditation (TM). Gives referrals on where to find a TM class nationwide.

CAUTION

People with some conditions should probably avoid meditation. Serious psychological conditions, such as severe depression and schizophrenia, can be worsened by meditation in some cases. Anyone with any doubts about whether meditation is advisable should talk to a health professional experienced with meditative practices.

MEDITATION TIPS

Find a quiet place and sit comfortably, with eyes closed and body relaxed. Pick a word, phrase, or image to focus on while you sit. Breathe slowly and naturally. If other thoughts, worries, and distractions come up, just gently brush them aside and return to your focus. Continue the meditation for about 20 minutes.

Here are a few general, basic ideas for helping you get the most out of your meditation:

- Make sure the place you pick is out of the way. It should be somewhere quiet, removed from distractions (at least the outer ones); for example, pick a place you can't hear the phone, or take it off the hook.
- Take on a comfortable physical position. It is not necessary to assume the lotus position to meditate; sitting or lying down is fine.
- Wear loose clothing.
- Relax and take on a passive attitude. Don't try to make something happen.

- Mind/Body Behavioral Medicine Clinic
  Deaconess Hospital
  Harvard Medical School
  1 Deaconess Rd.
  Boston, MA 02215
  617-632-9530
  Offers behavioral medicine programs designed to help people with chronic illness or stress-related physical symptoms better manage their condition.

- Mind/Body Health Sciences, Inc.
  393 Dixon Rd.
  Boulder, CO 80302
  303-440-8460
  Offers workshops on meditation and mind/body medicine. Publishes free annual newsletter and catalog listing mail order books and tapes.

- Stress Reduction Clinic
  University of Massachusetts Medical Center
  55 Lake Ave., North
  Worcester, MA 01655
  508-856-2656
  Specializes in mindfulness-based stress-reduction techniques. Offers training sessions.

Mind/Body Medicine

THE MIND AND THE BODY ARE VERY CLOSELY LINKED. IN FACT, THE IDEA THAT THE TWO ARE SEPARATE ENTITIES AT ALL IS A RELATIVELY RECENT CONCEPT IN HUMAN HISTORY. MAXIMIZING THEIR CLOSE RELATIONSHIP TO IMPROVE OVERALL HEALTH IS WHAT MIND/BODY MEDICINE IS ALL ABOUT. A DIVERSE GROUP OF THERAPIES FALL UNDER THE HEADING MIND/BODY MEDICINE, BUT THEY HAVE THAT ONE THING IN COMMON: THEY USE THE OFTEN UNTAPPED POWER OF THE MIND TO EFFECT A HEALING.

HISTORY

The Western world's recognition of the mind and body as distinct entities dates back to the 17th century, when Rene Descartes first formally postulated a difference between the two. Modern science has adhered to this artificial separation of mind and body ever since. But before the 1600s in the West and to this day in non-Western parts of the world, the whole human—mind and body—was and is considered one inseparable organism. Treating the whole being is truly the basis for mind/body therapies— therapies that have been around since the art of healing began.

WHAT IT IS

Scientists with fancy names like psychoneuroendocrinologists study the links between the brain, nervous system, and endocrine system that regulate the body's glands and hormones. Their counterparts, the psychoneuroimmunologists, study the relationship between the mind, nervous system, and immune system. No matter how big the words, however, the importance of the link between mind and body is gaining a new appreciation in Western science.

As modern scientists begin to unravel the mechanisms by which some mind/body interventions work, they are beginning to learn what traditional healers from around the world have known for centuries: We may not be able to explain exactly how, but there is an extraordinary interconnectedness between the mind and body. And each has the power to affect the other profoundly.

In recent years, modern Western science has been able to quantify physical changes and healing brought about by traditional healing systems such as meditation, qigong, and yoga. Despite advances in the understanding of some aspects of mind/body interactions, however, some Western medical practitioners still struggle with the concept that "psychosomatic" is not a dirty word.

Harder still for the mind trained in Western science to grasp is the idea that there is a consciousness or perhaps some form of energy out there that somehow links us all or connects us to a greater healing power. Researchers in the area of mind/body interventions stress that just because we don't know what it is or how it works does not mean that it isn't there. There are many therapies in conventional medicine that work without doctors' knowing exactly why. When penicillin was discovered, for example, doctors did not understand how it worked, just that it did.

Recognizing the power that the mind has over health, many organized therapies exist to tap into this potential. The range of disorders that these therapies can address is unlimited—as unlimited as the mind's power. Although it would be impossible to discuss all the therapies that could fall under the heading "mind/body," the following are some of the more prominent. Some require the guidance of a trained practitioner; others can be practiced privately without outside assistance, making mind/body medicine perhaps the most accessible method of healing.

ART THERAPY

Art is as old as the human race. Even before the first cave paintings of the Stone Age, people have expressed themselves through visual representations of their experiences. The art we create is a highly personal and unique translation of our sensory impression of the world.

HISTORY

Western medicine began to recognize the connection between art and mental health during the arrival of mental institutions in the late 1800s and early 1900s. *Artistry of the Mentally Ill*, published in 1922, focused attention on the use of art by mentally ill patients and helped bring about awareness that art could not only help in the diagnosis of patients but serve as a way to restore mental health. The modern field of art therapy was pioneered in the 1940s by Margaret Naumberg, who merged psychoanalytic techniques and art as a way to help individuals release their unconscious through the creation of spontaneous images.

WHAT IT IS

Art therapy is the use of art to help people express unspoken or unconscious concerns, foster self-awareness, and reconcile emotional conflicts. Art can be a valuable tool in assessing people, particularly children and psychiatric patients, who may not be able to talk about their concerns. Art therapy can help individuals express their emotions, discuss them, and learn to deal with them effectively.

Although teaching technique and appreciation of art can be a valuable part of art therapy, the main focus and most of the therapeutic benefit comes from the hands-on participation. Actually making art—expressing oneself—is thought to be the activity that can provide the greatest benefit. Painting, sculpture, pottery, printing, and even writing and making music all have potentially therapeutic application.

USES

Art therapy is particularly useful in working with children, who may not be able to remember or express emotions verbally. Before we learn to speak, many of our memories are visual or sensory. And in times of intense stress or terror, people of all ages may bypass the regular memory system. Art therapy's use of visual, sensory, and motor media can help children and people who have experienced severe trauma bring repressed traumatic memories to the surface. Studies on the effective use of art therapy have been published on a wide variety of situations and conditions including

- Alzheimer disease
- children who are dying
- children who are grieving
- mental illness

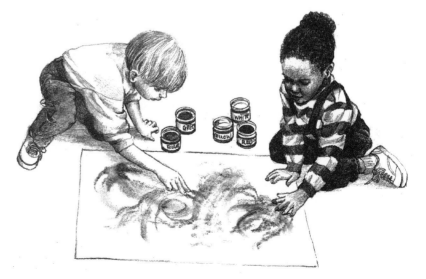

Psychological Problems in Children—Art therapy can be useful in working with children, adolescents, and adults who have repressed traumatic memories. In instances of sexual abuse, for example, art therapy can help children and adolescents to overcome resistance, build trust, reduce tension, and stimulate memory [1].

Art therapy has been found to be a helpful tool in adolescent group psychotherapy. The creative process stimulates expression, whereas the artworks and the verbal interaction about their meaning offer an opportunity to deal with group activity, individual conflicts, and difficulties related to adolescent development [2].

Multiple Personality Disorder—Sometimes the mind copes with abuse or trauma by creating an alternate identity system, which is intended to protect individuals from pain. The development of multiple personalities and dissociative disorders can result in significant problems in normal functioning due to amnesia and identity confusion. Patients with multiple personalities often have significant problems with issues such as control and trust and may be reluctant to join in structured groups. Many of these patients are, however, responsive to the opportunity to express themselves through art [3].

Post-traumatic Stress Disorder—Veterans suffering from post-traumatic stress disorder have been found to benefit from art therapy as well. Art therapy seeks to help these individuals improve coping patterns through individual and group interventions that promote expression of feelings, congruency between experience and self-concept, and feelings of effectiveness in behavioral change [4].

Schizophrenia—An Italian report on the use of art therapy in a group of institutionalized chronic schizophrenic patients found that art therapy helped to encourage the feeling of belonging and creative participation and that artistic expression can help restore communication to schizophrenic patients [5].

A Polish art therapy program in which participants were encouraged to exhibit their paintings found that patients with schizophrenia as well as people with chronic and terminal illnesses experienced positive changes in their family and social life [6].

WHO DOES IT

Art therapists are trained in studio arts, as well as in both diagnosis and helping patients with specific health problems. Registered Art Therapists (ATRs) have graduate training and a strong foundation in studio arts and therapy techniques. Therapists must complete a supervised internship with work experience.

DANCE THERAPY

Dance and movement therapists use movement and the body to bring about change, healing, and growth in the individual. Dance is a direct expression of the mind and body and can therefore be a powerful tool for healing and therapy.

HISTORY

Cultures throughout the world have traditionally used dance as a way to bond communities, celebrate major events, and heal the sick. The modern beginning of dance as a healing therapy can be traced to the 1940s when psychiatrists in Washington, D.C., noted that their patients were deriving therapeutic benefits from attending dance classes led by Marian Chace. Considered a pioneer of dance therapy in the United States, Chace was asked to work with psychiatric patients considered too disturbed to participate in group activities. On the West Coast, dancer and mime Trudi Schoop began working with patients in group dance therapy.

WHAT IT IS

The American Dance Therapy Association defines dance therapy as "the psychotherapeutic use of movement as a process that furthers the emotional, cognitive, and physical integration of the individual." Whereas conventional psychotherapy focuses on verbal communication, dance and movement therapy attempts to bring together the body, mind, and spirit.

HOW IT WORKS

Like other movement therapies (see pages 204–209), dance therapists hold that the process of changing how you move can affect total functioning. Dance therapists not only work with movement patterns but also focus on the interaction between mind and body to help people recognize and express feelings and develop attachments.

Dance therapy uses a variety of specific features that promote healing. For example, music, rhythm, and synchronous movement alter mood states, reawaken stored memories and feelings, organize thoughts and actions, reduce isolation, and establish rapport.

Total body movement stimulates functioning of the body's circulatory, neuromuscular, respiratory, and skeletal systems. And physical activity increases the level of endorphins, natural painkillers in the body that induce a state of well-being.

USES

Dance therapy is typically used for people with cognitive, emotional, and/or social concerns and problems. Therapy seeks to help emotionally disturbed patients express their feelings, gain insight, and develop healthy attachments.

Elderly persons can use dance therapy to enhance vitality, express fear and grief, develop relationships, and maintain a healthy body. Physically disabled persons can benefit from dance therapy as a way to help increase movement and self-esteem, have fun, and heighten creativity. And mentally retarded persons can use dance therapy to help develop better social skills, increase body awareness, and motivate learning.

Dance therapists work with people of all ages individually or in group settings. Therapists work in settings such as adult day-care centers, clinics, community mental health centers, correctional facilities, general and psychiatric hospitals, infant development centers, private practice, and schools and recreational facilities.

Dance therapy is believed to help reduce anxiety. A study of 84 college students compared anxiety before and after three months of dance class with students enrolled in exercise, music, and mathematics classes. The study found that students in the dance class had significantly lower levels of anxiety, but that students in the other groups had no significant reduction in anxiety [7].

In recent years, dance therapy is being used for disease prevention and health promotion among healthy people, and as a way to reduce stress in persons with AIDS, Alzheimer disease, and cancer, as well as individuals who care for them. Although extensive controlled scientific studies of dance therapy have not been conducted, it has been widely used in clinical practice for a variety of purposes:

- ameliorating depression
- decreasing fear and anxiety
- decreasing isolation
- decreasing bodily tension
- developing body image
- enhancing circulatory and respiratory function
- expressing anger
- facilitating attention
- increasing communication skills
- increasing feelings of well-being
- increasing and expanding self-concept and self-esteem
- increasing verbalization
- promoting healing
- reducing chronic pain
- reducing suicidal thoughts

WHO DOES IT

Although a variety of people use dance therapy, professional training is done on the graduate level. The American Dance Therapy Association approves five master's level programs. Students take courses in dance and movement therapy theory and practice, human development, observation and research skills, psychopathology, and psychotherapeutic theory, and they participate in a supervised internship in a clinical setting.

The ADTA offers two levels of certification: Dance Therapist Registered, or DTR, for people who have completed a master's level program in dance therapy, and Academy of Dance Therapists Registered, or ADTR, for registered dance therapists who have completed a requisite number of supervised employment positions in the field.

HORTICULTURAL THERAPY

As anyone who likes to putter in the garden can tell you, sometimes just putting your fingers in the dirt or tending to a plant can help relieve stress and make you feel a little more connected. Horticulture therapy uses this basic feeling in a variety of ways to promote health and well-being.

WHAT IT IS

Horticultural therapy uses plants and horticultural activities to improve people's social, educational, psychological, and physical adjustment and thereby improve their body, mind, and spirits. Therapy involves the patient in all phases of gardening and, sometimes, even the activity of selling the produce and plants grown.

HISTORY

The first known greenhouse for individuals with mental illnesses to use was built in 1879 by Pennsylvania's Friends Asylum for the Insane (today known as Friends Hospital). Modern-day horticultural therapy was fueled in part by its use in rehabilitating disabled veterans of World War II. The first undergraduate degree in horticultural therapy was awarded by Michigan State University in 1955.

HOW IT WORKS

As the American Horticultural Therapy Association likes to say, horticultural therapy harvests many benefits. Growing plants, whether indoors or out, can promote cognitive development, improve psychological outlook and status, promote social growth, and aid in physical rehabilitation.

USES

Cognitive Development—Growing plants teaches new skills and language, increases attention spans, raises concentration levels, and improves the ability to work independently, solve problems, and follow directions.

Psychological Development—Because plants depend on people for care, nurturing needs are met through responsibility for something living. Successful projects encourage creativity and promote self-esteem and feelings of usefulness and responsibility. Activities such as hoeing, weeding, repotting, and pruning help relieve aggressive feelings, anger, tension, and stress.

Social Growth—Working in a horticultural therapy group encourages learning to compromise and share work toward common goals. These therapy groups increase social interaction and heighten awareness of nature.

Physical Rehabilitation—Gardening activities can be adapted to the individual's limitations and can provide incentive to exercise and retrain muscles through gross and fine motor activities. This balance of work and relaxation for the mind and body provides a restorative setting.

Horticultural therapy can be beneficial for a wide variety of people, including people who are
- developmentally disabled
- elderly
- mentally ill
- physically disabled
- public offenders
- socially disadvantaged
- substance abusers

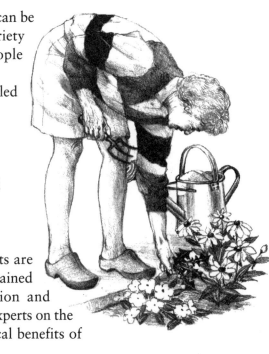

WHO DOES IT

Horticultural therapists are specially educated and trained members of rehabilitation and therapy teams who are experts on the medical and psychological benefits of gardening.

HUMOR THERAPY

It is often said that laughter is the best medicine. Ever since Norman Cousins described his dramatic recovery from a bizarre rheumatic condition by watching hours of funny movies, there has been growing interest in humor as an aspect of treating illness.

Humor can affect health on many levels. It can reduce or eliminate stress, ease discomfort, and generally stimulate the mind and body, producing a positive outlook and a healthy perspective. Laughter can increase the production of endorphins—chemicals that act as natural opiates—reducing pain and improving mood. It increases heart rate and improves circulation. There is also evidence that laughter can temporarily increase the amount of immunoglobulin A in saliva, a substance that can help fight the initial stages of infections such as the flu and the common cold.

NEUROLINGUISTIC PROGRAMMING

Pattern recognition is one of the hallmarks of thought and consciousness. Most of the time, this ability to learn and use complex patterns of information and events is beneficial to our functioning in social and physical challenges. However, certain patterns and modes of thinking can be negative, creating obstacles to the healing process and well-being in general. Neurolinguistic programming can replace the patterns of association that limit the body's natural healing ability with patterns that promote wellness.

HISTORY

Neurolinguistic programming was developed in the early 1970s by a student and a professor at the University of California at Santa Cruz. By studying certain communicative cues (verbal language, body language, eye movements, and others) of a few successful, healthy subjects, they were able to make out patterns of thinking that assisted in the success of the subjects. The two theorized that the brain can learn the healthy patterns and behaviors and that this would bring about positive physical and emotional effects.

HOW IT WORKS

Neurolinguistic programming uses self-image and attitudes toward illness to effect change and promote healing. When a person feels helpless in the face of a chronic disease, for example, the body can stop trying to heal itself and the disease goes on unabated. However, when the patient learns to see the situation and his or her own abilities differently, the body can respond with powerful healing tools.

The neurolinguistic programming practitioner uses the verbal and non-verbal cues of the patient to diagnose (recognize) patterns of thought and develop strategies to repattern the patient's attitudes. By focusing the patient's mind on a state of health, programming activates the body's immune system and endocrine system to a state of balance and health. Furthermore, when the mind is aligned with a state of health, destructive behaviors are also more likely to be avoided.

One strategy for examining belief systems and attitude patterns is to study what are called the *modalities* and *submodalities* of a person's thoughts. Modalities of memory and thinking are the way the brain stores information; the modalities coincide with the five senses. Submodalities are other aspects within the sense modalities. For example, when an old friend comes to mind, what point of view is the mental picture from? Is he young like when you first met or is it a later image? Is it his face smiling, or is it his whole body far away? These submodalities are all parts of the way the mind visualizes. There are, of course, submodalities for the other senses, too.

Neurolinguistic programming has several ways to deal with negative patterns. Reprogramming is often accomplished by guided imagery in which the practitioner guides the patient to a self-image of health and vitality, thus triggering the body to respond as if it were disease free. Another successful technique is memory imprinting, in which the submodalities that shade a certain memory and create confusion, worry, stress, and illness can be reassessed and relearned in a positive perspective.

USES

Neurolinguistic programming has had anecdotal successes in treating serious life-threatening diseases such as cancer and AIDS, but controlled scientific studies of its utility in this area are lacking. Certainly, the technique's ability to enhance the body's own defenses in these illnesses and promote a healthy mental attitude are advantages.

Perhaps the therapy's greatest successes have come in the realm of mental health. Trauma, for example, can have negative consequences on mental health for years after. Neurolinguistic programming can help a person examine the memories—including submodalities—of the event and change the harmful perceptions that continue to cause problems. One report describes the use of neurolinguistic programming in a group of adolescents who were in the hospital after an accident. The technique aided the patients in completing the healing and grieving process [8].

Another report of the technique's use involved an elderly patient diagnosed with clinical depression. By reviving positive memories and helping to build an imaginary photo album of the patient's life, the practitioners were able to create a more positive self-image for the patient [9].

WHO DOES IT

Practitioners receive certification from various organizations around the United States and Canada. There is no one governing body or one set curriculum, but most programs require the successful completion of a training course that usually involves some clinical experience.

PET THERAPY

Companionship doesn't even have to be human. Just as contact with living, growing things such as plants can help people connect with nature and provide a pathway for spirituality and connectedness, animals can play an important role in psychological and physical health and well-being. The therapeutic use of pets as companions has gained increasing attention in recent years for a wide variety of patients —people with AIDS or cancer, the elderly, and the mentally ill. Unlike people, with whom our interactions may be quite complex and unpredictable, animals provide a constant source of comfort and focus for attention.

A study of 92 patients hospitalized in coronary care units for angina or heart attack found that those who owned pets were more likely to be alive a year later than those who did not. The study found that only 6 percent of patients who owned pets died within one year compared with 28 percent of those who did not own pets [10].

Although people who own pets may have different personality traits than those who do not, the study notes that previous research has found that complex, varied, and interesting daily activity is the strongest social predictor of longevity. The researchers suggest that pet ownership may affect people physiologically through the soothing and relaxing effect of touch. And that speechless communication with a pet, or simply watching a cat or fish, may produce a relaxation response with little demand on the patient.

PRAYER

Praying for healing is practiced in almost all societies, whether to the Western Judeo-Christian God or another higher being or power. Although most Americans pray when they or a loved one is ill, there is little scientific evidence that prayer is beneficial.

However, one study of heart attack patients admitted to the coronary care unit of San Francisco General Hospital found that those who were prayed for had a better outcome than those who were not. The study involved 393 patients admitted to the coronary care unit—192 patients were assigned to a prayer group and 201 patients served as controls. Patients in the prayer group were prayed for by Christians outside of the hospital. These "intercessors" were given the first name of the patient, told of their diagnosis and condition, and were asked to pray daily for a rapid recovery, for prevention of complications and death, and for other concerns. Both groups of patients had no significant differences upon entry to the study. Neither the patients, staff, or doctors knew which patients were in which group.

Patients in the prayer group had a significantly better hospital course and an overall better outcome than those in the control group. Patients who were prayed for required less drug therapy, had fewer cardiac arrests and episodes of pneumonia, and were less likely to need a ventilator for breathing [11].

RELIGION AND SPIRITUALITY

The search for meaning and an understanding of how we fit into the world is central to the world's religions. While the names may differ, virtually all cultures and societies hold a belief in a higher power or universal life force. In the West, the most common religions are focused on the Judeo-Christian God. A number of cultures recognize a universal force or life energy, such as qi in China or prana in India. Whatever definition you choose, religion or spirituality can have profound effects on health.

Blood pressure is an excellent example. A review of nearly 20 studies conducted over a 30-year period concluded that religion "probably" has a beneficial effect on blood pressure. Overall, the studies reviewed indicate that persons who report higher levels of religious commitment seem to be at lower risk of illness and death. The following are some examples:

- People in Evans County, Georgia, who reported at least weekly religious attendance had lower blood pressure than those who did not.
- Significant protective effects against high blood pressure are associated with religious attendance among rural Zulus and church membership among urban female Zulus.
- Buddhist priests have significantly lower mortality due to hypertension than laypeople.
- American Baptist male clergy have significantly lower mortality due to hypertension with heart disease than laymen.
- Mormons in Utah have significantly lower rates of hypertensive heart disease than non-Mormons.

There are a number of hypotheses for why religion is associated with decreased rates of hypertension [12]:

- *Belief Systems*—Religious belief systems can help bring about a greater sense of peacefulness, self-confidence, and purpose. In some cases, however, they may also bring about feelings of depression, guilt, and self-doubt. For example, people who believe they are bewitched are at greater risk of high blood pressure.
- *Healthy Behavior*—Many churches prohibit or discourage the use of alcohol, tobacco, caffeine, and other harmful substances.
- *Psychosocial Effects*—Religion fosters a sense of belonging, participation, and social cohesiveness that can positively influence health.
- *The Use of Ritual*—Private and public rituals can help alleviate anxiety and fear, while helping to alleviate depression, loneliness, and tension.

SELF-HELP GROUPS

The past few decades have seen a tremendous rise in the advent of self-help groups for people with a variety of ailments and conditions. These groups provide an important opportunity for individuals to express their emotions and concerns, exchange information, and learn new ways of coping with their problem.

A survey of 232 people in 65 different self-help groups found that self-help groups can offer significant help to people suffering from chronic diseases and other problems. Researchers found that more than 80 percent of people interviewed said they felt an improvement in at least one aspect of their health [13].

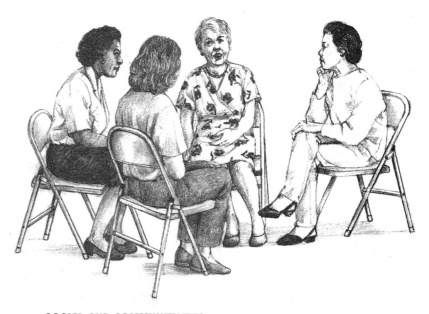

SOCIAL AND COMMUNITY TIES

A number of studies have shown that socially isolated people have higher rates of illness and death. For example, unmarried people, particularly men, have consistently higher death rates from all causes than those who are married. People who have close ties with family and friends are less likely to die than those with few close contacts. And attendance at church and participation in organizations can contribute to health as well.

Marital disruption has been linked to a number of diseases. For example, separated or divorced individuals have higher rates of mortality from infectious diseases, including as much as six times the deaths from pneumonia. Research shows that the stress from the breakup of a marriage can result in alterations in immune function and, therefore, susceptibility to disease.

A study of 38 married women and 38 separated or divorced women found that those who were recently separated or divorced had significantly poorer immune function than married women. Among the 38 separated or divorced women, the 16 who had been separated one year or less had decreased numbers of important immune cells such as helper T lymphocytes and natural killer cells [14].

A study of nearly 7,000 adults in Alameda County, California, found that people who lacked social and community ties were more likely to die in the nine-year follow-up period than those who had more extensive contacts [15].

THE ROSETO STORY

The importance of close family and community ties can be illustrated by the town of Roseto, Pennsylvania. Researchers in the mid-1950s to early 1960s found a remarkably low incidence of deaths from heart attack in the close-knit Italian-American community despite risk factors such as lack of exercise, high fat intake, obesity, and smoking. At this time, the townspeople of Roseto still embraced "Old World" values such as close family and community ties, a secure and respected place for elders, and a low level of social competitiveness. In 1965, the death rate from heart attacks among people in Roseto was half that of people in the neighboring community of Bangor. But, as traditional family and community ties loosened in Roseto, the death rate from heart attacks began to climb. By 1975, the death rate from heart attacks in this now "Americanized" and "modern" town had reached the same level as that of Bangor and closely resembled that in the United States at large [17].

A number of theories exist on how social networks and support promote health. Such support may help promote behavior or neuroendocrine responses that adapt to stress or other health hazards. Close family and or community ties may help reinforce positive health habits, such as appropriate use of alcohol, proper diet, regular exercise, healthy sleep patterns, and prompt medical care.

Noting that Americans are less likely to be married, have children, and participate in voluntary organizations than they were in the 1950s, there may be reason for concern about the potential impact of such a decline now that we have recognized the importance of such relationships [16].

OTHER MIND/BODY THERAPIES

In a sense, all of the therapies included in this book could be considered mind/body. An adequate discussion of mind/body therapies is beyond the scope of this book and even a set of encyclopedias. Some of the more prominent and extensively researched mind/body therapies are discussed in separate sections, including

- biofeedback (see page 188)
- hypnotherapy (see page 272)
- guided imagery (see page 237)
- meditation (see page 276)
- sound therapy (see page 354)
- yoga (see page 360)
- qigong (see page 342)
- homeopathy (see page 260)

RESOURCES

- American Art Therapy Association
  1202 Allanson Rd.
  Mundelein, IL 60060
  847-949-6064

Founded in 1969, the Association is dedicated to the use of art therapy and the development of professional standards of practice for art therapists and research. Provides information on approved programs of art therapy education and clinical programs, serves as an information clearinghouse, and disseminates publications and audiovisual materials.

- American Association for Therapeutic Humor
1163 Shermer Rd.
Northbrook, IL 60062-4538
847-291-0211
Promotes the use of humor as an adjunct to treatment and publishes the bimonthly newsletter *Lighten It Up*.

- American Dance Therapy Association
10632 Little Patuxent Pkwy.
2000 Century Plaza, Ste. 108
Columbia, MD 21044
410-997-4040
fax 410-997-4048
http://www.citi.net/ADTA/
Founded in 1956, the Association is the national professional support organization for dance and movement therapists. Publishes a journal, fosters research on dance therapy, monitors standards for professional practice, and maintains a registry for dance therapists.

- American Horticultural Therapy Association
362A Christopher Ave.
Gaithersburg, MD 20879
301-948-3010
800-634-1603
fax 301-869-2397
http://aggiehorticulture.tamu.edu/horther/ahta.html
Founded in 1973, the Association seeks to advance the practice of horticulture as therapy to improve human well-being. Administers a voluntary professional registration program, sponsors continuing education programs, publishes reports and periodicals, and hosts an annual conference.

- Institute for the Advancement of Health
16 East 53rd St.
New York, NY 10022
212-832-8282
Publishes several journals and sponsors seminars and lectures in the field.

- Institute for the Advancement of Human Behavior
P.O. Box 7226
Stanford, CA 94306
415-851-8411
fax 415-851-0406
Sponsors conferences designed to facilitate communication among professionals in both conventional and alternative health care fields.

Naturopathic Medicine

NATUROPATHIC MEDICINE IS NATURAL MEDICINE IN THE FULLEST SENSE OF THE WORD. NATUROPATHIC PHYSICIANS TREAT PATIENTS BY RESTORING OVERALL HEALTH INSTEAD OF SUPPRESSING A FEW KEY SYMPTOMS. PRACTITIONERS SEEK TO FIND THE UNDERLYING CAUSE OF A CONDITION AND APPLY A VARIETY OF TREATMENTS THAT ARE INTENDED TO WORK WITH THE BODY'S NATURAL HEALING MECHANISMS.

HISTORY

Naturopathy celebrated its 100th anniversary in 1996, but in truth, the principles on which it's based and the methods it employs are much older, many dating to ancient times. Once a thriving area of practice throughout most of the United States around the turn of the century, naturopathic medicine fell on hard times with the rise to prominence of allopathic institutions. However, more and more states are now recognizing its value, and naturopathy seems to be once again on the rise.

WHAT IT IS

Naturopathic physicians treat disease and restore health using a wide variety of therapies that are combined and tailored to meet the needs of an individual patient. For the most part, naturopathic physicians are primary health care providers and are equipped to handle most medical conditions, but they routinely refer patients to other practitioners for diagnosis or treatment when appropriate. Although some practitioners specialize in particular modes of treatment, such as acupuncture, or particular medical areas, such as pediatrics or obstetrics, most naturopathic physicians are in general practice.

PRINCIPLES OF NATUROPATHIC MEDICINE

Naturopathy operates on the basis of six principles of healing. These precepts circumscribe a time-tested approach to healing that spans many traditions and still has room to grow and incorporate new therapies as they arise.

The Healing Power of Nature—Naturopathy believes that nature acts powerfully through healing mechanisms in the body and mind to maintain and restore health. Naturopathic physicians seek to restore and support these inherent healing systems through medicines and techniques that are in harmony with natural processes.

Find the Cause—Whereas allopathic medicine has a tendency to address symptoms, naturopathic physicians are trained to find and remove the underlying cause of a disease. Symptoms are the body's reaction to a disease state; they are not the disease itself. In fact, symptoms are often part of the body's way to heal itself. Therefore, suppressing them would inhibit the natural healing process. Naturopathic medicine focuses on finding the underlying cause so it can be addressed without hindering the body's healing power.

First Do No Harm—First mentioned by Hippocrates—the ancient Greek "father of medicine"—and still a part of allopathic medicine's Hippocratic oath, this principle seems straightforward and obvious. But in these days of high-tech possibilities, conventional medicine can, and often does, lose sight of this most basic axiom. Naturopaths prefer noninvasive treatments that minimize the risks of harmful side effects.

Treat the Whole Person—Health involves every part of a person's being, and disease affects every aspect also. Naturopathic physicians treat the whole person, taking into account the complex interaction of dietary, emotional, environmental, genetic, lifestyle, physical, and social factors. Healing cannot be fully realized unless all of the areas of imbalance or distortion are addressed.

The Physician Is a Teacher—A doctor is not a mechanic who fixes things when broken. A physician should be a partner with the patient, both with health and healing as their common goal. Naturopathic physicians share information with their patients and teach their patients to take responsibility for their own health.

Prevention—Most people see the doctor only when they're ill. However, naturopathic medical schools focus on the study of health and disease prevention almost as much as they study disease states. While healing is a vital part of the naturopathic practice, not getting sick in the first place should be the true first goal of all medicine. Naturopathic practitioners seek to prevent illness—and to keep minor illnesses from developing into more serious or chronic degenerative diseases—by providing education and care to patients who are well.

THERAPIES USED IN NATUROPATHY

There are many treatment options open to a naturopath, enabling the practitioner to address health problems on many levels. Naturopathic physicians are trained in conventional diagnostic techniques and therapies and in a variety of natural therapies. Treatments are combined and tailored to meet the needs of an individual patient.

The following therapies form the core of the naturopathic discipline, but many other diagnostic and treatment methods—both conventional and alternative—are also included in naturopathic practice depending on the practitioner's training and expertise.

Nutritional Therapy—A cornerstone of naturopathic medicine, nutrition and the therapeutic foods are used to treat many medical conditions. Naturopathic physicians receive at least 140 hours of classroom instruction in nutrition compared with the fewer than 20 hours that most allopathic physicians receive.

Nutritional counseling can often be as effective as drug therapy but with fewer complications and side effects. For example, conventional allopathic treatment for arthritis generally includes the use of nonsteroidal anti-inflammatory drugs that can cost up to $1,000 per year and may cost far more in both side effects and further illness for patients. Nutritional treatment for rheumatoid arthritis, however, may include a variety of approaches such as fasting and special additions to the diet—none of which has significant side effects or costs.

Nutritional supplementation can also have significant therapeutic benefit. Naturopathic physicians are trained to prescribe appropriate vitamin and mineral supplements as well as lesser-known supplements such as amino acids and enzymes. (For more on Nutritional Therapy, see pages 303–333.)

Botanical Medicine—Also called phytomedicine, botanical medicine is the use of plants to treat various conditions and promote well-being. Naturopathic physicians receive training in preparing and prescribing herbs in various forms—teas, tinctures, capsules, and topical preparations. Herbs are well suited to the practice of naturopathic medicine because of their natural origins and general lack of side effects, upholding the principle, "First do no harm." (For more information on Herbal Medicine, see pages 241–259.)

Homeopathy—The science of homeopathy is a prominent part of many naturopathic practices. Homeopathy uses small amounts of natural substances that bring about healing actions in the body. Homeopathy is another therapy that dovetails well with the naturopathic philosophy of the healing power of nature and treating the whole person. (For more information on Homeopathy, see pages 260–264.)

Bodywork—Depending on their specific training, naturopathic physicians can employ a full range of physical therapeutics. Massage, therapeutic naturopathic manipulations (similar to chiropractic and osteopathic techniques), movement reeducation, Therapeutic Touch, and other hands-on techniques are often incorporated into naturopathic practice. (For more information on Bodywork, see pages 192–213; on Chiropractic Medicine, see pages 217–221; on Osteopathy see pages 334–337.)

Oriental Medicine—Naturopathy has a great deal in common with oriental healing philosophies. Naturopathic physicians use aspects of acupressure, acupuncture, Ayurvedic medicine, qigong, traditional Chinese medicine, yoga, and other therapies of Asian origin. The oriental concept of life force, or qi, and the naturopathic concept of the healing power of nature are similar in theory if not in language. (For more information on Acupressure, see pages 169–172; on Acupuncture, see pages 173–177; on Ayurvedic Medicine, see pages 182–187; on Qigong, see pages 342–345; on Traditional Chinese Medicine, see pages 346–353; on Yoga, see pages 360–364.)

Psychological Medicine—In keeping with the tenet "treat the whole person," naturopathy recognizes the nonphysical components of health and disease. The mind and the spirit are part of the healing equation, and ignoring psychological or spiritual troubles can only lead to a deterioration in mental *and* physical well-being. Naturopathic physicians receive extensive training in counseling and stress management, and many practitioners have additional training in hypnotherapy, mind/body medicine, guided imagery, and social medicine. (For more information on Mind/Body Medicine, see pages 282–293; on Hypnotherapy, see pages 272–275.)

Minor Surgery—Naturopathic practitioners are equipped to cope with minor surgical procedures such as stitches, deep splinters, and boil or cyst removal.

Other Therapeutic Techniques—The seven major therapeutic areas mentioned above are not the full extent of naturopathic practice. Hydrotherapy, hyperthermia, wave therapy, environmental medicine, biofeedback training, and other treatment modalities can also be part of the naturopaths practice. Different practitioners have various amounts of training in these fields and choose to use them on an individual basis.

Diagnostics usually thought of as allopathic, such as high-technology imaging (X rays, magnetic resonance imaging, computed tomography, ultrasonography, and so on), are often employed by naturopaths. Naturopathic medicine is, by no means, frozen in time, either. Practitioners follow advances in science and technology and regularly incorporate new techniques in their practices as long as they are in keeping with the philosophy of naturopathy. In addition, as primary health care providers, naturopathic physicians can make referrals to other therapists, both conventional and alternative.

Naturopathic obstetrics is a growing part of many naturopathic practices. As more and more women choose natural childbirth over the medicalized version, naturopaths have stepped up to meet the needs of their patients in the arena of prenatal care, perinatal care (many naturopaths deliver babies), and referrals to midwives and other practitioners in the field. (For more on natural childbirth, see Appendix 2.)

USES

Naturopathic physicians diagnose, treat, and work to prevent the entire range of human disease. They are primary health care providers in the fullest sense, and unlike many other alternative therapists, they are not limited to specialized applications of their art. Nevertheless, a few examples of how naturopaths treat common conditions will serve to show the range and depth of naturopathy's practice and the difference between the naturopathic and allopathic approaches.

CHRONIC OTITIS MEDIA
(MIDDLE EAR INFECTION)

About 30 percent of children under the age of six suffer from chronic infections and blockage of the middle ear. Conventional treatment generally includes repeated treatment with antibiotics, although recent clinical studies suggest they may be ineffective. Because chronic ear infections can result in hearing loss, conventional practitioners often resort to surgery to open the pathway through the eardrum when antibiotic treatment fails. Of more than one million such operations that are performed each year, about 30 percent must be repeated.

True to one of its basic tenets, naturopathic treatment seeks to identify and eliminate underlying causes—allergies, food sensitivities, or nutritional deficiencies—that bring about the chronic disorder, rather than simply eliminating the acute symptoms. Instead of using conventional antibiotic therapy, naturopathic physicians may prescribe botanicals that have antimicrobial properties, such as garlic, goldenseal, licorice, and myrrh. Homeopathic medicines and other botanicals, such as echinacea, may be used to enhance general immune resistance to infection, empowering the body's own mechanisms to heal and ward off future occurrences.

Hydrotherapy and physical therapy may include heat or alternating heat and cold massage, or eustachian tube massage to manage symptoms during treatment.

Naturopathic physicians report that they can successfully manage most cases of otitis media and that they refer less than one case in five back to surgery. This nonsurgical, cause-oriented approach to managing chronic ear infections not only prevents complications such as permanent scarring that may occur with surgery but is also significantly less expensive than conventional treatment. The cost of treatment for chronic ear infections by a conventional practitioner ranges from $144 to $7,137, with an average cost of $1,093. Naturopathic treatment for the same condition ranges from $208 to $668 [1].

HIGH BLOOD PRESSURE

Approximately 60 million Americans have high blood pressure, a disease that plays a contributing role in most heart attacks and strokes. Although conventional medicine recognizes the usefulness of some dietary and lifestyle changes, treatment is generally focused on drug therapy, usually starting with diuretics, beta blockers, or calcium channel blockers. Although drug therapy is effective in treating most cases of high blood pressure, about half of all patients stop treatment because of side effects, and most can look forward to taking the prescribed medication for life.

Naturopathic treatment emphasizes diet, exercise, and lifestyle factors and uses nontoxic blood pressure–lowering herbal medicines. Although standard blood pressure medication may be used when necessary, naturopaths continue to encourage patients to modify their diet and lifestyle. Research suggests that 40 percent of people with mild to moderate hypertension may be able to control their disease simply by maintaining normal weight and reducing alcohol and sodium intake.

Naturopathic physicians encourage patients with high blood pressure to reduce smoking and alcohol use, to lose weight if necessary, and to decrease the amount of salt, cholesterol, and fat in their diet. Patients are also screened for adequate levels of potassium, calcium, and magnesium, and, when necessary, treated with supplements (see pages 330–331).

Botanical and food therapy may include substances that naturally lower blood pressure, such as garlic and onions, and the herbs cayenne, hawthorn, skullcap, taraxacum, and valerian. Patients are also instructed in stress management techniques.

WHO DOES IT

Naturopaths are primary care physicians who are clinically trained in a wide variety of medical systems, both conventional and natural medicine. Their training is similar to that for conventional physicians: four years of postgraduate education at naturopathic medical colleges. Naturopaths study a standard medical curriculum plus course work in natural therapeutics such as acupuncture, botanical medicine, homeopathy, hydrotherapy, natural childbirth, naturopathic manipulative therapy, therapeutic nutrition, and mind/body connections. The

---

CAUTION

Some persons who identify themselves as "NDs" have degrees from programs that do not require clinical training. These "NDs" are generally not licensable in any state. Make sure your practitioner is licensed, a graduate of an accredited naturopathic medical college, or a member of the American Association of Naturopathic Physicians.

---

first two years of training are in basic medical science, with the last two years emphasizing clinical training in naturopathic therapeutics in a primary care outpatient setting.

There are currently three colleges of naturopathic medicine in the United States:

- John Bastyr University of Naturopathic Medicine in Seattle
- National College of Naturopathic Medicine in Portland, Oregon
- Southwest College of Naturopathic Medicine and Health Sciences in Scottsdale, Arizona.

Canada has the Canadian College of Naturopathic Medicine in Toronto.

Naturopaths practice in all states, sometimes under other types of licensure, but currently, 11 states license naturopathic physicians:

- Alaska
- Arizona
- Connecticut
- Hawaii
- Maine
- Montana
- New Hampshire
- Oregon
- Utah
- Vermont
- Washington

More than 90 insurance carriers cover naturopathic medicine in the United States and Canada. Three states—Alaska, Connecticut, and Washington—have mandated insurance reimbursement for medically necessary and appropriate naturopathic medical services. And these numbers will surely increase as issues of prevention and cost-cutting become increasingly important in public health care policy debates.

RESOURCES

- American Association of Naturopathic Physicians
2366 Eastlake Ave. East, Ste. 322
Seattle, WA 98102
206-323-7610
fax 206-323-7612
http://infinite.org/Naturopathic.Physician

The AANP is the professional association for naturopathic physicians. It publishes a listing of naturopathic physicians in the United States. The Web site provides consumer information and helpful hints on everything from cooking (with recipes for healthy eating) to an extensive listing of self-care information on a wide variety of conditions and ailments.

Neural Therapy

ALTHOUGH LITTLE KNOWN IN THE UNITED STATES, NEURAL THERAPY IS WIDELY PRACTICED IN EUROPE, ESPECIALLY GERMANY. IT'S A HEALING TECHNIQUE THAT INVOLVES INJECTING ANESTHETICS AT SPECIFIC POINTS IN THE BODY TO RELIEVE HEALTH PROBLEMS. NEURAL THERAPY HAS BEEN FOUND ESPECIALLY USEFUL IN TREATING CHRONIC PAIN.

HISTORY

The development of neural therapy is credited to Ferdinand Huneke, a German physician, who discovered that injecting a patient's lower leg scar with an anesthetic immediately cleared chronic shoulder pain that had failed to respond to other medical treatment. Occurring in 1940, this was the first documented example of what came to be known as the "Huneke phenomenon."

THE THEORY BEHIND THE THERAPY

Understanding neural therapy involves a comprehension of physiology, electrophysiology, physics, and neurology. Simply, neural therapy can be thought of a technique for restoring balance in the body's electrical system. All cells in the body conduct electricity. When a cell's conductivity is skewed outside of its normal range, abnormal signals get sent through the body. The flow of biological energy gets disrupted, and illness results.

INTERFERENCE FIELDS

The concept of interference fields is key to neural therapy. As neural therapists see it, 30 to 45 percent of illnesses and bodily pains can be traced to interference fields. These interference fields disrupt the normal flow of electromagnetic energy in the body. For example, an interference field might be the site of an old injury, scar or illness, or it might be a condition that has shown no symptoms and has gone undetected, such as a tooth abscess.

The interference field emits abnormal signals into the autonomic nervous system. Dysfunction may result even at some place in the body away from the location of the interference field. An upper respiratory infection, for instance, can leave the sinuses as a long-lasting interference field even after a person has recovered from the original infection. The sinus interference field then can spark symptoms such as chronic neck pain, migraines, chronic fatigue, and premenstrual syndrome.

Any part of the body that has been traumatized or ill can become an interference field—even the teeth and intestines, which some neural therapists indicate are the two interference fields most frequently overlooked.

ACTIVE AND INACTIVE INTERFERENCE

Interference fields can lie dormant for some time, only to be eventually activated by malnutrition, emotional stress, eating incompatible foods, and so on. For successful recovery, both the triggering condition and the interference field need to be treated.

INTERFERENCE FIELDS AND ILLNESS

Neural therapists believe there are certain common relationships between interference fields and illnesses. They consider these relationships when attempting to find the root source of an illness. Examples include
- tonsils—knee joint
- abdominal scars—large joints and lower back
- leg scars—sciatica
- tonsils and teeth—migraines
- prostate, stomach, and sinuses—neck and upper back

- gallbladder scar—shoulder
- pelvic scars—premenstrual syndrome, depression, and arthritis

WHAT IT IS

A neural therapist essentially has to function as a sleuth to determine first whether an interference field is, indeed, the culprit behind an illness. Indicators that suggest this include the following:

- The illness does not respond to other therapies.
- The illness or condition was unexpectedly made worse by another treatment.
- All symptoms are on one side of the body only.
- A patient's condition begins to accumulate—for example, after an appendectomy, the patient develops arthritis, indicating that a chain of interference fields might now be strong enough to cause illness.

Once an interference field is suspected as the root cause of an illness, the next step is for the neural therapist to find it and treat it. Treatment consists of injecting local anesthetics, such as procaine and lidocaine, which break down easily and are readily eliminated from the body. Often, immediate pain relief occurs, but follow-up injections may be needed to bring permanent results. Neural therapists also are now using alternative approaches that use electricity or light instead of needle injections.

Sometimes one interference field can on its own cause illness or pain. But most often, one interference field is just a link in a chain of interference fields. Writing the *Journal of Neurology and Orthopedic Medicine and Surgery* in 1993, internationally recognized neural

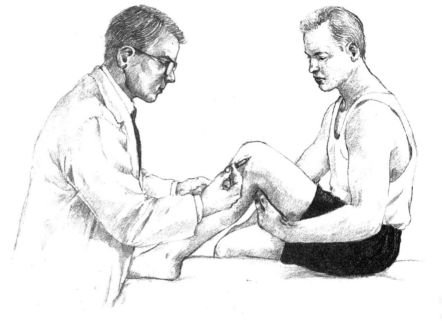

therapist D.K. Klinghardt related the following case study illustrating the phenomenon of chain interference fields. A patient experienced severe neck pain for one year. An injection was given at the site of a scar from surgery for removing the gallbladder. A day later, the patient reported no change in the neck pain and, in addition, she developed a sore throat. As it turned out, the patient had had recurring bouts of strep throat prior to onset of the neck pain. The next injection was done in the tonsils, which brought some relief in the neck pain, but now the patient reported pelvic pain. She had had a pelvic infection three years before. The pelvis was given an injection, which brought some improvement in symptoms, but also triggered itching at the site of an old appendix scar, which dated back to the woman's childhood. The scar area was treated next. All symptoms then subsided, including the original major complaint, neck pain.

The process of pinpointing interference fields depends to a great extent on therapist–patient communication. In the first place, the neural therapist relies on complete health history information from the patient to aid in detecting all interference fields. Once therapy is under way, patient feedback is crucial in guiding treatment, as the above case study clearly illustrates. The person undergoing neural therapy must pay close attention to changes and responses in his or her body to give clues as to what the next step should be in the neural therapy process.

USES

Neural therapy has been shown effective in treating hundreds of health problems. One distinguishing feature of neural therapy is that it is a treatment that often works to relieve chronic pain or illnesses that were unresponsive to other forms of treatment. Although neural therapy is still fairly unknown in the United States, it has become one of the most widely used methods for treating chronic pain and illness in Europe, especially in Germany. Some of the many conditions that neural therapists say they can successfully treat are

- allergies
- circulatory disorders
- ear, nose, and throat disorders
- lower-back pain
- migraines
- neck pain
- pelvic pain
- premenstrual syndrome
- sciatica
- sports injuries
- temporomandibular disorder
- ulcers

Neural therapists also emphasize that there are illnesses for which neural therapy is not advised. These include

- cancer—lymphatic spread could be facilitated by neural therapy
- genetic disorders
- nutritional deficiencies
- diabetes
- tuberculosis
- psychiatric illness, except depression
- end-state chronic illness, during which the patient is too weak to respond to therapy

In addition to the above, neural therapy will have no effect on conditions such as fractures, infectious diseases, or organ disorders.

RESOURCES

- American Academy of Neural Therapy
  2442 Cerrillos Rd., Ste. 270
  Santa Fe, NM 87505
  505-988-3086

Provides training in neural therapy and pain management techniques to physicians. Referrals to neural therapists nationwide also available.

Nutritional Therapy

HEALTHFUL DIETS HELP PEOPLE OF ALL AGES FEEL AND PERFORM THEIR BEST. OUR FOOD CHOICES CAN HAVE A PROFOUND IMPACT ON WELL-BEING AND LONGEVITY. SIMPLY EATING RIGHT IS CERTAINLY A PART OF NUTRITIONAL THERAPY, BUT THERE'S MORE, TOO. WITH THE LUXURY WE NOW HAVE OF EASILY MEETING OUR MINIMUM REQUIREMENTS FOR MOST NUTRIENTS, WE CAN BEGIN TO CONSUME THE OPTIMAL LEVELS OF HEALTHFUL NUTRIENTS THROUGH FOOD AND SUPPLEMENTS.

Our "affluent" meat-based diet often contains more calories than we can use from an excess of energy-dense foods rich in animal fat, partially hydrogenated vegetable oils, and refined carbohydrates. Yet it tends to lack the whole grains, fruits, and vegetables our bodies need.

While Americans' diets may be rich in calories, too often many of these are empty calories from refined carbohydrates and sugar. The processed foods that line our grocery store shelves are deficient in many micronutrients and other important components that are in the original unrefined foods.

In recent years, we have all heard about the benefits of a low-fat and high-fiber diet. The good news is that by simply eating more grains, fruits, and vegetables, you are well on your way. Plant foods are naturally low in fat and high in fiber. So increasing your consumption is an easy and natural way to get what you need and avoid what you do not.

A HEALTHFUL DIET

The basics of a healthy diet are no secret. Whole unprocessed foods, such as grains, vegetables, fruits, beans, nuts, and seeds are all good food choices and are easy to incorporate in the diet.

In 1992, the Department of Agriculture released its new Food Guide Pyramid. The Pyramid has a broad base consisting of bread, cereal, rice, and pasta, indicating that these should be eaten the most. The next layer consists of vegetables and fruits, then dairy products and meat. The smallest layer is the tip of sweets, fats, and oily foods, meaning that these should be consumed only in small amounts.

Both government officials and alternative practitioners agree on the basic foundation of a healthy diet. Although agreeing with the recommendation that Americans should eat more grains, vegetables, and fruits, some people think it doesn't go far enough. The Physicians Committee for Responsible Medicine, for example, says if the top two tiers (representing meat, dairy products, and fats and oils) were removed, we'd all be healthier.

GENERAL GUIDELINES

CHOOSE A DIET LOW IN FAT

Choosing a diet with low levels of cholesterol, total fat, and saturated fat is important to your health and reduces your risk of cancer, heart disease, and many other conditions. Fat, whether from plant or animal sources, contains more than twice the number of calories

The modern American diet is linked to a wide range of ailments—cancer, cerebrovascular disease, coronary heart disease, dental cavities, diabetes, gallstones, gastrointestinal disorders, and osteoporosis, to name a few. A healthy diet can reduce risk factors such as high blood pressure and high cholesterol levels and can even reverse heart disease.

Food Guide Pyramid
A Guide to Daily Food Choices

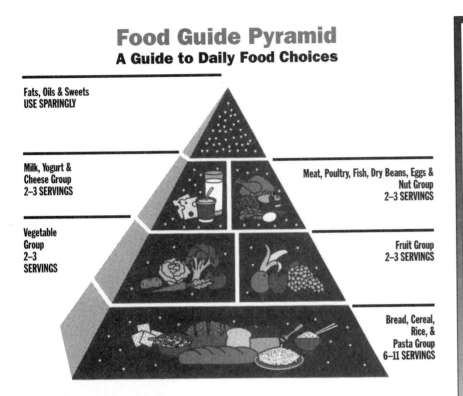

**Fats, Oils & Sweets
USE SPARINGLY**

**Milk, Yogurt &
Cheese Group
2–3 SERVINGS**

**Meat, Poultry, Fish, Dry Beans, Eggs &
Nut Group
2–3 SERVINGS**

**Vegetable
Group
2–3
SERVINGS**

**Fruit Group
2–3 SERVINGS**

**Bread, Cereal,
Rice, &
Pasta Group
6–11 SERVINGS**

KEY

◯ Fat (naturally occurring
and added)

▽ Sugars (added)

These symbols show fats, oils,
and added sugars in food.

THE PYRAMID EXPLAINED

Grain Products (6–11 servings) Eat products made from a variety of whole grains, such as wheat, rice, oats, corn, and barley. Eat several servings of whole-grain breads and cereals daily.

Vegetables (2–3 servings) Choose dark-green leafy and deep-yellow vegetables often. Eat starchy vegetables, such as potatoes and corn.

Fruits (2–3 servings) Choose citrus fruits or juices, melons, or berries regularly. Eat fruits as desserts or snacks. Drink fruit juices.

Meat, Poultry, Fish, Eggs, Beans, and Nuts (2–3 servings) Use meats labeled "lean" or "extra lean." Trim fat from meat, and take the skin off poultry. Most beans and bean products are almost fat-free and are a good source of protein and fiber. Limit your intake of processed meats such as sausages, organ meats such as liver, and egg yolks.

Milk and Dairy Products (2–3 servings) Choose skim or low-fat milk, fat-free or low-fat yogurt, and low-fat cheese. If you do not eat dairy products, make sure to eat other calcium-rich foods.

Fats and Oils (Use sparingly) Use small amounts of salad dressings and spreads such as butter, margarine, and mayonnaise. Consider using low-fat or fat-free dressings for salads. Choose vegetable oils such as canola or olive oil most often because they are lower in saturated fat than solid shortenings and animal fats, even though their caloric content is the same.

of an equal amount of carbohydrate or protein. The government recommends that you choose a diet that provides no more than 30 percent of total calories from fat. Many health advocates would go much lower, and numerous studies show that the lower your fat intake, the lower your risk of disease.

Low-fat cooking is easier than you think, and there are many delicious and easy ways to prepare alternatives to high-fat foods. Many favorites such as lasagna can be modified to a low-fat version.

Saturated Fat—Fats contain both saturated and unsaturated (monounsaturated and polyunsaturated) fatty acids. Saturated fat raises blood cholesterol more than other forms of fat—even more than eating cholesterol itself. Fats from meat, milk, and milk products are the main sources of saturated fats in most diets. Many bakery products may also contain large amounts of saturated fat.

Vegetable oils supply smaller amounts of saturated fat. Olive and canola oils are particularly high in monounsaturated fats; most other vegetable oils, nuts, and high-fat fish are good sources of polyunsaturated fats. While these are better for your cholesterol level than saturated fats, they are still fats. And polyunsaturated oils may not be the best choice for heating; when heated they tend to form free radicals that can increase your risk of several diseases, including cancer. Use monounsaturated oils (olive and canola) for heating.

Cholesterol—Our bodies make all the cholesterol we need. Dietary cholesterol comes from animal sources such as egg yolks, fish, meat, milk products, and poultry. Many of these foods are also high in saturated fat, which raises our cholesterol level. Eating foods with low or no cholesterol can help lower your blood cholesterol levels.

CHOOSE A DIET WITH PLENTY OF VEGETABLES, FRUITS, AND GRAINS

Vegetables, fruits, and grains are the most nutrient-dense foods you can eat for the calories. They are low in fat but loaded with vitamins, minerals, complex carbohydrates, and—perhaps most important—fiber.

Eating the American Cancer Society's five servings of fruit and vegetables daily may significantly reduce your risk of certain forms of cancer. And when you consume that many vegetable, fruit, and grain products, you have little room for the higher-fat foods, leading to a generally lower-calorie diet.

USE SUGARS ONLY IN MODERATION

For several reasons, it's a good idea to limit the amount of sugar in your diet. Sugars add calories to the diet often without contributing any nutrients. By spending calories on sugars, you have fewer opportunities to consume quality nutrient-dense foods. Sugar contributes to tooth decay, heart disease, and osteoporosis, and even relatively low amounts of sugar may decrease immune function.

Sugar goes by many names. Watch for the following on food labels:
- corn sweetener or syrup
- fructose
- fruit juice concentrate
- glucose
- dextrose
- maltose
- sucrose
- honey
- lactose
- molasses

USE SALT AND SODIUM ONLY IN MODERATION

Sodium plays an essential role in regulating fluids and blood pressure. Numerous studies have shown that a high sodium intake is associated with high blood pressure. Most Americans consume too much salt. The body only needs about one teaspoon per day.

Many processed foods, such as canned goods (meats, soups, and vegetables), frozen dinners, packaged mixes, salad dressings, and snack foods, contain high levels of sodium. Condiments such as soy and many other sauces, pickles, and olives are also high in sodium. Ketchup and mustard, when eaten in large amounts, can also contribute significant amounts of sodium to the diet. Check the food content label. Experiment with using spices and herbs instead of salt to season foods.

Plant foods are naturally lower in sodium, which can help lower your blood pressure. Fruits and vegetables also contain potassium, which may help reduce blood pressure as well.

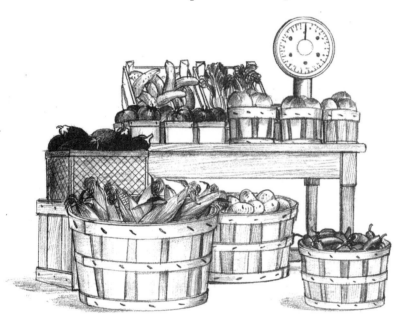

DRINK ALCOHOLIC BEVERAGES ONLY IN MODERATION

People have enjoyed alcoholic beverages for centuries. And current research suggests that moderate drinking may be associated with a lower risk for heart disease. Higher levels of alcohol, however, increase the risk of

- accidents
- birth defects
- certain forms of cancer
- cirrhosis of the liver
- heart disease
- high blood pressure
- pancreatic disease
- stroke
- suicide
- violence

Although not a nutrient, alcohol supplies energy—about seven calories

EAT WITH THE SEASON

Try to eat fresh foods that are in season. In today's global economy, consumers are greeted by a staggering array of fruits and vegetables flown in from literally around the world. Grapes may come from Chile. Those vine-ripe tomatoes may have traveled across the ocean all the way from Holland. And exotic fruits are appearing in grocery stores across the nation.

The ability to move vast quantities of produce quickly means we can get foods that do not match our region's growing season and climate. Eating foods that correspond with the season, however, both saves money and makes sense for our body and its needs. Think of what foods we associate with summer, for example. Fresh watermelon and cantaloupes, cucumbers, summer squash, tomatoes, and fresh tender greens are light foods with a high water content—just what our bodies need on hot days.

In addition, buying at your local farmers market fresh greens and vegetables picked that morning will give you more nutrients at a lower price than making a run to the local grocery chain. When possible, choose organically grown produce to avoid potential problems with pesticides and food irradiation.

per gram. This puts heavy drinkers at risk of malnutrition because they may substitute the calories in alcohol for those in more nutritious foods.

Alcohol should be avoided by women who are trying to conceive or who are pregnant. Persons taking prescription and over-the-counter medications should check with their doctor or pharmacist to see if alcohol may alter the effectiveness or toxicity of the medication.

NATURE VERSUS NURTURE

Modern medical science is learning more and more about the importance of genetics. Scientists find genes responsible for various diseases on a regular basis these days. And while it is true that we may have a family history of say, heart disease or cancer, it is not just genes that we inherit from our family.

What we eat is a complex blend of our personal history, environment, and culture. And, if you grew up in the United States, odds are you grew up eating a diet that centered on meat as the main course. Study after study has shown a correlation between diet and diseases such as cancer. A number of studies have shown that these differences are not due solely to genetic differences.

For example, women in Japan have a much lower rate of breast cancer than do women living in the United States. Japanese women eat significantly less fat than do Americans. When Japanese women move to Hawaii and adopt a Western diet, though, they have an incidence of breast cancer more than twice that of their sisters back home.

DIET AND DISEASE

Epidemiologic research has repeatedly shown the benefits of traditional diets that are rich in fruits and fiber and low in animal fat. The incidence of cancer and a number of chronic diseases such as heart disease and high blood pressure are lower in populations where the traditional diet is low in animal fat and high in plant foods.

As a sort of meeting ground between the East in West, Hawaii offers some particularly useful insights into the role of diet in disease. In contemporary society, Native Hawaiians have high rates of death from heart disease and related risk factors, such as diabetes, high blood pressure, and obesity. In fact, Native Hawaiians have the second highest prevalence of obesity of any ethnic group in the United States. And while overall, residents of the Hawaiian Islands have the greatest longevity of any Americans, Native Hawaiians have one of the shortest lifespans of all ethnic groups in the United States.

Native Hawaiians have not always been plagued by such problems. Before adopting Western dietary habits, Native Hawaiians were described in historical accounts as being on the thin side by Western standards. The traditional Hawaiian diet was low in cholesterol and fat and high in fiber, complex carbohydrates, and the ratio of polyunsaturated to saturated fatty acids.

Research shows that a return to the traditional Hawaiian diet can return people to good health. A study of 20 Native Hawaiians found that eating a traditional Hawaiian diet for 21 days resulted in significant weight loss, lower blood pressure, and decreased blood cholesterol and blood sugar levels. The diet consisted of foods such as taro (a starchy rootlike potato), poi, sweet potatoes, yams, breadfruit, greens, fruit, seaweed, fish, and chicken. In three weeks, participants lost an average of 17 pounds, lowered their cholesterol levels by an average of 17 percent, and had significant drops in blood pressure and blood sugar levels [1].

CANCER

A high intake of animal fat is known to increase the risk of certain cancers. A number of studies have suggested that the higher your fat intake, the greater your risk of developing breast cancer. For example, the increased risk of breast cancer in Japanese women after they move to Hawaii is believed to be associated with their increased fat intake. Women who eat high-fat diets produce high levels of estrogen, which translates into a higher risk for breast cancer [2].

Another factor in the increased risk may be the women's decrease in soy-product intake. Tofu and other soy products may provide some protection from breast cancer.

Colon cancer is another concern. A six-year study of 88,751 female nurses found that those who reported daily consumption of beef, lamb, or pork had a 2.5 times higher risk of developing colon cancer than women who reported eating such meals less than once a month. Increased risk for colon cancer was also associated with eating processed meats and liver. However, women who reported eating unprocessed chicken without the skin two or more times a week instead of other meats had half the risk of colon cancer of women who ate it less than once a month. A low intake of fiber from fruits also appeared to contribute to the risk of colon cancer [3].

Numerous studies have suggested that fruits and vegetables can reduce the risk of a variety of cancers, including cancer of the bladder, cervix, colon, esophagus, larynx, mouth, pharynx, rectum, and stomach. Some, such as cancer of the cervix and esophagus, may be linked to overall poor nutrition and multiple micronutrient deficiencies. Others, such as lung cancer, may be linked to a lack of beta-carotene, an antioxidant found in fruits and vegetables that may protect against cancer. A review of 11 studies of diet and lung cancer found that all showed an increased intake of vegetables and fruit was associated with decreased risk of cancer.

Researchers have sought to determine whether beta-carotene itself is protective or whether another constituent of these vegetables and fruits might act to protect against lung cancer. One study showed that total vegetable intake was more strongly associated with a lower risk of lung cancer than the intake of the group of nutrients called carotenoids (see page 321). And other vegetables, such as tomatoes, dark-green vegetables, and cruciferous vegetables, seem to be as protective as carrots, which are rich in beta-carotene [4].

This idea that there may be something more than beta-carotene that protects against cancer has become increasingly important in the second half of the 1990s (see The CARET Trial, page 320).

DIABETES

Low-fat diets that are primarily vegetarian may also help control newly diagnosed cases of adult-onset diabetes without drugs. An analysis of 652 patients with non–insulin-dependent diabetes mellitus enrolled in an intensive three-week diet and exercise program found that lifestyle modification can control diabetes and reduce vascular risk factors. Patients in the lifestyle program had reductions in their fasting glucose levels. Of the patients on drug therapy, 71 percent were able to discontinue their medication. More than a third (39 percent) of the patients taking insulin were also able to discontinue their medication.

Because the program was far more effective in controlling diabetes in patients taking no medication or oral agents compared with patients taking insulin, the researchers believe there is a need for an early emphasis on lifestyle modification in the treatment of diabetes [5].

HEART DISEASE

Diet plays a major role in the development of heart disease, which is the leading cause of death in the United States. The typical American diet—high in fat and sodium and low in fiber—significantly contributes to the risk factors for heart disease, including obesity, high blood pressure, and high blood cholesterol levels.

A 20-year study of 25,153 Seventh-Day Adventists in California found that men who ate meat daily had three times the risk of fatal heart disease that those who did not eat meat had. As part of their beliefs, Seventh-Day Adventists are encouraged to limit their consumption of meat, fish, coffee, alcohol, and tobacco [6].

While the bad news is that the mainstream Western diet can cause heart disease, the good news is that changing your diet can actually reverse heart disease. A low-fat, vegetarian diet in combination with other lifestyle changes—stopping smoking, reducing stress, and getting regular exercise—has been shown to reverse severe coronary artery disease after only one year, even without the use of medication.

In a famous study by Dean Ornish, M.D., the effects of lifestyle modification in 48 patients with coronary atherosclerosis (clogged arteries) were examined. The 28 patients in the experimental group were asked to eat a low-fat vegetarian diet, exercise, stop smoking, and practice stress-reduction techniques such as breathing techniques, imagery, meditation, progressive relaxation, and stretching exercises. The diet included fruits, vegetables, grains, legumes, and soybean products, with no animal products allowed except for egg whites and one cup per day of nonfat milk or yogurt. The diet contained approximately 10 percent of calories as fat, 15 to 20 percent protein, and 70 to 75 percent predominantly complex carbohydrates. Caffeine was eliminated, and participants were asked to limit alcohol intake to no more than two drinks a day. A semiweekly group discussion provided social support to help patients adhere to the lifestyle change program.

After one year, the researchers performed angiograms on the patients to compare the percentage of blockage in their arteries with their condition at the beginning of the trial. They found that 82 percent of patients in the experimental group showed regression of their coronary blockage, whereas heart disease progressed in 53 percent of the patients in the control group who made no modifications. Patients in the lifestyle modification group reported a 91 percent reduction in the frequency of angina (chest pain), a 42 percent reduction in the duration of angina, and a 28 percent reduction in the severity of angina. Persons in the control group, however, reported a 165 percent increase in the frequency of angina, a 95 percent rise in the dura-

tion of angina, and a 39 percent rise in its severity [7].

SWITCHING TO A HEALTHFUL DIET

Many health care educators and professionals believe that it is easier to make small changes in diet and other habits. That's the basis of big health education campaigns such as efforts to reduce fat intake or increase consumption of fruits and fiber. But a growing body of evidence suggests that it's both easier and more effective to make a big change. Trying a new diet for just two or three weeks can make you feel so much better that you won't want to go back.

Minor changes in diet, such as reducing fat intake from 40 percent to 30 percent, take effort. Although they may help slightly reduce your cholesterol and, therefore, somewhat reduce your statistical odds for heart disease, you are not likely to feel much different.

A review of research trials using different diets to reduce the risk of heart disease found those that set stricter limits on fat intake achieved a higher degree of dietary change than those with more modest goals. For example, one study of men at high risk for coronary artery disease limited fat intake to 35 percent and cholesterol to 250 mg per day. Fat intake only dropped from 38 percent to 34 percent, and cholesterol intake was reduced from 451 to 267 mg per day.

A research study using stricter fat limits, however, not only reached its goal of 10 percent fat intake, but decreased fat consumption to an average of 7 percent. Other factors that contributed to a lower fat intake included initial residential treatment, family in-

---

THE HIGH COST OF MEAT

One study estimates that medical costs attributable to meat consumption may be as high as $60 billion per year. Based on the different rates of illness reported between vegetarians and meat-eaters, the authors estimated that direct health care costs associated with meat consumption ranged from $28.6 to $61.4 billion in 1992.

Health care costs estimated for specific diseases were:
- Cancer: up to $16.5 billion
- Diabetes: $14 to $17.1 billion
- Food-borne illness: $0.2 to $5.5 billion
- Gallbladder disease: $0.2 to $2.4 billion
- Heart disease: $9.5 billion
- High blood pressure: $2.8 to $8.5 billion
- Obesity-related musculoskeletal disorders: $1.9 billion

These estimated costs do not include nonmedical costs, such as lost productivity [9].

---

volvement, group support, monitoring dietary intake at least monthly, provision of food, the use of vegetarian diets, and the presence of symptoms of heart disease [8].

VEGETARIANISM

Nutritional therapy has many options for healthy eating. As discussed above, the government recommends moderation in certain dietary areas, but nutritional therapists believe that some even more restricted and specific diet plans can be even more effective at promoting health as well as preventing and even treating disease.

By now, almost everyone can think of a couple of reasons why meat is not good for you. Some avoid it on moral or environmental grounds, but many others have only health in mind. The high fat content of meat and its specific links to diseases have turned many toward the vegetarian lifestyle.

COMPLEMENTING

When vegetarianism started to take off in the United States during the 1970s, there was concern that the diet would not provide adequate nutrition. No one vegetable contains all the amino acids required to create "complete" protein. People were advised to pair up vegetables with complementary amino acids so that the body would get the complete set. This idea that vegetables and grains must be combined in a special way to get the nutrients we need was the "complementary protein" theory.

Many of these recipes for complementing were traditional combinations such as rice and beans, but the rigors of always following the formula for

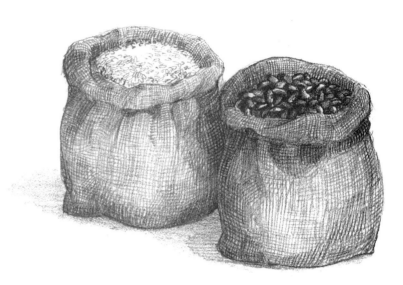

combining the proper foods led more than a few people to become disheartened and give up. This version of vegetarianism created confusion and the wrong impression that vegetarianism is hard.

It turns out that vegetarians needn't have worried. The body has the ability to store a type of amino acid until its complement arrives. But despite the confusion, the early days in American vegetarianism did help create a growing awareness that humans cannot only survive without eating animal products, but they can thrive.

HEALTH BENEFITS

Adopting a vegetarian diet can benefit your health and well-being on many levels. First, the vegetarian diet is almost always a low-fat diet. Plant products, though they can contain fat, are generally much leaner than meat products, and what fat they do have is usually unsaturated—the kind that does not stimulate a rise in blood cholesterol level. Nonanimal food sources also contain no cholesterol (milk and eggs do, though). Combine these factors with the fewer calories that a vegetarian diet usually entails and you have the formula for a healthy heart and vascular system.

Second, when meat is no longer around to focus on, the menu must rely on grains, vegetables, fruits, and legumes. These foods are great choices for more reasons than just not being meat. These plant-based foods have soluble and insoluble fiber and contain thousands of compounds—from vitamins and minerals to phytochemicals—that may have protective effects. Certainly, fiber has been shown to improve gastrointestinal health including constipation, diverticular disease, hemorrhoids, and irritable bowel syndrome, but it can also lower the risk of colorectal cancers and lower levels of blood cholesterol. Vitamins and minerals, essential to metabolism, can also have protective effects as antioxidants. And phytochemicals are just beginning to be researched for potentially powerful disease-fighting potential.

Third, avoiding meat also means a general reduction in the amount of protein in the diet. Although protein is an important nutrient vital to the growth and repair of body tissues, an excess is starting to be recognized as a potential hazard. Researchers have found that excess protein—animal proteins, in particular—may play a role in diseases such as non–Hodgkin lymphoma [10].

Excess animal protein may also play a role in the development of kidney stones. People prone to calcium oxalate kidney stones should avoid excess animal protein. A nationwide survey in Britain showed that stone formation in vegetarians was approximately half of what would normally be predicted in the general population [11]. Excess protein is hard on the kidneys in general and should be avoided by people with compromised kidney function, including people with diabetes.

Switching to a vegetarian diet has also helped ease the symptoms of rheumatoid arthritis. Although the exact mechanism by which the vegetarian diet helps is unclear, a study of people with rheumatoid arthritis in Norway showed that avoiding meat after a short period of fasting could produce significant clinical improvement [12]. The fatty acid, arachidonic acid, found in meat, eggs, and dairy products may be the problem for people with arthritis. In the body, this fatty acid converts to inflammatory substances that can contribute to arthritic processes. Allergic reactions to concentrated proteins may be another mechanism.

WHAT ABOUT FISH?

Like so much in nutrition and science these days, the news about fish is confusing. Not everyone considers fish in the same category as other meat because in some ways it doesn't seem to have the same effects as other animal

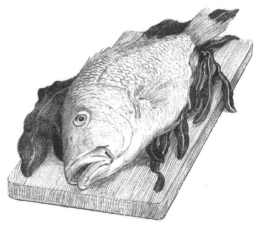

products. For example, there have been many reports about the beneficial effects of consuming a diet with plenty of the fatty acids found in fish—fatty acids called omega-3. These compounds may help prevent heart attacks or ease the symptoms of rheumatoid arthritis.

A study of 334 patients with heart attacks examined differences in fatty acid intake with that of control cases of the same age and sex. The study estimated that levels equal to eating one fatty fish meal per week were associated with a 50 percent reduction in the risk of heart attack [13].

A study of 2,033 men who had recovered from a heart attack found that those who increased their intake of fatty fish had a 29 percent reduction in death from all causes two years later, whereas those who slightly decreased their fat intake, or increased intake of cereal fiber had no difference in mortality [14].

Eating cold-water fish such as mackerel and salmon is often recommended for patients with arthritis. Recent research shows that fatty acids may help alleviate symptoms of the disease and decrease the need for pain medication. A study of 66 patients with rheumatoid arthritis found that those who took fish oil supplements had improved activity and significant decreases in the number of tender joints, the duration of morning stiffness, and pain, whereas patients who took placebo capsules containing corn oil had no improvement. Some of the patients taking fish oil supplements were able to stop taking anti-inflammatory medication without experiencing a flare-up of their arthritis [15].

MACROBIOTICS

Macrobiotics, derived from the Greek words *macros* (great or long) and *bios* (life), is a dietary system based on the traditional Chinese philosophy of yin and yang.

HISTORY

The macrobiotic diet was introduced to the United States in the late 1950s by Georges Ohsawa, the pen name for Yukikaza Sakurazawa. Ohsawa was a Japanese teacher who reportedly cured himself of a serious illness by eating a traditional diet of brown rice, miso soup, and sea vegetables.

Having studied the writings of a late 19th century Japanese physician Sagen Ishikuzuka, Ohsawa developed a philosophy of macrobiotics. Ohsawa outlined ten stages of diet with varying percentages of animal products, cereal grains, vegetables, and soups.

In the 1970s, Ohsawa's leadership of the macrobiotic movement in the United States was taken over by one of his students, Michio Kushi, who replaced the ten-phase dietary levels with

MACROBIOTICS AND B$_{12}$

One of the main nutritional concerns when following a macrobiotic diet is getting enough vitamin B$_{12}$, especially if you don't consume fish. A deficiency of this vitamin can cause a form of anemia, among other problems. If you go the macrobiotic route, you may want to have the diet supervised by a practitioner familiar with macrobiotics, and you should probably take vitamin B$_{12}$ supplements.

what is now the general or standard macrobiotic diet.

WHAT IT IS

The standard macrobiotic diet emphasizes whole cereal grains and vegetables, with minimal consumption of animal products except for fish. The diet is, therefore, low in fat and high in complex carbohydrates and fiber—factors associated with a lower risk of cancer and heart disease. By weight, the proportions of food in the daily diet should be

- 50 percent whole grains
- 20 to 30 percent vegetables
- 5 to 10 percent legumes and sea vegetables
    - 5 to 10 percent soups of various kinds

From this breakdown, it's obvious that the macrobiotic diet is a vegetarian one, but that is not technically true. Macrobiotic prescriptions for food choices are not strict guidelines on what to eat when, but rather theoretical guidelines on how to balance a diet between yin and yang. Foods are categorized into yin-producing and yang-producing foods. Yin-producing foods include those that are

- grown in a hot climate
- high in water content
- grown above the ground
- sour, bitter, hot, or aromatic
- fruits and leaves

Yang producing foods include those that are

- grown in cooler climates
- drier
- grown below ground
- salty or sweet
- stems, roots, and seeds

All foods have a combination of yin and yang, but they can have a preponderance of one or the other. Animal products are more yang and fruit products are more yin; however, the yin or yang energy of a particular food can vary even within a given species. A smaller, drier apple can be more yang than an apple growing on the opposite side of the same tree.

Although balancing strong yin foods with strong yang foods is possible, it is not recommended. The majority of food choices should be from the middle ground; that is, foods that are balanced themselves. Whole grains, beans and bean products, round root vegetables, leafy greens, nuts and seeds, fruit from temperate climates, vegetable oils, and springwater are among the more balanced foods. Meat, poultry, and other animal products are, therefore, to be avoided not because they are forbidden but because they have a significant potential to create an unhealthy balance.

STRONG YANG FOODS

- Eggs
- Meat
- Cheese
- Fish

STRONG YIN FOODS

- White rice
- Tropical fruits and vegetables
- Spices
- Alcohol
- Coffee and tea

HEALTH BENEFITS

With its focus on whole grains and various vegetables, a macrobiotic diet provides plenty of vitamins, minerals, and fiber with little or no fat, saturated fat, or cholesterol. The benefits for weight control, blood pressure, and cardiovascular health are great.

Macrobiotic diets are also used as an alternative treatment for cancer. A patient's illness is classified according to whether it is mainly yin or yang or a combination of both (see Traditional Chinese Medicine, pages 346–353). Although patients use the standard macrobiotic diet, foods with the character opposite that of the cancer are emphasized. The use of macrobiotic and other dietary approaches to cancer therapy has been met with extreme skepticism by the mainstream medical community because of fears that it could delay standard treatment, but as an adjunct to conventional therapy, macrobiotics may prove very useful.

A published review of studies on the use of a macrobiotic diet in cancer patients found evidence for increased survival in patients with nutritionally linked cancers. Patients with metastatic prostate cancer (prostate cancer that has spread to other organs) who modified their diet had a longer survival and improved quality of life than those who did not. Among patients with pancreatic cancer—a particularly fast and deadly type of cancer—those who modified their diets had a higher rate of survival at one year. Although the design of the studies has been criticized, the idea that such a diet may help control cancer is gaining a little more attention, if not actual support, from the scientific community [16].

ENZYME THERAPY

Enzymes are proteins that break down food substances into a form that the body can use and absorb. All living things make enzymes to transform the nutrients they ingest into a usable form. Enzyme therapy involves supplementation with external enzymes to ease digestive stresses and treat conditions from digestive problems to heart disease.

TYPES OF ENZYMES

Enzymes made in the body are called *endogenous* enzymes. Enzymes from a source outside the body are called *exogenous* enzymes. Enzyme therapy involves supplementing the body's supply of endogenous enzymes with exogenous versions.

Plant Enzymes—Although exogenous enzymes can be acquired from other species of animals, plant enzymes are of particular interest in enzyme therapy. Plants make four kinds of enzymes:

- amylase—to break down carbohydrates
- protease—to break down protein
- lipase—to break down fat
- cellulase—to break down fiber

The human pancreas produces enzymes similar to the first three but cannot produce an enzyme like cellulase. Humans cannot digest fiber.

When taken orally (usually in capsule form), plant enzymes begin to digest food in the stomach before the body's own enzymes begin their work. This predigestion alleviates the stresses on the pancreas and other digestive organs by taking some of the digestive workload. The addition of these extra enzymes also ensures that all of the available nutrients are broken down into an absorbable form and no undigested food will contaminate the lower bowels.

Pancreatic Enzymes—These enzymes are derived from animal sources and include amylase, protease, lipase, and sometimes cellulase. In general, these enzymes do not function as predigestive aids as plant enzymes do. The environment of the stomach is too acidic for these enzymes to function. However, they do play a role beyond the digestive tract. Some of the enzyme molecules are absorbed into the bloodstream and actually track down and destroy (digest) foreign substances in the blood, such as viral particles, scar tissue, and allergens.

HOW IT WORKS

Therapy with enzymes involves an initial consultation with a practitioner who will take a complete history with particular attention given to any history of food allergies or sensitivities. Diagnostic blood tests may be in order, and a breath test, in which expired air is tested for certain chemicals, may be used for certain conditions. This information helps the therapist determine the proper formula of enzymes to be used.

Plant enzyme therapy usually involves taking capsules of a mixture of enzymes. The capsules are usually administered around mealtimes so that they can be present in the stomach at the same time as the food. Pancreatic enzymes used for digestive purposes are taken with meals. When used for other purposes, they are administered in between meals so that they can be absorbed into the bloodstream without

interference. Intravenous administration of both types of enzymes is also used in select cases.

Enzymes are often used in combination with other remedies. Many herbalists, naturopaths, and homeopaths use enzymes as an adjunct to their other prescriptions, taking advantage of the improved nutrient absorption and the detoxification effects brought about by enhanced digestion.

USES

Malabsorption—Many conditions, such as chronic pancreatitis and cystic fibrosis, can cause the pancreas to function improperly, leading to an insufficiency of the enzymes it secretes. This insufficiency can lead to malnutrition as food passes undigested through the digestive tract. People having undergone bowel surgery may also experience similar malabsorption problems. Enzyme supplementation can improve nutrient absorption in all these cases and prevent the weight loss and deficiency syndromes that accompany malabsorption [17].

Food Allergies and Intolerances—Enzyme therapy can significantly reduce problems with allergies and intolerances. Food allergies are triggered when large molecules from the digestive tract "leak" into the bloodstream where the immune system reacts to them as invaders. Enzymes break down the molecules either before they leave the stomach or before the immune system reacts.

The same application works for intolerances such as lactose intolerance. When administered at the same time as milk or dairy consumption, the enzyme lactase effectively eliminates the symptoms of maldigestion. In one study, enzyme therapy proved to be as effective as—and less expensive than—treating milk to eliminate the lactose content through prehydrolyzation [18].

Celiac disease is an intolerance to the protein gluten found in wheat, oats, barley, rye, and some other grains. This condition can cause severe gastrointestinal symptoms as well as broader disorders such as weight loss and anemia resulting from malabsorption. Plant enzymes have been shown to eliminate symptoms when administered with meals. A study of four individuals with celiac disease who were symptom free after following a gluten-free diet reintroduced gluten to their diet. Three also took enzyme supplements; one did not. The three treated with enzymes remained free of symptoms, whereas the untreated control subject experienced a return of the signs and symptoms [19].

Vascular Disease—Numerous studies have shown enzyme therapy to be very effective in treating and even reversing the progression of vascular disease. Intravenous administration of proteolytic enzymes (enzymes that target proteins) can clear narrowed areas in arteries that may otherwise progress to blockages that can cause heart attacks and strokes, among other problems. A study of enzyme therapy involving intravenous administration of an enzyme derived from a fungus showed that the enzyme improved circulation significantly better than no therapy and standard anticoagulant therapy [20].

Cancer—Enzymes have been used in cancer treatment for various functions. Although the mechanism is unclear, it has been suggested that the way enzymes react with the surface of tumor cells can aid in standard treatment. The enzymes may help make the surface antigens of the tumor more recognizable to therapeutic agents, thus enhancing their effectiveness. Another, as yet unproved assertion is that enzymes may decrease the chance of tumors spreading (metastasis) by making the outer surface less likely to stick to a new location.

Viral Infections—Some suggest that pancreatic enzyme therapy can slow or even halt the course of viral infections by scavenging the virus in the bloodstream and digestive tract. The outer coating of a virus is protein; therefore, proteolytic enzymes can destroy the virus's protective armor and leave it vulnerable to the immune system. This theory remains unproved.

NUTRITIONAL SUPPLEMENTS

Over the years, scientists have been able to isolate individual nutrients in the diet and analyze their particular functions. By no means has every nutrient important to health been identified, but progress toward understanding the roles of many vitamins and minerals has shown that certain nutrients may be valuable therapeutically— both to treat diseases and prevent them.

The recommended dietary allowances (RDAs) are a breakdown of the amount of each known nutrient necessary for basic health requirements. They represent the amounts of nutrients that are adequate to meet the needs of most healthy people. However, a number of nutritionists and health care practitioners believe that the RDAs set by the government are too low. While these levels may keep people from developing overt nutrient deficiencies, they may not be the right level for optimal health.

With some exceptions, a healthy diet with a variety of foods can provide adequate amounts of nutrients. Nutritional supplements may be needed by some people and for some conditions. But an overreliance on nutrition through pills is not a good idea. Because foods contain many nutrients and other substances that promote health, the use of supplements cannot substitute for proper food choices. And supplements of some nutrients, particularly some fat-soluble vitamins and some minerals, may be harmful if taken regularly in large amounts.

WHO NEEDS SUPPLEMENTS?

More than 20 percent of Americans take supplements on a daily basis. A few groups in particular may benefit the most from supplement use.

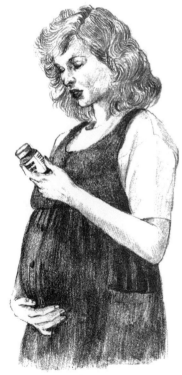

Elderly—Nutritional deficiencies are common in the elderly for a variety of reasons, including a poor diet and decreased absorption of dietary nutrients. Elderly people and people with little exposure to sunlight may need a vitamin D supplement. As we age, our immune responses tend to weaken and we become more susceptible to infection. In fact, infection is the fourth leading cause of death among the elderly. Research shows that modest amounts of nutritional supplements can improve immunity and decrease the risk of infection in old age.

A one-year study of 96 independently living, healthy elderly people compared those who took nutritional supplements with those who did not. After one year, the group that took supplements had higher numbers of certain immune cells—natural killer cells and T cells that fight infection—and had higher antibody responses. They were also significantly less likely to become ill due to infection and, when they did, required fewer days of antibiotic therapy. The study used modest amounts of essential vitamins and trace elements. Large doses were not used, as very large doses of certain micronutrients may actually impair immunity [21].

Pregnant Women and Women of Childbearing Age—The increased nutritional requirements of pregnancy are no surprise; after all, a pregnant woman is "eating for two." Many practitioners recommend a high-potency multivitamin-mineral supplement designed for pregnant women (sometimes called a prenatal vitamin), but here are some of the particular nutritional concerns.

Iron supplements are recommended for pregnant women. The developing fetus needs a great deal of iron because it is in the process of making its own blood and hemoglobin—the iron-based, oxygen-carrying component of blood.

Women of childbearing age must also be careful to get enough of a few nutrients because of the possibility of becoming pregnant. Women of childbearing age may reduce the risk of certain birth defects, called neural tube defects, by consuming folate-rich foods or folate supplements (usually in the form of folic acid). Folate's role in preventing neural tube defects occurs so early in pregnancy that a woman may not even be aware that she is pregnant before a folate deficiency has already caused problems. Therefore, maintaining adequate folate intake is vital throughout a woman's childbearing years.

Adequate amounts of protein and calories are vital for a healthy pregnancy. Between 75 and 95 grams of protein daily is generally recommended and may help prevent toxemia during pregnancy.

In addition to getting enough of certain nutrients, it is also important to limit one's intake of certain others. For example, vitamin A can be toxic in high doses; daily intake should not exceed 10,000 IU.

Vegetarians—People who eat no animal products of any kind, including milk, eggs, or dairy products, are known as vegans. Because meat, fish, and poultry are major contributors of iron, zinc, and B vitamins, vegans should pay special attention to eating plant foods rich in these nutrients.

Most Americans obtain vitamin D and calcium from milk products; vegetarians who avoid dairy products should make sure their diet includes plant foods high in calcium and also expose their skin to some sunlight each day to produce vitamin D. The only essential nutrient that is found only in animal foods is vitamin B_{12}, so vegans need to take this supplement.

Although nutritional supplements may be an important part of treatment for a variety of conditions and for everyday needs, you can generally get adequate amounts of the nutrients you need by eating a variety of fresh, unprocessed foods. However, adequate does not always mean optimal, and

---

CAUTION

Like any substance, excessively high levels of vitamins can be toxic.

- Fatal poisoning has occurred in children who have taken large doses of iron and vitamins A and D. Store vitamins in child-proof containers and keep out of the reach of children.
- People taking blood thinners should avoid high doses of vitamin E, which can cause prolonged bleeding.

---

that's where supplementation comes in. Here are the basic nutrients in the diet, their functions, and their food sources.

AMINO ACIDS

Amino acids are the body's building blocks for proteins. Some evidence suggests that certain amino acids may be useful in the treatment of psychiatric conditions. For example, the amino acids methionine and L-tyrosine have been used to treat depression, and glycine has been used to treat schizophrenia. More controlled clinical trials need to be done to assess the effectiveness of amino acid therapy in these areas.

N-Acetyl-cysteine, a form of the amino acid cysteine, is useful in reducing the viscosity of mucus in chronic bronchitis. It may also have a role in detoxification, aiding in the removal of harmful substances from the body.

The amino acid carnitine is used by some athletes in an effort to enhance performance. Studies have shown that supplementation with L-carnitine (one form of the amino acid) can result in

THE CARET TRIAL

Eager to find a way to protect people at high risk of lung cancer against developing the deadly disease, the National Cancer Institute launched a massive trial of beta-carotene and vitamin A supplements to protect against lung cancer. Studies had shown that people who eat a diet rich in these nutrients generally have a lower rate of lung cancer, but actual supplementation had not been well studied.

Called the Beta Carotene and Retinol Efficacy Trial, or CARET, the study involved 18,314 people at high risk for lung cancer due to smoking or asbestos exposure. Half were given supplements, the other half a placebo.

In early 1996, a regular review of study data found that more people in one group were developing and dying of lung cancer than in the other. The study was immediately "unblinded"—stopped to ensure that both groups would benefit from the better treatment. However, researchers were stunned and confused to learn that, contrary to their expectations, it was the people in the vitamin group who had the highest rates of cancer. People in the group who took beta-carotene and vitamin A supplements had 28 percent more lung cancer and 17 percent more deaths [24].

The failure of beta-carotene supplements to protect against cancer could be due to some other components in these foods rather than the single element beta-carotene. So, while the scientists try to figure out exactly what is in carotenoid-rich foods that protects against cancer, eat a few carrots each day, and reduce your risk the natural way.

---

significant improvement in cardiovascular functioning, exercise intensity and duration, and energy metabolism in muscle tissue [22, 23]. Carnitine has also been used extensively in cardiovascular disorders to lower high blood cholesterol levels and improve heart function after a heart attack.

An outbreak in the late 1980s of the severe and sometimes fatal inflammatory disorder eosinophilia myalgia syndrome (EMS) was linked to the use of the amino acid L-tryptophan for insomnia and mood disorders. Although the cases were clearly linked to contamination in the amino acid made by one Japanese manufacturer, the Food and Drug Administration removed the amino acid from the market and has refused to allow its reintroduction in the United States except for veterinary use.

ANTIOXIDANTS

These compounds prevent the oxidation of substances in food or in the body. Oxidation is a process caused by molecules called free radicals which are by-products of several normal metabolic processes. Free radicals are highly reactive molecules that cause damage to the body by reacting with other molecules, such as cell membranes and DNA. Antioxidants neutralize free radicals, rendering them inactive.

Most free radicals are a result of normal metabolic processes such as energy production. Environmental factors also contribute to the amount of free radicals in the body. For example, smoking increases the body's load of free radicals. Alcohol, air pollutants, fried foods, pesticides, ultraviolet radiation, and solvents also increase free radicals in the body. Free radicals are believed to be involved in the aging process and the development of atherosclerosis and cancer.

Antioxidants chemically react with free radicals and, therefore, can block the damage they can cause. Scientists believe that high enough levels of antioxidants in the tissue can reduce damage from free radicals. By neutralizing free radicals, these compounds prevent them from attaching to cell membranes and causing damage.

Natural antioxidants include vitamins C and E, beta-carotene, and selenium. A number of studies have shown a relationship between diets high in these nutrients and a lower rate of cancer and other diseases.

Carotenoids—Although beta-carotene is the best-known carotenoid, there are hundreds of different types, many of which have not yet been well studied. Beta-carotene converts to vitamin A in the body, so it is often lumped together with vitamin A in nutrition discussions, but there is mounting evidence that beta-carotene may have special properties separate from vitamin A.

A few fresh carrots can provide as much as 20 to 30 mg of beta-carotene. But the average American takes in less than 2 mg of beta-carotene a day.

Carotenoids function as pigments in plants. Therefore good food sources can be recognized by their dark color or red-orange-yellow shade. Some good sources of carotenoid, including beta-carotene, are

- broccoli
- carrots
- pumpkin
- red peppers
- sweet potatoes
- tomatoes
- dark-green leafy vegetables (such as chard, collards, kale, mustard greens, spinach, and turnip greens)
- mango
- papaya
- cantaloupe

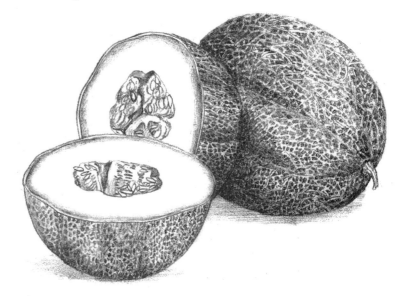

Although many physicians may encourage supplementation with antioxidants, there is a growing awareness that eating a diet high in these compounds may be better than taking supplements. Natural carotenoids offer more protection than supplements, and concentrated plant extracts are probably the next best choice.

Despite earlier reports of beta-carotene's ability to protect against lung cancer, the government's CARET trial showed that beta-carotene and vitamin A supplements failed to protect against cancer. We still do not know enough about exactly what is in these compounds that offers protection (see The CARET Trial, page 320).

Flavonoids—Another group of plant pigments, flavonoids, is what gives fruits and flowers their colors. These compounds also act as antioxidants and free-radical scavengers and appear to help modify the body's response to foreign compounds such as allergens and viruses.

Flavonoids tend to work against a variety of free radicals. Various flavonoids are also partial to certain tissues. This makes certain botanical compounds useful for specific conditions. For example, the herb milk thistle (*Silybum marianum*) contains flavonoids that protect the liver. Milk thistle has been used to treat toxic mushroom poisoning and has been shown to increase survival in people with cirrhosis of the liver.

VITAMIN A

Vitamin A is needed for reproduction and vision, to promote bone growth, and to maintain the body's epithelial tissue (gastrointestinal, lung, and skin tissue). Vitamin A deficiency is linked to night blindness and increased rates of infection. The best source of vitamin A is beta-carotene, which converts to vitamin A in the body. (Some people, such as those with impaired thyroid function, do not convert beta-carotene to vitamin A efficiently. For these people and in some other instances, preformed vitamin A may be a better supplement choice.)

RDA—The RDA for Vitamin A is 1,000 retinol equivalents (RE) or 5,000 international units (IU) for men; 800 RE or 4,000 IU for women; and 400 to 1,000 RE or 2,000 to 5,000 IU

for children, increasing from infancy to 14 years of age.

Toxicity—Vitamin A has been associated with birth defects, so women who are pregnant or who are trying to become pregnant should check with their physician before taking vitamin A supplements. Vitamin A toxicity in adults is rare in persons taking less than 100,000 IU per day, but acute toxicity has been seen in children who have ingested a single high dose.

Symptoms of acute toxicity include anorexia (loss of appetite), headache, fatigue, and muscle and joint pain. Chronic toxicity can result in dry cracking skin, hair loss, fatigue, nausea, and irritability. Prolonged doses of excessive vitamin A can result in bone fragility. Because the vitamin is stored in the liver, the main toxicity of prolonged use occurs in this organ. Toxicity symptoms normally disappear when excessive vitamin A intake is stopped.

Therapeutic Uses—Although vitamin A is an effective treatment for a number of skin conditions—ranging from acne to psoriasis—the high doses used for treatment may result in the development of toxicities. Supervision by a health care professional is a necessity.

Recent research has found that vitamin A therapy can help reverse cervical dysplasia, a precancerous condition of the opening to the uterus. The study involved 301 women—151 with moderate dysplasia and 150 with severe dysplasia. The women inserted cervical caps with sponges containing either retinoic acid (vitamin A) or a placebo. Women with moderate cervical dysplasia who were in the vitamin A treatment group had a complete histologic regression rate (the rate at which laboratory tests showed no more cancerous changes) of 43 percent compared with only 27 percent of those in the placebo group. Among women with severe dysplasia, there was no difference in treatment [25].

THE B VITAMINS

The B complex vitamins are found in foods such as whole-wheat bread, fruits, green and yellow leafy plants and animal sources such as eggs, dairy products, and liver.

Vitamin B$_1$ (Thiamine)—Thiamine acts as a coenzyme to remove carbon monoxide from the body. Some research suggests that high levels of thiamine may be associated with fewer degenerative diseases and less illness. Thiamine deficiency can cause beriberi, a disease marked by mental confusion, paralysis, and swelling.

The RDA for thiamine is 1.5 mg for men and 1.1 mg for women. Because thiamine is vital to carbohydrate metabolism, people who eat large amounts of refined carbohydrates may require thiamine supplementation. Supplements can be taken at levels of 5 to 15 mg per day. No toxicities have been associated with thiamine intake.

Alcoholics are the main group that develops thiamine deficiency. The metabolism of alcohol and the general lack of good nutrition depletes the body's supply. Often during detoxification, very high doses of thiamine are given by injection.

Good sources of thiamine include
- bread
- dairy products
- fruits
- vegetables

Vitamin B$_2$ (Riboflavin)—Riboflavin is needed for the blood, tissue repair, and vision. Riboflavin may help prevent the development of cataracts. Riboflavin deficiency can cause cracks at the corner of the mouth and sensitivity to light. Riboflavin is found in milk, meat, whole grains, and vegetables.

The RDA for riboflavin is 1.7 mg for men and 1.3 mg for women. There are no known toxicities associated with riboflavin. Very high doses of riboflavin in combination with vitamin B$_6$ may have therapeutic value in the treatment of carpal tunnel syndrome. Doses in the neighborhood of 25 mg are not uncommon for therapeutic use.

Vitamin B$_3$ (Nicotinic Acid, or Niacin)—Niacin is important in body processes such as energy and lipid metabolism. Some research has shown that nicotinic acid can help lower low-density lipoprotein (LDL) cholesterol—the "bad" cholesterol—and increase high-density lipoprotein (HDL) cholesterol—the "good" cholesterol.

The RDA for niacin is 19 mg for men and 15 mg for women. High doses of niacin (more than 1,000 mg) can cause a variety of problems ranging from heart irregularities to nausea, stomach pain, and diarrhea.

Niacin's cholesterol-lowering effects only occur at levels high enough that it has begun to act like a drug rather than a nutrient. At those levels, niacin can cause serious side effects. Do not use niacin supplements without a health care professional's supervision. People with diabetes should avoid niacin supplementation at high doses because of niacin's tendency to increase blood sugar levels. It is necessary at lower doses for people with diabetes, though, because it is part of a substance called glucose tolerance factor.

Vitamin B₆ (Pyridoxine)—Vitamin B_6 is needed for the metabolism of amino acids and for a wide range of body functions, from the metabolism of fatty acids to the production of neurotransmitters. Vitamin B_6 deficiency can cause abnormal brain activity, skin soreness, and a smooth tongue. Some studies suggest that low levels of vitamin B_6 may play a role in the development of heart disease. Vitamin B_6 may also be helpful in maintaining immune function, particularly in the elderly. Therapeutically, the vitamin has been used in the treatment of various conditions, including carpal tunnel syndrome, premenstrual syndrome (PMS), kidney stones, and morning sickness.

The RDA for vitamin B_6 is 2 mg for men and 1.6 mg for women. However, optimal doses are 25 to 100 mg. Extremely high doses of vitamin B_6 (500 to 1,000 mg) may cause sensory and motor impairment, which can also be caused by a deficiency of the vitamin. It is thought that large doses may actually block the activated form of the vitamin from working, resulting in a deficiency state.

Folate (Folic Acid)—Folate, or folic acid, is a B vitamin that, among its many functions, reduces the risk of birth defects called neural tube defects. Folate deficiency can cause anemia, diarrhea, and a smooth tongue. Research also suggests that low levels of folate may lead to higher rates of cancer (particularly cervical cancer) and cardiovascular disease.

The RDA for folic acid was recently lowered to 180 µg per day for women, but research suggests that an intake of 400 µg per day may reduce cancer risk. A level of 400 µg per day by pregnant women may also reduce the risk of neural tube defects in their babies. Because this is most effective in the earliest weeks after conception, women who are trying to become pregnant should discuss vitamin B supplementation with their physician. Despite revisions to the RDA, most therapists still recommend for pregnant women 800 µg daily—the amount found in most prenatal vitamin formulas.

Scientists have found that people with high dietary levels of folate have a lower risk of cancer of the colon. One study looked at the incidence of colon cancer in 15,984 women and 9,490 men. The analysis found that high dietary folate was associated with a lower risk of colon cancer in both men and women. Persons with low folate intake were more likely to develop cancer of the colon, and those who had low folate levels and drank two or more alcoholic drinks per day had a three times greater risk for cancer of the colon than people who had low alcohol and high folate intake [26].

Good sources of folate include
- dry beans (such as red beans, navy beans, and soybeans)
- lentils
- chickpeas
- cow peas
- peanuts
- leafy greens (spinach, cabbage, brussels sprouts, romaine, loose leaf lettuce)
- peas
- okra
- sweet corn
- beets
- broccoli

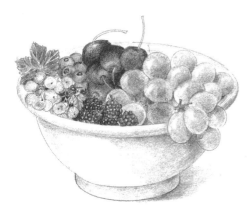

- berries
- kiwi fruit
- orange juice (fortified with folate)
- plantains

Vitamin B₁₂ (Cyanocobalamin)—Vitamin B_{12} is needed for central nervous system functioning and for enzymes involved in the metabolism of amino acids, folic acid (folate), nucleic acid, and fatty acids. Deficiencies can result in anemia, as well as cerebral, neurologic, and psychiatric abnormalities. Some evidence suggests that vitamin B_{12} may help prevent some types of cancers and may reduce the risk of atherosclerosis.

The RDA for vitamin B_{12} is 2 µg daily for adults. This vitamin is considered safe in amounts as much as 1,000 times the RDA.

Because vitamin B_{12} is found only in animal products (meat, poultry, fish, eggs, and dairy), strict vegans often need to take vitamin B_{12} supplements. Vitamin B_{12} deficiency is common among elderly persons, in part because they poorly absorb the vitamin from the intestinal tract.

VITAMIN C

Vitamin C is probably the most studied of the vitamins and, subsequently, the most often taken supplement. Vitamin C is needed to form connective tissue and bones and to maintain a healthy immune system.

RDA—The government's RDA for vitamin C is 60 mg per day. Although a diet rich in fruits and vegetables can provide 250 to 500 mg per day, an estimated 25 percent of women consume less than 40 mg per day. There is no government approved protective range, but proponents advocate 1,000 mg or more per day. In cases of acute infection, some practitioners may recommend vitamin C totaling as much as 6,000 mg per day to boost immune functioning.

Some other conditions for which vitamin C supplementation can be beneficial include

- allergies
- asthma
- cancer
- injuries (for wound healing)
  Good sources of vitamin C include
- citrus fruits
  brussels sprouts
- dark-green vegetables
- strawberries
- bell peppers

Toxicity—Vitamin C is generally safe. Being a water-soluble vitamin, excessive amounts are excreted through the kidneys, but extremely high doses have been linked to iron overload because the vitamin facilitates the absorption of iron (see page 330). Some suggest that vitamin C could be associated with the formation of urinary stones, but this has not been shown conclusively. Diarrhea is the main symptom experienced with very high doses.

Therapeutic Uses—Elderly people may benefit from increased vitamin C intake. People who smoke need to take three to four times the amount of vitamin C of a nonsmoker. Heavy drinkers may also require increased levels of vitamin C. Vitamin C may help reduce the risk of cancer, cataracts, and heart disease.

Some vitamin C advocates, like pioneer Linus Pauling, recommend the use of high doses of vitamin C as an adjunct in the treatment of cancer. Vitamin C given along with vitamin B_{12} to mice who are implanted with experimental cancer has been shown to increase survival [27].

Vitamin C is important for maintaining healthy teeth, gums, bones, muscles, and blood vessels. Some scientists believe it can prevent and cure the common cold. Studies have not proved that vitamin C can prevent colds but suggest it may reduce their severity.

Recent research on the use of vitamin C in asthma and allergy has found a number of promising and positive re-

sults, but specific recommendations require more study [28].

VITAMIN D

Vitamin D helps bones and teeth take up calcium to grow and stay healthy. Vitamin D deficiency can cause lax muscles, rickets (bowed legs or other bone deformities), osteoporosis, and tooth decay. Vitamin D may also play a role in keeping blood pressure under control. Some research suggests that vitamin D and calcium may reduce the risk of colon cancer.

Vegetarians and people who have limited exposure to sunlight may need to take special care to get enough vitamin D. The elderly are also at risk of vitamin D deficiency because they tend to have decreased exposure to sunlight, and their skin produces less vitamin D after exposure to sunlight than that of a younger person. Elderly people may have a limited calorie intake and decreased absorption of vitamin D from foods.

RDA—The RDA for vitamin D is 200 IU (400 IU for pregnant and lactating women), but few studies exist to show that this is an optimal dose. Vitamin D is synthesized by exposure to sunlight, but persons who get little or no sun may have deficiencies. Milk is fortified with vitamin D and is the major source of the vitamin for most Americans.

Therapeutic Uses—Vitamin D may help protect against the development of cataracts. A study of 112 people looked at the relationship between nutritional status and cataracts. The study found a very strong association between vitamin D levels and the risk of cataracts [29].

CAUTION

Use caution in taking supplements of fat-soluble vitamins. These vitamins are stored in the body's fat tissues and certain organs, and unlike water-soluble vitamins such as vitamin C, excess amounts are not excreted by the body. High doses of some fat-soluble vitamins, particularly vitamins A and D, may be toxic. Fat-soluble vitamins include
- vitamin A
- vitamin D
- vitamin E
- vitamin K

VITAMIN E

Vitamin E is an important antioxidant that protects cell membranes from damage by free radicals. Vitamin E is important for healthy red blood cells, the repair of cell membranes and DNA, and maintaining immune function. A low intake of vitamin E may be linked to an increased risk of certain cancers, cataracts, and heart disease.

RDA—The current RDA for vitamin E is 8 IU for women and 10 IU for men, a reduction from an earlier RDA of 30 IU for both men and women. Although a diet with numerous servings of fruits and vegetables, nuts, whole-grain breads, and vegetable oils can provide 30 IU, the median intake of vitamin E in the United States is only 5 IU. Vitamin E is naturally found in plant oils such as corn oil.

Safety Concerns—People taking blood-thinning medications should take vitamin E supplements with caution. For the general population, vitamin E appears to be safe in doses as high as 3,200 IU. Supplementation may also elevate blood pressure in people who already have hypertension. Introduce the supplements gradually and monitor blood pressure regularly.

Therapeutic Uses—Levels of vitamin E of 100 IU or higher have been found to be associated with reduced risks of cataracts, oral cancer, and heart disease. A study comparing the vitamin supplement intake of 1,114 people with oral and pharyngeal cancer with 1,268 people of the same age and sex found that those who took vitamin E supplements had a lower risk of cancer. Persons who took vitamin E supplements had a reduced risk of cancer regardless of tobacco and alcohol use.

Overall, the use of vitamin E supplements was associated with approximately half the risk of cancer. Vitamin A supplementation was also associated with a reduced risk of oral and pharyngeal cancer [30].

Research also suggests that high doses of vitamin E may reduce the risk of heart disease. Two large studies have found that people who had used vitamin E supplements for two or more years had approximately 40 percent lower rates of coronary heart disease. Vitamin E supplementation of less than 100 IU per day or for shorter periods had no significant effect on the rate of heart disease [31].

A study comparing the use of vitamin supplements by 175 cataract patients with that of 175 individually matched cataract-free subjects suggests that vitamins C and E may reduce the risk of cataracts by at least 50 percent [32].

VITAMIN K

In adults, vitamin K is produced by normal intestinal bacteria. Vitamin K helps form the protein thrombin, which the body needs to form blood clots to stop bleeding. Vitamin K is also involved in the development of bones. Supplementation is rarely needed except in women who have extremely heavy menstrual bleeding. It is also routinely given to newborns because they do not yet have the normal intestinal bacteria. Vitamin K and vitamin C together have been shown to be effective in the treatment of morning sickness.

RDA—The RDA for vitamin K is 80 mg for adult men and 65 mg for adult women. Most people get well over the amount of vitamin K they need. Much of the vitamin K the body needs is formed by bacteria that live in the intestinal tract.

CALCIUM

Calcium is the most abundant mineral in the body. It's stored in the bones, providing our skeleton with structural strength. It is also needed for a number of important body functions, including the digestion of fat and protein, energy production, neuromuscular activity, and the absorption of other nutrients.

RDA—The RDA for calcium is 800 mg per day for adults. Some experts recommend that women consume 1,000 to 1,500 mg of calcium per day to maintain bone health and prevent osteoporosis. While it is possible to take in this much calcium per day in

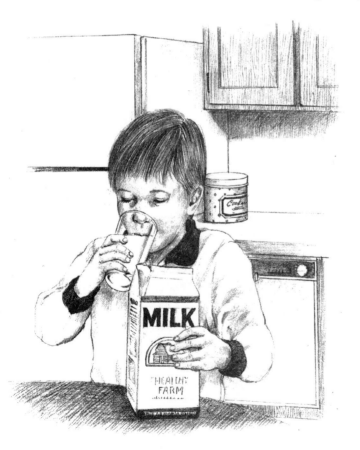

your diet, the median calcium intake among American women is only 600 mg per day. Calcium deficiency can contribute to osteoporosis (a disease of later life that causes fragile bones) and stunted growth.

Your need for calcium depends on how much protein you eat. High levels of protein require a higher calcium intake. Although there has been much attention in recent years about the role of calcium in preventing osteoporosis, the fact is your body needs an optimal intake of all nutrients to maintain healthy bones.

Thanks to urging by the Dairy Council, most of us think automatically of milk and dairy products as a quick and easy way to get the calcium we need. Plant foods can also provide a rich source of calcium—10 dried figs contain 269 mg, and a cup of broccoli contains 178 mg of calcium. Other good sources include

- dark-green leafy vegetables, such as kale, mustard greens, bok choy, and turnip greens
- canned fish with the soft bones packed in such as sardines, anchovies, and salmon
- most foods in the milk group, including cheese and yogurt
- tofu, if it's processed with calcium sulfate
- tortillas made from lime-processed cornmeal

Adequate calcium intake may have a protective effect against colon cancer. It is also useful therapeutically in the treatment of conditions such as high blood pressure (when combined with magnesium supplementation) and muscle cramps including those associated with menstruation.

CHROMIUM

Chromium is a trace element needed to metabolize glucose and lipids and helps regulate insulin. Some studies suggest that low chromium levels may be associated with heart disease. Processed foods are often low in chromium. Although there is no RDA for chromium, the National Research Council (the organization that decides the RDAs) set the safe and adequate range for chromium intake at 50 to 200 µg for all ages.

Chromium shows promise in the fight against heart disease. It appears that supplementation with chromium in various forms can lower blood cholesterol levels. One study examined the effects of daily supplementation with 200 µg of chromium on the blood cholesterol levels of 34 men. The researchers found that the total blood cholesterol in the subjects dropped an average of 14 percent, and perhaps more important, the ratio of HDL cholesterol level to LDL cholesterol level improved by an average of 7 percent [33].

Chromium may play a role in regulating insulin's effectiveness in people with non–insulin-dependent diabetes. Chromium can increase the number of cell receptors for insulin, which may explain why the mineral seems to help with blood sugar control. In a study of 17 people with glucose intolerance (a precursor condition to adult-onset diabetes), supplementation with 200 µg of chromium daily improved the subjects' ability to handle an intake of sugar [34].

COPPER

Copper is an essential element needed by all tissues, and especially by the liver. Copper is important for healthy red blood cells and helps the body maintain the myelin covering of nerves.

The RDA for copper is 1.5 to 3 mg per day for all ages. Because copper produces free radicals, supplements should be taken with caution. A balance between copper and zinc enables these compounds to act against free radicals. A ratio of 8 to 1 (or as much as 15 to 1) of zinc to copper is recommended for good health. Excessive copper can result in immune suppression, anemia, bone and joint problems, neurologic problems, and heart disturbances.

IODINE

Part of the thyroid hormone thyroxin, iodine helps control the body's metabolic rate. The RDA for iodine is 150 µg. Iodine is found naturally in seafood. Before the introduction of iodized salt, some people living in inland areas had iodine deficiencies, the main symptom of which is goiter, or enlarged thyroid gland. This condition is now very rare in the United States.

IRON

Iron is the main constituent of hemoglobin, the part of blood cells that carries oxygen through the body. Small amounts of iron are needed to replace blood cells that are destroyed in the body processes.

The most common problem associated with iron deficiency is iron-deficiency anemia. This is characterized by fatigue, intolerance to cold, irritability, malaise, and paleness. Iron deficiency affects about 8 percent of low-income women and between 10 and 20 percent of low-income children. Young children, teenage girls, and women of childbearing age should eat enough iron-rich foods, such as lean meats and whole-grain bread, to keep the body's iron stores at adequate levels.

In men, iron overload is likely to be more of a problem than deficiency. Iron overload may contribute to heart disease. Although iron from plants and supplements is not absorbed efficiently if your body's stores of iron are adequate, iron from red meat continues to be absorbed. For this reason, some scientists believe that men should avoid daily consumption of red meat. High levels of iron have also been associated with arthritis, cancer, and liver disease.

The RDA for iron is higher for women of childbearing age (15 mg per day) than for men (10 mg). Research shows that calcium can decrease the absorption of iron; vitamin C increases absorption. Good sources of iron include

- legumes (dry peas and beans)
- yeast-leavened whole-wheat breads
- bread, cereals, pasta, and rice
- leafy greens of the cabbage family, such as broccoli, kale, and greens
- fish, meats, and poultry (especially dark meat)

MAGNESIUM

Magnesium is important for the health of arteries and the heart. Magnesium deficiency interferes with fat metabolism and allows levels of LDL cholesterol and triglycerides to increase, while decreasing the levels of HDL cholesterol, which removes fat deposits from artery walls.

RDA—The RDA for magnesium is 350 mg per day for men and 280 mg for women, but most Americans get less than half this amount. Magnesium is found in cereals, chocolate, dark-green vegetables, nuts, legumes, and seafood.

Therapeutic Uses—Magnesium may be helpful in reducing risk factors for heart disease. A study of 430 patients compared the effects of a magnesium-rich diet with that of a usual diet for 12 weeks. Persons in the group eating a diet rich in magnesium (about 1,142 mg per day) had a significant decrease in levels of total serum cholesterol, LDL cholesterol, and triglycerides than those in the usual diet group. Blood HDL cholesterol levels increased slightly in the group eating a magnesium-rich diet [35].

Magnesium has been shown to reduce mortality in people with heart attacks. A study of 2,316 patients with suspected acute myocardial infarction (heart attack) found that immediate intravenous administration of magnesium sulphate significantly reduced mortality. People in the magnesium group had a 24 percent lower rate of death than those who received a placebo injection of saline [36].

Two years later, those treated with magnesium had a 21 percent reduction in mortality from ischemic heart disease and a 16 percent reduction in mortality from all causes [37].

Animal studies show that chronic magnesium deficiency causes damage to the arteries and heart. Magnesium has also shown promising results in the treatment of conditions such as

- asthma
- migraine
- premenstrual syndrome
- muscle cramps

POTASSIUM SUPPLEMENT WARNING

It is best to get your potassium from food or from the small amounts (100 mg or so) found in multimineral supplements. Large doses of potassium in supplement form can cause electrolyte imbalances, resulting in dangerous heart-rhythm abnormalities (arrhythmias). Dietary potassium will not have this effect. However, people taking diuretic medications may need to take supplemental potassium because the diuretic causes potassium loss, and a deficiency of potassium can also cause arrhythmias. In either case, follow your practitioner's advice closely regarding potassium supplementation.

- high blood pressure
- kidney stones

POTASSIUM

Potassium is found in a wide variety of vegetables and fruits and may help reduce the risk for high blood pressure. Good sources of potassium include

- legumes (dried peas and beans)
- vegetables, especially potatoes (with skins) and sweet potatoes, spinach, Swiss chard, broccoli, winter squashes, and parsnips
- fruits, especially dried apricots, dates, bananas, cantaloupes, mangoes, plantains, prunes, orange and grapefruit juice, and raisins
- milk and yogurt

Numerous studies have shown that adequate potassium intake, especially when paired with adequate magnesium intake, can lower blood pressure and may even have a beneficial effect on blood cholesterol levels. A British study of 37 people with mild hypertension showed that potassium supplements lowered the subjects' blood pressure and total blood cholesterol levels [38]. Another study of 47 patients being treated for hypertension with various medications showed that increasing dietary potassium reduced the need for antihypertensive medication by as much as 76 percent [39].

SELENIUM

Selenium is an antioxidant that may help protect against certain cancers. Some evidence suggests that selenium and vitamin E can help improve mental functioning in elderly people.

RDA—The RDA for selenium is 70 µg for adult men and 55 for adult women. High doses (more than 10 times the RDA) may be harmful. Selenium is a mineral found in the soil, so it is contained in a wide variety of foods.

Therapeutic Uses—A British study of 50 people found that those taking a 100 µg selenium supplement had a general elevation of mood and decreased anxiety compared with those taking a placebo [40].

The antioxidant properties of selenium seem to have a protective effect against certain cancers. As early as the 1960s, studies began to show that adequate selenium intake lowered the risk of cancers of the gastrointestinal tract and the breast [41].

A study of 1,110 men in Finland found that concentrations of selenium in the blood seemed to have a protective effect against heart disease and stroke. Men with lower levels of selenium were about one and a half times more likely to die from cardiovascular causes than men with higher blood levels [42]. Low levels of the mineral may also be a risk factor for the heart condition called cardiomyopathy.

ZINC

Zinc is needed for central nervous system and immune function, growth and development, and the metabolism of carbohydrates, fats, and proteins. Zinc deficiency can result in decreased immune function, a loss of sense of smell and taste, and retarded growth.

RDA—The RDA for zinc is 15 mg for adult men and 12 mg for adult women. Doses within two to eight times the RDA are considered safe.

Toxicity—Excessive intake of zinc may result in low copper levels, impaired immune function, negative changes in the ratio of good to bad cholesterol, and gastrointestinal irritation.

Therapeutic Uses—Besides generally boosting immune function, zinc supplementation may have therapeutic value in the following:

- enlarged prostate
- wound healing
- acne
- arthritis

ORTHOMOLECULAR MEDICINE

Orthomolecular medicine is the use of high-dose vitamins to treat disease. Nobel Prize winner and well-known vitamin C proponent Linus Pauling first introduced the term "orthomolecular medicine" in a 1968 article in the journal *Science.*

In recent years, there has been an increased interest in orthomolecular therapy. High-dose vitamin therapy is used to treat a wide variety of conditions. For example, niacin is used to lower cholesterol. A number of uses for high-dose vitamin or mineral therapy are described in the Nutritional Supplements section above.

PSYCHIATRY

Early work in orthomolecular medicine centered around the use of high-dose vitamins to treat psychiatric disorders. As Dr. Pauling defined it: "the treatment of mental disease by the provision of the optimum molecular environment for the mind, especially the optimum concentration of substances normally present in the human body." He proposed that the optimum molecular concentration of such substances may differ from that provided by the diet and from the minimum amount required for life, or the recommended daily amounts [43].

Dr. Pauling noted that mental symptoms of vitamin deficiency may occur before physical symptoms and that a variety of deficiency disorders are associated with mental symptoms. For example, depression accompanies scurvy, a deficiency of vitamin C. And pellagra, a deficiency of niacin (vitamin B_3), can cause psychosis.

In the 1950s and 1960s, two Canadian psychiatrists, Abram Hoffer and Humphrey Osmond, began treating schizophrenic patients with high doses of vitamin B_3, vitamin C, and other vitamins. Their reports of success, however, were criticized by the American Psychiatric Association. Proponents of vitamin therapy said the criticism focused on therapy in chronically ill patients and that vitamin therapy was only effective in the early stages of schizophrenia.

CANCER

In the 1970s, Dr. Pauling and Ewan Cameron, M.D., reported that large doses of vitamin C could prolong the life of cancer patients. Government-funded studies conducted at the Mayo Clinic did not find any impact on the survival of cancer patients, leading to criticisms of the study designs by vitamin C proponents. Many practitioners and researchers consider the studies flawed.

RESOURCES

- American Association of Naturopathic Physicians
2366 Eastlake Ave. East, Ste. 322
Seattle, WA 98102
206-323-7610
fax 206-323-7612
http://infinite.org/Naturopathic.Physician
The AANP is the professional association for naturopathic physicians. Publishes a listing of naturopathic physicians in the United States. The Web site provides consumer information and helpful hints on everything from cooking (with recipes for healthy eating) to an extensive listing of self-care information on a wide variety of conditions and ailments.

- American Board of Nutrition Secretariat Office
1675 University Blvd.
Webb Building, Rm. 234
Birmingham, AL 35294-3360
205-975-8788
fax 205-934-7049
Composed of medical doctors who have had additional training in nutrition, the Board certifies physicians and has a directory of practitioners for referral.

- Physicians' Committee for Responsible Medicine
5100 Wisconsin Ave. NW, Ste. 404
Washington, DC 20016
202-686-2210
fax 202-686-2216
The Physicians' Committee for Responsible Medicine has a free brochure on healthy eating available by calling 1-800-US-LIVES. Promotes a vegan diet with no dairy or egg products and offers a "Vegetarian Starter Kit" for a small fee.

Osteopathy

FUNDAMENTAL TO THE PRACTICE OF MANY OSTEOPATHIC PHYSICIANS IS THE USE OF MANUAL DIAGNOSIS AND MANIPULATIVE TREATMENTS BASED ON THE CONCEPT OF THE BODY AS AN INTERCONNECTED SYSTEM OF NERVES, MUSCLES, AND BONES—ALL OF WHICH NEED TO FUNCTION AS AN INTEGRATED WHOLE. PROBLEMS IN THE MUSCULOSKELETAL SYSTEM OFTEN AFFECT THE HEALTH OF UNDERLYING ORGANS. DOCTORS OF OSTEOPATHY (CALLED O.D.s) ARE ALL TRAINED TO USE OSTEOPATHIC MANIPULATIONS TO RELEASE PHYSICAL BLOCKAGES TO ENABLE THE BODY TO REGAIN ITS INNATE ABILITY TO HEAL ITSELF.

HISTORY

Hippocrates in the fifth century B.C. used some form of manipulation. More recently, physicians commonly used it until the 18th century. Dr. Andrew Taylor Still originated the practice in the Midwest, first teaching it in 1892 when he opened the American School of Osteopathy in Kirksville, Missouri. The practice initially grew out of his understanding of the use of magnetism and bone-setting manipulations and his skepticism of medicines that had become standard, although they had not been proved effective. He believed that obstruction or imbalance of body fluids was caused by misplaced bones, especially in the spinal column.

ROAD TO CREDIBILITY

Early osteopathic physicians faced numerous legal challenges, often contesting their right to practice medicine. Conventional medical doctors (M.D.s) frequently appealed to state legislatures to prohibit the practice of osteopathy.

By 1920, though, the profession had gained considerable recognition nationwide. Nearly all states had regulations governing the practice of osteopathic therapy, and more than half had laws stipulating the formation of independent boards of osteopathic examination and registration to regulate the practice. In addition, osteopathic colleges mandated a four-year period of study, the same as for conventional medical colleges.

The difference between modern osteopathic physicians and conventional M.D.s has narrowed significantly, though, as the profession has grown to more than 38,000 osteopathic physicians in the United States. Since the 1960s, the Civil Service Commission and the Department of Defense have accepted both M.D.s and O.D.s on an equal footing. In Europe, osteopathy became the first alternative health care system to gain legal statutory recognition when Queen Elizabeth signed the Osteopaths Bill in 1993.

In the United States, osteopathic physicians are fully licensed to practice medicine in all 50 states. For that reason, much of the osteopathic profession considers itself within the mainstream of organized medicine. For many osteopathic physicians, osteopathic manipulation is an option they do not choose to include in their practice. In 1994, an estimated 10 percent of osteopathic physicians used manual diagnosis and treatment a great deal and 60 percent of them used it in selected cases. It is the aspect of osteopathic medicine that continues to be misunderstood and underappreciated for its therapeutic benefits and the part of osteopathy that many in the profession consider alternative medicine.

The practice of osteopathic medicine has grown from a traditional emphasis on primary care and attention to underserved areas to a system of overall patient care. More than 60 percent of osteopathic physicians are primary care physicians, all are trained to be family physicians, and most practice in smaller towns and rural areas. In recent decades, osteopathic physicians increasingly have turned to specialty areas of medicine, from psychiatry to neurosurgery and geriatrics.

This greater emphasis on specialty medicine has led some within the osteopathic community to criticize osteopathic medicine, calling for it to return to its original mission of primary care and to abandon specialty training or restrict it to those who have completed primary care residencies.

Still, even when osteopathic physicians do not employ manipulative therapies, organized osteopathy maintains its unique contribution in that osteopathic physicians treat the whole person, not just the disease, emphasizing the interconnectedness of structure and function. For example, removal of a gallbladder may solve the immediate problem, but osteopathic physicians also consider the nerve and blood supply and chemical balances of body fluids that may have contributed to the diseased gallbladder. They consider the patient's mental and emotional state and pay attention to the home environment, job, and other factors that affect health.

WHAT IT IS

Osteopathic physicians use a variety of manipulative approaches. They can choose from about 25 techniques, although eight are most commonly used. Generally, these differ slightly from the approaches used by most chiropractors and naturopathic physicians, but individual styles sometimes overlap.

The following are some of the most common techniques used by osteopathic physicians.

Soft-Tissue Technique—Commonly applied to the musculature surround-

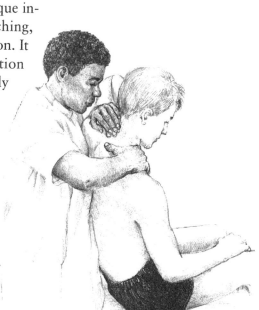

ing the spine, this technique involves rhythmic stretching, deep pressure, and traction. It enhances muscle relaxation and the circulation of body fluids.

Myofascial Release— In these techniques, the myofascial tissues—fibrous layers surrounding and separating individual muscle tissues—are guided along a path of least resistance until free movement is achieved.

Thrust Technique— The physician applies a high velocity, low-amplitude thrust to restore specific joint motion. The joint regains its normal range of motion and resets neural reflexes.

Muscle Energy Technique—This technique involves gently teasing and releasing specific muscles to produce relaxation, restore motion, and decrease muscle and tissue changes. The physician directs a patient to use muscles from a precise position and in a specific direction against a counterforce applied by the physician.

Cranial Techniques—Also called craniosacral techniques, these involve manual techniques to assess and release tensions in the head and tailbone. Considered a specific approach within the osteopathic concept, cranial techniques influence the structure and fluid surrounding the central nervous system (see also Craniosacral Therapy, pages 222–224).

Counterstrain Technique—In this technique, the physician locates tender points that relate to specific patterns of abnormal joint movement. The tenderness is turned off by moving the body or limb to a treatment position that quiets the pain. The technique results in improved movement and decreased pain.

USES

Most early patients of osteopathy had spinal, bone, or joint problems, but Dr. Still believed that the therapy could have wider applications. For example, he asserted that manipulative therapy shortly after occurrence of a lesion—a disorder within the musculoskeletal system—would reduce the chance of an infection becoming established. Osteopathic medicine has a much broader application now. Osteopathic manipulative therapy has been used to aid patients with

- spinal and joint conditions
- arthritis
- allergies
- cardiac diseases
- breathing dysfunctions
- chronic fatigue syndrome
- hiatal hernia
- high blood pressure
- headaches
- sciatica
- neuritis
- hyperactivity, mood disorders, dizziness, or dyslexia (in young children)
- carpal tunnel syndrome
- menstrual cramps
- neurologic problems (in children)

Research has demonstrated that osteopathic manipulation and manual diagnosis do appear to have some health benefit. Published reports since 1981 have shown manipulation eased lower-back pain, neurologic development problems in children, carpal tunnel syndrome, postoperative collapsed lung, and burning in an extremity.

BACK PAIN

Trials studying osteopathic treatments for back and neck pain have consistently shown the procedures to improve pain and range of motion. One study conducted on 95 patients with lower-back pain compared osteopathic manipulations with massage. The ones who had manipulative therapy reported more immediate relief after the first treatment than the massage group and showed substantial improvement when discharged [1].

PAIN IN THE EXTREMITIES

Reflex sympathetic dystrophy is characterized by swelling and deep burning pain in a limb. The condition can be caused by a stroke or heart attack or by a minor injury to the area. This pain can be notoriously difficult to treat, but certain osteopathic manipulative treatments have shown promise in stopping the pain and reversing the condition [2].

CARPAL TUNNEL SYNDROME

The conventional treatment of carpal tunnel syndrome often involves the use of drugs and/or surgery, but recent studies of an osteopathic technique called myofascial release manipulation show its promise as a nonpharmaceutical, nonsurgical alternative. Several studies have shown the osteopathic approach to be effective in improving symptoms, the outcome of nerve-conduction studies, and the width of the carpal tunnel. Osteopathic treatment also seems to lessen the need for surgery in mild to moderate cases [3,4].

NEUROLOGIC DEVELOPMENT

Osteopathic manipulations have found a use in the management of childhood developmental impairment. One study of children with neurologic impairments aged 18 months to 3 years showed that 6 to 12 osteopathic manipulative treatments resulted in significant neurologic improvement [5].

DIAGNOSIS OF OTHER DISORDERS

One study showed the potential of osteopathic palpation (investigating by feeling) at identifying internal difficulties. In a comparison of patients with normal and high blood pressure, researchers found those patients with high blood pressure to have a certain pattern of musculoskeletal findings in the neck and upper back.

RESOURCES

- American Academy of Osteopathy
  3900 DePauw Blvd., Ste. 1080
  Indianapolis, IN 46268-1136
  317-879-1881

The mission of the Academy, one of the affiliates of the American Osteopathic Association, is to teach, explore, and advance the science and art of total health care management, emphasizing osteopathic principles, palpatory diagnosis, and osteopathic manipulative treatment.

- American Osteopathic Association
  142 East Ontario St.
  Chicago, IL 60611
  312-280-5854
  800-621-1773

The parent organization of the osteopathic profession with 22 practice affiliates, one of which is the American Academy of Osteopathy. Primarily a professional organization, the Association is organized to advance the philosophy and practice of osteopathic medicine by promoting excellence in education, research, and the delivery of quality and cost-effective health care in a distinct, unified profession.

Oxygen Therapy

OXYGEN THERAPY INVOLVES THE USE OF DIFFERENT FORMS OF OXYGEN TO PRO-MOTE HEALING BY ALTERING THE BODY'S CHEMISTRY. THERE ARE SEVERAL TYPES OF OXYGEN THERAPY: OXYGENATION USING HYPERBARIC (HIGH-PRESSURE) OXY-GEN CHAMBERS; THE ADDITION OF HYDROGEN PEROXIDE OR OTHER COMPOUNDS TO CAPTURE ELECTRONS FROM FOREIGN SUBSTANCES IN THE BODY IN A NATURAL PROCESS CALLED OXIDATION; AND OZONE THERAPY, WHICH AIDS IN BOTH OXIDA-TION AND OXYGENATION.

HISTORY

The first book on medical applications of oxygen therapy dates back to 1796, but the age of hyperbaric oxygen therapy began in 1937 when researchers reported using it for treatment of decompression sickness. Use of peroxide dates back to at least 1884, and reports of clinical research on medical uses go back to at least 1914.

HYPERBARIC OXYGEN THERAPY

WHAT IT IS

The value of hyperbaric oxygen in medicine, debated for decades, got an especially public and unfavorable airing when a picture of singer Michael Jackson spending time in a hyperbaric oxygen chamber appeared in a tabloid newspaper in the 1980s. However, recent findings have found that oxygen therapy can help patients suffering from a variety of conditions. Hyperbaric oxygen therapy has

- saved failing liver transplants
- prevented amputation in severe frostbite
- treated eye diseases
- been used for patients after stroke

Hyperbaric oxygen therapy is the short-term inhalation of pure (100 percent) oxygen at pressures up to two atmospheres (the equivalent of 33 feet of seawater). Normally, the air we breathe is 21 percent oxygen. Patients can receive the treatment in a multi-place chamber (usually a large steel cylinder) pressurized with air while the patient breathes 100 percent oxygen via a mask, head tent, or endotracheal tube (patients on ventilators only). Alternatively, a monoplace (one-person) chamber pressurized entirely with 100 percent oxygen is sometimes used.

The therapy can last 60 to 90 minutes. In some chambers, the patient has clear visibility beyond the chamber, can maintain constant communication with an attendant, and can be removed at any time.

HOW IT WORKS

Normally, oxygen is transported through the body by red blood cells. Hyperbaric oxygen causes the oxygen to dissolve in all the body's fluids—white blood cells, spinal fluid, brain fluid, and others. This extra oxygen can, therefore, reach much more of the damaged tissue to aid the body's own healing. Other gases are eliminated as the body is flooded with pressurized oxygen, thus reducing any damage caused by toxic gases such as carbon monoxide.

USES

Hyperbaric oxygen is the treatment of choice for decompression sickness ("the bends") and arterial gas embolism (the formation of bubbles that can block blood flow to critical areas). It has also been useful in the treatment of several other conditions, including

- gas gangrene
- osteomyelitis (bone infection)
- radiation damage

- severe carbon monoxide poisoning
- anaerobic infections
- immune compromising conditions

Proponents also contend that the therapy can help patients with circulatory problems and strokes, when adequate oxygen cannot reach the damaged area. Medicare coverage of the therapy includes treatment for gas gangrene, diabetes with peripheral circulatory disorders, chronic ulcer of skin, a variety of crushing injuries, the toxic effect of carbon monoxide, air embolism, and decompression illness. The American College of Hyperbaric Medicine lists more than 60 uses, including stroke, vegetative coma, burns, frostbite, migraine, near hanging, and near electrocution.

AIDS—Hyperbaric oxygen is increasingly being used to treat some of the symptoms associated with HIV infection and AIDS. Two to three one-hour treatment sessions seem to alleviate the chronic fatigue, wasting, and anorexia that can accompany the disease by interfering with certain biochemical reactions. Anemia associated with AIDS can also be managed with hyperbaric oxygen therapy [1].

Carbon Monoxide Poisoning—One of the well-established uses for hyperbaric oxygen therapy is in cases of carbon monoxide poisoning, which accounts for half of all fatal poisonings in the United States. Carbon monoxide binds to the blood's hemoglobin more readily than oxygen does; so in cases of poisoning, too much hemoglobin is taken up by carbon monoxide and not enough is free to transport oxygen to body tissues. Although the exact mechanism is not well understood, hyperbaric oxygen therapy may displace the

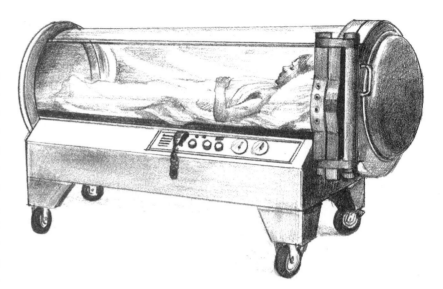

carbon monoxide and force oxygen on the hemoglobin molecules. The therapy remains one of the few treatment options for this condition [2].

Stroke—The Ocean Hyperbaric Center tells how the therapy helped a man who was bedridden and progressively failing due to an ischemic stroke. After 14 treatments, the patient began speaking for the first time in four years. Ultimately, the man was able to push himself in a wheelchair.

Tissue Necrosis—This term refers to the death of cells in any part of the body. Necrosis can occur as a result of infections, loss of blood supply (because of crushing injury, for example), or frostbite. Hyperbaric oxygen holds promise for all of these problems.

Infection with clostridial bacteria (also known as gas gangrene) can occur when the organisms enter a wound or cut. The infection can be life threatening, and treatment of severe cases usually involves surgical removal of the tissue (sometimes meaning amputation). Hyperbaric oxygen therapy can be a valuable adjunct to antibiotics and surgery—in some cases, decreasing mortality and improving the results of surgery [3].

The results of hyperbaric oxygen therapy for frostbite also can be dramatic. An anecdotal report from a doctor at the State University of New York Health Science Center at Syracuse told the story of an 18-year-old high school student, numbed by alcohol, who wandered barefoot for hours during a freezing night. The teenager might have lost as many as five toes, but instead of surgery, hyperbaric oxygen was used. In frostbite, tissue dies as oxygen fails to reach the cells. In the teenager, early tests showed almost no blood flow into the compromised tissues. After a week of 60-minute hyperbaric oxygen treatments, the patient was discharged—all toes intact—with pink skin.

Radiation Damage—Hyperbaric oxygen therapy can be effective in treating damage caused by radiation exposure (often from radiation therapy in cancer cases). This tissue damage can affect soft tissue, bones, and even vision. Hyperbaric oxygen therapy can be a helpful adjunct to conventional approaches on all of these fronts. The therapy can encourage tissue to vascularize (form new blood vessels), thus causing grafts to take more easily and making reconstructive surgery more effective [4].

OZONE THERAPY
WHAT IT IS

Although oxygen is an element that can exist one atom at a time, it tends to be found in the air we breathe in its diatomic form—that is, a molecule of two oxygen atoms bound together. In contrast, ozone has three oxygen atoms for each gas molecule, in which one of the oxygen atoms is relatively loosely bound to the other two. The result is a more reactive molecule that both contributes the diatomic oxygen gas that we normally breathe, plus adds an extra oxygen atom that, when it breaks with the ozone molecule, becomes available to attract electrons from harmful substances in the body.

In clinical practice, ozone can be administered in a number of ways. It can be mixed with blood drawn from a patient and then returned to the patient. It can be blown into the vagina or rectum. It can be applied topically as a gas or mixed in water or olive oil. Some practitioners recommend ozone therapy as part of a combined approach that may include antioxidants to limit any damage caused by ozone's oxidative qualities.

USES

Public health uses of ozone can be traced to 1870 in Germany where one researcher reported using it to purify blood. Ozone was used successfully by the military during World War I to treat infections. Now an estimated 7,000 physicians and naturopathic doctors use ozone therapy. The therapy has been used as a treatment for

- AIDS and AIDS-related illnesses
- dissolving arteriosclerotic plaque
- fungal infections in the intestine
- allergies
- inflammatory infections
- chronic infections
- multiple sclerosis
- cancer
- arthritis
- disinfection during surgery
- poor healing wounds
- burns

Some advocates of the therapy are vocal supporters of ozone's use as a treatment for AIDS, believing that ozone selectively destroys viruses, which have no protection against oxidants, whereas healthy human cells do have antioxidants to ward off any damage caused by ozone. Laboratory tests have been promising, but small human trials have not been successful against AIDS.

However, a trial for AIDS-related diarrhea did prove intriguing. When ozone gas was given rectally in a study of five AIDS patients with intractable diarrhea, the diarrhea disappeared in three patients, and the fourth patient improved [5].

OXIDATION THERAPY
WHAT IT IS

Oxidation therapy involves the administration of hydrogen peroxide to treat and prevent various conditions. Hydrogen peroxide is required for the metabolism of protein, carbohydrates, fats, vitamins, and minerals. Infection-fighting cells called *granulocytes* produce the substance—known chemically as H_2O_2—as a first line of defense against all invading organisms. Reports of successful treatment of diphtheria with a peroxide nasal spray date back to 1898, and intravenous hydrogen

---

CAUTION

Avoid taking hydrogen peroxide orally. It can be dangerously toxic. Oxidation therapy should not be self-administered; seek the advice of a trained professional.

---

peroxide reduced mortality rates of a 1919 flu epidemic. Hydrogen peroxide can be administered intravenously or orally (in very dilute solution).

Some of hydrogen peroxide's reputed treatment successes include
- viral infections
- allergies
- tumors
- migraine headaches
- Alzheimer disease
- emphysema
- chronic fatigue syndrome

Although there is not much research supporting the claims of practitioners in the field and there are many skeptics, anecdotal evidence and practitioners' own experience have been promising enough to keep the therapy growing in the United States.

RESOURCES

- Ocean Hyperbaric Center
  4001 Ocean Dr.
  Lauderdale-by-the-Sea, FL 33308
  800-552-0255
  954-776-5800
  fax 954-776-0670
  Conducts research and provides referrals worldwide.

- Hyperbaric Oxygen Institute
  1455 N. Waterman Ave., Ste. 125
  San Bernardino, CA 92404
  909-884-1790
  fax 909-884-6853

- Oxygen and Ozone Therapies Area
  on the World Wide Web
  http://www.oxytherapy.com
  Lists practitioners and clinics worldwide, as well as research and testimonials. Provides basic information on therapies and links to other Web sites.

Qigong

A COMPONENT OF TRADITIONAL CHINESE MEDICINE, QIGONG (PRONOUNCED CHEE-GONG) HAS BEEN PRACTICED FOR SEVERAL THOUSAND YEARS. QIGONG PROMOTES HEALTH, LONGEVITY, AND HEALING THROUGH EXERCISES DESIGNED TO CIRCULATE AND BALANCE QI, OR VITAL ENERGY, IN THE BODY.

Like yoga and other practices that combine physical exercise with mental effort and meditation, qigong reestablishes or rebalances the flow of vital energy and revitalizes the body and all of its systems.

Among the many techniques employed by qigong are

- breathing exercises
- deep relaxation
- meditation
- visualization
- body postures
- movements
- self-applied massage techniques

WHAT IT IS

Qigong exercises combine repetitions of slow, gently flowing movements of the arms, legs, and torso with mental concentration to allow for the movement of qi within the body. Qigong exercises involve moving the entire body (hands, shoulders, hips, feet, and so on) and breathing in such a way as to create movement patterns that are called forms. The exercises are to be performed for 30 to 60 minutes every day.

During exercise, the practitioner focuses on moving qi through the body's pathways, but describing the moving of the qi as something that the individual "does" through his or her own effort is misleading. The mental effort can be more accurately defined as mentally getting out of the way so the qi can move freely through the body. The movements, the breathing, and the mental "effort" bring the entire being more and more toward balance, harmony, and peace.

TAOIST UNDERPINNINGS

Qigong is related to the philosophy of Tao, or "The Way." Taoists believe that we are all an integral part of nature, and Taoists seek to harmonize with nature and draw on its beneficial energy.

Deng Ming-Dao, who has written several books on Taoism, says in his book *The Scholar Warrior* that Taoists "believe that it is humanity's refusal to regard itself as part of a greater order that causes confusion, ignorance, and sorrow. They feel that if human beings could balance themselves with this order, they would live a simple life of happiness and understanding." Some Taoist masters are said to have lived for well over 100 years.

EXERCISES

This effort to achieve balance with nature led to the development of exercises based on patterns observed in nature, such as the qualities and behavior of animals. The earliest written record of these exercises was by Huao Tuo in the first or second century and were based on the movements of five animals—bears, cranes, deer, monkeys, and tigers.

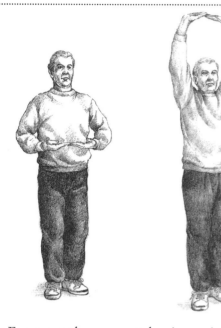

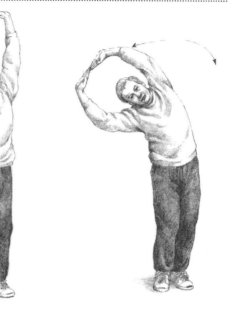

For example, crane-style qigong incorporates a set of movements that emulate those of a crane—the gentle opening and folding of its wings, its preening, its skimming flight along the water, and its meditative one-legged stance. While these movements are performed, the practitioner evokes the image of the graceful crane. These images combine with deep breathing and physical movement to open the energy channels in the body.

The source of qi is in the dan tian, located just below the navel. Therefore, each stance begins with hands placed just below the navel at the dan tian and ends with the return of qi to its storehouse. As practitioners carry out the movements, they feel the building and the flow of qi throughout the body before it is returned to the dan tian.

Qigong's slow, circular, and symmetrical movements are similar to those used in internal martial arts, such as Tai chi, or tijijuan. Qigong uses shorter movement groups that are repeated many times, whereas Tai chi employs dancelike movements that flow from one position to another. Like qigong, Tai chi combines physical exercise with meditation.

MENTAL EFFORT

There are more than 100 different forms of qigong exercise, but all consider the mental effort that goes with the exercises to be crucial. This mental effort is coordinated with the specific movements. As discussed earlier, the "effort" is not so much an exertion as it is a mental centering and relaxation. Just as water tends to find equilibrium, qi flows where it needs to go, back to balance if allowed and encouraged.

In addition to physical movements, practitioners are taught techniques for
- centering
- deep breathing
- achieving a state of physical balance
- meditating

Many of these are key components used in Western relaxation techniques.

Qigong may also incorporate the use of sounds and visualization. For example, for healing sounds qigong employs the repetition of specific sounds

This exercise is good for nourishing the dan tian (the souce of qi in the body): 1) Facing the east, place both hands in front of you at waist level, palms facing up. 2) Inhale while lifting the palms. When you reach the throat, turn your palms outward and continue lifting over your head, all the while continuing the same inhalation. 3) Lean to the side while exhaling and lean to the other side while continuing the same exhalation. Lower your hands and repeat the exercise six times. Eventually, work up to 21 repetitions.

and the visualization of colors associated with specific organs.

USES

Because of its gentle movements, qigong is good for increasing or maintaining flexibility in middle age or later years of life. But in addition to promoting health and longevity, qigong is widely used in China for a variety of ailments; it is used as an adjunct to cancer therapy and in the treatment of high blood pressure. The therapy is gaining increasing popularity in the United States, as well.

In China, qigong exercises have been under study for their long-term effects on a number of medical conditions:

- Cancer
- Coronary artery disease
- Paralysis and spinal cord injuries
- High blood pressure
- General health promotion
- Longevity
- Relaxation and stress reduction

Persons who practice qigong exercises have had good results in therapy for hypertension, cancer, and coronary artery disease. Qigong exercise has also been shown to affect the blood chemistry and immune system of individuals who practice it.

One of the reasons qigong has had a slow start in the West is that most of the scientific papers on the topic are written in Chinese. However, some review articles have been published in English, and hundreds of research papers have been presented at international conferences in recent years, suggesting that qigong is gaining acceptance especially as a valuable adjunct in the treatment of cancer, high blood pressure, and other chronic diseases.

EXTERNAL QIGONG

Obviously, qigong can be practiced on oneself, but it can also be practiced on someone else. Qigong exercises practiced by individuals to promote health and well-being are sometimes called internal qigong. External qigong, on the other hand, is practiced by qigong masters who have studied for many years. These masters can emit their qi to balance that of the patient and promote health and healing.

Researchers have been able to measure infrasonic energy in the emissions from external qigong practitioners. Studies have shown it can affect such diverse physical phenomenon as the germination rate of seeds and the electroencephalograms (a measurement of electrical activity in the brain) of persons who received qigong treatment from a qigong master.

CANCER

Advanced cancer patients who practice daily qigong in addition to their drug therapy have dramatic improvements in strength, appetite, and weight increase. In one study, 82 percent of 97 patients receiving a combination of qigong and chemotherapy reported regained strength compared with only 10 percent of 30 patients who received drugs alone [1].

CORONARY HEART DISEASE

Qigong was shown to improve brainwave patterns, heart rhythm, clinical symptoms, and laboratory values in 88 coronary heart disease patients. Researchers believe qigong stimulates blood flow and decreases the blood agglutination that can lead to heart attack [2].

HIGH BLOOD PRESSURE

Patients who practiced qigong in combination with small amounts of blood pressure medication fared better than those who took higher does of blood pressure medication alone. After six months, the qigong group in one such study had beneficial changes in plasma cholesterol, blood viscosity, and platelet aggregation abnormalities—all key factors in the development of the complications associated with hypertension. At six years, the qigong group also had significantly fewer strokes and deaths from stroke than the control group (17.3 percent and 11.5 percent versus 32 percent and 23 percent, respectively) [3].

GENERAL HEALTH

Qigong also appears to help boost the immune system. Studies have found that persons who practice qigong have higher levels of CD4 lymphocytes (important cells that fight off infection) and immune systems that respond faster to foreign cells [4]. Qigong also appears to have positive effects on cell functions such as the rate of cell growth and DNA synthesis [5].

Other studies have shown that qigong may improve the efficiency of oxygen uptake. Research suggests that qigong has a beneficial effect on enzyme and hormonal balance and can decrease heart and respiratory rates.

WHO DOES IT

Qigong and Tai chi are taught throughout the country in sites ranging from oriental health centers to recreation departments and senior centers. Contact the organization listed below for help in finding an instructor or practitioner in your area. You can also try contacting traditional Chinese medicine practitioners in your community. Many instructors teach on an informal basis or by referral. As always, ask about training and experience.

RESOURCES

- Qigong Institute, East-West Academy of Healing Arts
  450 Sutter St.
  San Francisco, CA 94108
  415-788-2227

Provides general information, hosts regular meetings, and provides English reviews of scientific studies of qigong.

Traditional Chinese Medicine

Practiced for thousands of years, traditional Chinese medicine includes a vast array of preventive and therapeutic techniques still in use in China today. The practice has spread throughout Asia and the world. Other Asian countries, such as Korea, Japan, and Vietnam, have built on its foundations to create their own systems of healing, and many traditional Chinese practices have gained considerable attention in the West.

HISTORY

Traditional Chinese medicine has been practiced for more than 2,000 years. The oldest Chinese medical text is the *Yellow Emperor's Classic* (also known as the *Nei Jing*), written around 200 B.C.

WHAT IT IS

PHILOSOPHY

The fundamental concepts of traditional Chinese medicine are rooted in the philosophies of Buddhism, Confucianism, and Taoism. A brief understanding of the major principles underlying these philosophies and how they differ from those in the West can help explain the Oriental approach to life and to medicine.

Modern Western thought emphasizes the separation of mind and body. Eastern philosophies, on the other hand, consider the mind and body to be inextricably linked and believe that the individual and nature are fundamentally interrelated. Chinese medicine seeks ways to learn from and harmonize with nature and draw on its beneficial energy.

Like other traditional medicines with a long history, traditional Chinese medicine focuses on the individual and what imbalances may be contributing to or causing illness or disease. Traditional Chinese medicine places primary emphasis on the balance of qi (pronounced CHEE), or vital energy. There are 12 major meridians, or pathways, for qi, and each is associated with a major vital organ or vital function. These meridians form an invisible network that carries qi to every tissue in the body.

This vital energy comprises two parts: yin and yang. Simply speaking, yin and yang can be considered opposites—active and passive, masculine and feminine, heavenly and earthly—but in many ways they are one, like two sides of the same coin. The concept is probably best described by the traditional yin-yang symbol. The yin-yang symbol is a circle divided by a curved line into a white and black side, each of which contains a smaller circle of the opposite color. The curve represents the ever-changing balance between yin and yang, and the smaller circles demonstrate that each contains elements of the other. This coincides with the Chinese belief that the universe is forever

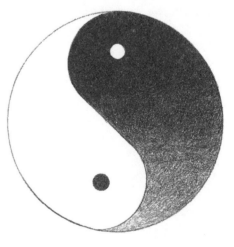

changing. And as an integral part of the universe, so are we.

The two—yin and yang—must be balanced with each other in an individual for the body to function normally. Therefore, diagnosis aims to detect patterns of disharmony or imbalance in vital energy. Accordingly, treatment seeks to help individuals rebalance this vital energy and restore harmony and health.

In traditional Chinese medicine, treatment is highly individualized, so that two patients coming in with the same problem are not necessarily treated alike. Practitioners instead focus on correcting the root cause of the imbalance that is contributing to or allowing illness and disease.

DIAGNOSIS

Traditional Chinese medicine practitioners use relatively simple but very effective tools, including

- listening
- looking
- palpation (touching and feeling)
- pulse diagnosis
- questioning

Most of the features of an examination by a practitioner of traditional Chinese medicine will seem familiar to Westerners. One diagnostic tool, however—pulse diagnosis—is unique to traditional Chinese medicine.

In the West, a pulse reading is a calculation of the number of times the heart beats. It's simple and is performed in a matter of seconds. A pulse *diagnosis* by a practitioner of traditional Chinese medicine, however, takes considerably longer and is used to assess the body's overall status and to detect disharmonies.

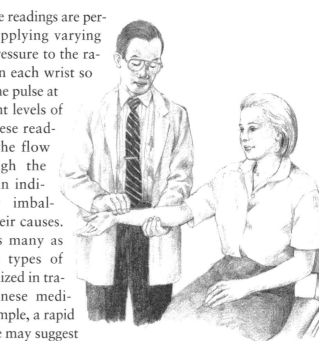

These pulse readings are performed by applying varying degrees of pressure to the radial artery on each wrist so as to assess the pulse at three different levels of pressure. These readings reveal the flow of qi through the body and can indicate energy imbalances and their causes. There are as many as 30 different types of pulses recognized in traditional Chinese medicine. For example, a rapid floating pulse may suggest a deficiency of yin.

Another aspect of traditional Chinese diagnosis is the tongue diagnosis. The physician notes different color, thickness, and "fur" distributions on the tongue.

All of these methods are used to assess the eight principal patterns. These consist of the balances between the following four pairs of opposites:

- yin and yang
- heat and cold
- deficiency and excess
- interior and exterior

PERNICIOUS INFLUENCES OR EVILS

Traditional Chinese medicine recognizes six external factors that can play a part in disease: wind (which usually brings along another pernicious influence); cold; heat; dampness; dryness; and summer heat.

ORGAN SYSTEMS AND THEORY

Western and traditional Chinese thought both ascribe specific functions to the various organs of the body, but traditional Chinese medicine tends to use a broader classification that looks more at an organ's relationship to other organs rather than its specific function alone. For example, the heart in traditional Chinese medicine refers not just to the blood-pumping machine of Western medicine but also to blood vessels and the circulation of blood, as well as the storage place of the spirit, or "shen."

THERAPIES

A wide range of therapies are used in traditional Chinese medicine to correct physical symptoms, restore energetic balance, and redirect and normalize a person's qi. Some of the treatment options used are

- acupuncture
- cupping
- herbal medicine
- massage
- moxibustion
- qigong

Acupuncture and Acupressure—Acupuncture is the insertion of tiny, hair-thin needles into specific points of the body. Acupuncture is used to correct the flow of qi to restore health by stimulating specific points along these pathways (see Acupuncture, pages 173–177). Acupressure is similar, but involves putting pressure on the points rather than needles in them (see Acupressure, pages 169–177).

Cupping—Cupping is the application of suction over specific points or zones in the body to relieve local congestion. Practitioners warm the air in a bamboo or glass jar, then overturn it onto the body. As the air cools, it contracts, causing the suction. This technique is often used to treat arthritis, bronchitis, and sprains.

Diet and Nutrition—Diet and nutrition programs are individualized according to the patient's needs and illness. Foods are classified according to their energetic properties, such as cooling, drying, dispersing, heating, moistening, and toning. Chinese cultural and medical practice emphasizes eating foods that are in harmony with the seasons and with life activities.

Some common elements of the traditional Chinese diet may also help protect against disease. Green tea, for example, may have certain anticancer effects and certain heart benefits. An analysis of 1,016 patients with esophageal cancer compared their green tea consumption with an equal number of persons who did not have cancer but were the same age and sex. The study suggests that drinking green tea may

Much of the Western world's recent interest in traditional Chinese medicine can be traced to the early 1970s when President Richard Nixon visited China in an effort to reestablish diplomatic relations. One of the reporters covering the story, James Reston of *The New York Times,* was stricken with appendicitis. His story about how acupuncture was used to treat his pain after an emergency appendectomy sparked an interest in this and other forms of traditional Chinese medicine that continues today.

have a protective effect against the development of esophageal cancer [1]. Studies in mice show that a component of green tea has a protective effect against experimentally induced skin cancer.

A study of 137 men found that blood levels of cholesterol and triglycerides were lower in those with higher consumption of green tea. This suggests that green tea may have a protective effect against cardiovascular disease. Green tea displayed protective benefits for the liver as well [2].

Herbal Medicine—Herbs remain the backbone of traditional Chinese medicine as practiced in China and Asia today. Herbal remedies are used as both tonics to maintain health and as treatments for a wide range of ailments, such as breathing difficulties, chronic debilitating illnesses, infections, and pain. China's traditional materia medica contains some 3,200 herbs and 300 animal and mineral extracts. The *Encyclopedia of Traditional Chinese Medicinal Substances* (*Zhong yao da ci dian*) published in 1977 contains nearly 6,000 entries.

Herbal compounds used in traditional Chinese medicine are usually complex mixtures that include many ingredients. Herbal preparations are classified according to their energetic qualities, such as heating, cooling, drying, or moisturizing. Medicines are prescribed for their action on energy balance and flow, organs, or seasonal physical disturbances.

These prescriptions are developed to have more than one effect, such as affecting the disease or disharmony, balancing out any side effects of the principal therapy, and directing the

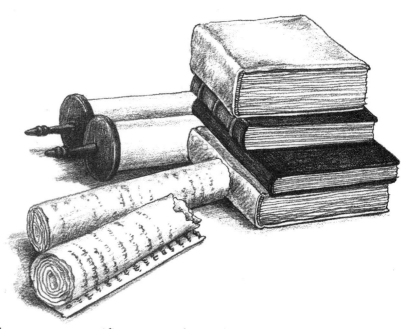

therapy to a specific area or physical process in the body.

Massage—Traditional Chinese medicine has an ancient history of massage. Practitioners use a complex series of hand movements called the eight *kua* on specific parts of the body. The two traditional massage systems used are *an-mo* and *tuina*. *An-mo* is used to tone the system through pressing and rubbing hand motions. *Tuina* is used to soothe and sedate through thrusting and rolling hand motions.

Massage is used to maintain well-being, like the traditional "Keep-Fit Massage for Health Preservation" routine, which includes techniques for massaging the eyes, ears, brow, and all the body to improve blood circulation and adjust and harmonize the function of various parts of the body.

> A typical hospital in China today is likely to go through more than one ton of herbs a day.

Massage may also be used to treat specific disorders, such as ulcers. One study involving 98 patients with peptic ulcers reported that traditional Chinese massage of the stomach and stimulation of key points resulted in a 75 percent cure rate, and an additional 21 percent showed improvement [3].

Moxibustion—Moxibustion is the use of heat on energetically active points of the body to stimulate the flow of qi. Practitioners burn the crushed leaves, or moxa, of a daisylike plant, *Artemisia vulgaris,* in loose or stick forms to release a radiant heat that penetrates deeply and restores the balance and flow of qi. In moxibustion, the lit end of a piece of burning *Artemisia* is held near the acupuncture point (not close enough to burn the skin, though). The use of heat to stimulate points on the body works on the same principles as acupuncture and is believed to predate the use of needles to stimulate the flow of qi.

A study of 71 persons with hypothyroidism found that moxibustion along with the application of Chinese medicinal powder to specific points led to recovery of thyroid function and better immune function [4].

Qigong—Qigong is used to promote health, longevity, and healing through exercises designed to circulate and balance qi, or vital energy, in the body. Qigong includes breathing exercises, deep relaxation, meditation, visualization, body postures, movements, and certain self-applied massage techniques (see Qigong, pages 342–345).

USES OF CHINESE HERBAL PREPARATIONS

Chinese government officials intent on "modernizing" China after the revolution in 1949 sponsored numerous studies of various aspects of traditional Chinese medicine. The results of these studies led them to conclude that traditional Chinese medicine deserves equal status with "modern" Western medicine.

Despite the many studies on the effectiveness of traditional Chinese medicine, information is lacking in the West because many of these have been published only in Chinese. In recent years, however, a growing number of well-designed studies have been published in English that show the promise of this traditional approach for the treatment of a wide variety of conditions.

CORONARY HEART DISEASE

A study of 80 persons with coronary heart disease found that traditional Chinese herbal remedies resulted in marked symptomatic relief in 38 percent of patients and improvement in the symptoms of 58 percent, for an overall effectiveness rate of 92 percent. Therapy consisted of the same basic herbs to activate blood, but other ingredients were added according to specific diagnoses of what deficiencies (yin or yang) were present in the individual patients [5].

HIGH BLOOD CHOLESTEROL

At least one Chinese herbal preparation has shown great promise in reducing blood cholesterol levels—a key risk factor in the development of heart disease. A study of 130 persons with high cholesterol found that treatment with yi shou jiang zhi tablets was 87 percent effective in lowering blood cholesterol levels and 81 percent effective in lowering the level of triglycerides. This herbal preparation contains five different Chinese herbs [6].

HYPERACTIVITY

Hyperactivity is a problem for many children; it can lead to learning problems and delayed development. A Chinese study of 66 hyperactive children found that treatment with yizhi ("wit-increasing") syrup resulted in an 85 percent improvement in behavior, school records, and symptoms [7].

INFECTIOUS DISEASES

A wide variety of herbal preparations are used in traditional Chinese medicine to treat infectious diseases. Recent studies show that some of these do not necessarily have specific antiviral or antibiotic effects, but rather they help fight infection by boosting the body's immune system. Many studies in animals show that Chinese herbal preparations can stimulate immune system functioning. These actions include increases in a wide variety of immune mechanisms that fight infection and disease, including increases in
- antibody production
- levels of helper T cells
- immunoglobulin A production
- interferon production
- interleukin-6 secretion
- lymphocyte production
- levels of natural killer cells

ACUTE BRONCHIOLITIS

A study of 96 children with acute bronchiolitis compared the use of Chinese herbs combined with antibiotic therapy, Chinese herbs alone, and antibiotics alone. Children who received herbs alone or in combination with an-tibiotics had a significantly shorter course of illness and faster improvement of symptoms such as coughing and wheezing than those who received antibiotics alone.

The herbal preparation used, shuang huang lian, consists mainly of the herbs huangqin, lianqia, and shuanghua. Huangqin is known to boost immune function, specifically lymphocyte transformation and macrophage function—two important microbiological processes in the immune system. The other two herbs are known to act as anti-inflammatories. The study used an intravenous preparation of the herbs, a method of administration that is not practical for use in the United States where hospital stays are much shorter than in China. Researchers are now studying an aerosol form of shuang huang lian, which seems to be equally effective and may be a more practical form of administration [8].

KIDNEY FAILURE

A study of 50 persons suffering from chronic kidney failure found that 37 improved after treatment with a preparation of rhubarb, dandelion, and oyster shell [9].

ULCERS

Chinese medicine holds great promise in the treatment of gastric and peptic ulcers. A study of 80 children with peptic ulcers reported that those treated with a Chinese herbal preparation known as wang pengfei had a cure rate of 81 percent after six to eight weeks of treatment. Another 11 percent of the patients showed improvement after more than eight weeks of therapy [10].

STROKE

A review of studies of traditional Chinese medicine approaches in the treatment of strokes found that herbal preparations intended to improve blood circulation in the brain can lead to significant improvements in stroke patients, such as recovery from paralysis [11].

OTHER AREAS

Promising areas of research in traditional Chinese medicine include

• asthma
• chronic hepatitis
• migraines
• osteoporosis
• pain
• Parkinson disease
• scleroderma

WHO DOES IT

Most physicians trained in China today learn both Western medicine and traditional Chinese medicine. Like any different systems based on different beliefs and philosophies, each offers certain advantages over the other. Western medicine, for example, is much more adept at high-tech areas such as emergency trauma care. Traditional Chinese medicine practitioners, on the other hand, are more likely to look at the whole person and focus on prevention, making their success with chronic health problems more substantial.

In the United States, many conventional practitioners learn elements of traditional Chinese medicine, and naturopathic colleges provide training in traditional Chinese medicine. Most states require that a practitioner have a license to perform acupuncture.

RESOURCES

- American Association of Acupuncture and Oriental Medicine
433 Front St.
Catasauqua, PA 18032
610-266-1433
Provides lists of state-licensed or NCCA certified providers.

- National Acupuncture and Oriental Medicine Alliance
14637 Starr Rd. SE
Olalla, WA 98359
206-851-6896
Operates a referral service for certified practitioners. Provides lists of national organizations and offers information on health insurance organizations. Sponsors annual conferences and conventions and an ongoing list of events.

- National Commission for the Certification of Acupuncturists
P.O. Box 97075
Washington, DC 20090
202-232-1404
Certifies practitioners in both acupuncture and Chinese herbology.

Wave Therapy

SOUND WAVES, LIGHT WAVES, AND MAGNETIC FIELDS ALL HAVE BENEFICIAL HEALTH EFFECTS WHEN APPLIED APPROPRIATELY. MUSIC THERAPY, FOR EXAMPLE, HAS BEEN USED TO REDUCE PAIN AND ANXIETY, STEMMING FROM ITS ABILITY TO AFFECT PHYSIOLOGIC PROCESSES SUCH AS RESPIRATORY RATE, BLOOD PRESSURE, AND CARDIAC OUTPUT. WHEN LIGHT ENTERS THE EYE, IT TRIGGERS A CASCADE OF NERVE AND ENDOCRINE (GLANDULAR) ACTIVITIES THAT ULTIMATELY INFLUENCE MOST BODILY FUNCTIONS, INCLUDING SEXUAL FUNCTION, IMMUNITY, AND SLEEP. MAGNETIC FIELD THERAPY MAY STIMULATE METABOLISM AND INCREASE THE AMOUNT OF OXYGEN TO THE CELLS.

HISTORY

The essence of the three wave therapies has been around since the beginning of time. There has always been sound and light to soothe, magnetism in the form of the Earth's magnetic field, and naturally occurring magnetic rocks.

Incantations for healing the sick are mentioned in the oldest known written account of medical practices, the *Kahum* papyrus. Aristotle considered several instruments, but especially the flute, to be very powerful facilitators of healing. But despite this early recognition, the first accounts of music's significant influence on breathing, blood pressure, digestion, and muscular activity were documented during the Renaissance.

The medical uses of light can be traced to the Greeks, Romans, and Egyptians who recognized its unique power to influence the human psyche. In modern times, the medical value of light was observed in the 1890s by Danish physician Niels Finsen, the father of photobiology; he successfully treated skin tuberculosis with ultraviolet light.

About 1000 B.C., a Persian physician used magnets to relieve muscle spasms and gout. In Greece, in 22 B.C., the Greek physician Galen found that natural magnets relieved pain. Magnetic field therapy has been used in China for thousands of years. It also was used in ancient Egypt.

MUSIC THERAPY
WHAT IT IS

Of the three forms of wave therapy, music therapy is perhaps the best developed. Music therapy is the use of music to accomplish therapeutic aims: the restoration, maintenance, and improvement of mental and physical health. Therapists work with individuals of all ages who need assistance because of behavioral, social, learning, or physical disabilities.

Therapy can include creating music, singing, moving to music, or listening. In addition, when combined with guided imagery, music can be used to evoke imagery in the form of symbols, memories, or feelings. During those guided imagery and music sessions, a trained facilitator encourages the client to engage in spontaneous speech, movements and insights to create an opening for healing and change (see Guided Imagery & Creative Visualization, pages 237–240).

Music therapy is recognized by federal law as a service that can enhance a child's ability to benefit from special education. The Joint Commission on the Accreditation of Healthcare Organizations also recognizes music therapy as one of the creative arts therapies. In the United States, there are more than 5,000 registered music therapists. Many are registered with the National Association for Music Therapy, which offers a professional registration program for individuals who have met rigorous education and clinical training requirements.

USES

Applications for music therapy are constantly expanding as new benefits get reported from many different specialties and disciplines. The following are some of the uses for music therapy:

- To stimulate, physically or emotionally, those with chronic pain or impaired movement.
- To help those with autism communicate.
- To help the mentally ill with emotional expression.
- To help evoke memories or times, places and persons for those with Alzheimer disease and other dementias.
- To ease pain and anxiety for dental procedures or during childbirth.
- To improve weight gain and increase movements of hospitalized newborns.
- To help cancer patients improve their ability to discuss their feelings about the trauma of the disease.
- To distract burn patients from constant pain.
- To reduce the neurologic problems of children with cerebral palsy, when used with physical therapy.

Alzheimer Disease—Both listening to and actively making music seems to help patients with Alzheimer disease.

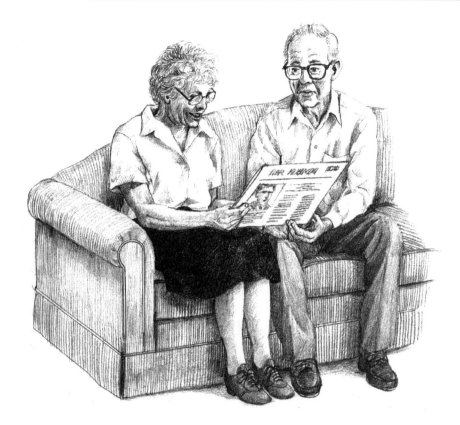

Music therapy has several benefits to offer the Alzheimer patient. It can improve mood, reduce the need for medication, and may stimulate centers of the brain that would otherwise be subject to progressive deterioration [1].

Depression—People with varying degrees of depressive disorder may benefit greatly from music therapy. One study examined the effect of music therapy on 30 older adults diagnosed with depressive disorder. Those assigned to the treatment group who underwent at-home music therapy on a weekly basis performed significantly better on standardized tests for depression and also reported less distress, a better mood, and more self-esteem than the untreated control group [2].

Insomnia—Listening to music before bed can have a relaxing effect on both body and mind. A study of music therapy in 25 elderly people with sleep disturbances revealed that music therapy improved sleep patterns in 24 of the subjects [3].

Psychosis—Music therapy's effect on 76 people with schizophrenia showed that after only one month of treatment, those undergoing the therapy experienced a decrease in negative symptoms. They were better able to communicate with others and showed more of an interest in external events [4].

An Adjunct to Other Therapy—Medical procedures—everything from dental appointments to minor surgery—can be difficult for any number of reasons. Several studies have examined music therapy's ability to lessen both the anxiety and the sensation of pain involved in medical procedures. A study of 38 adults who arrived in the emergency room with cuts large enough to require stitches were randomly assigned to undergo the procedure with or without music. The group with music reported significantly less pain during the procedure [5].

Music therapy seems to have an effect on patients' mood and relaxation during recovery from surgery. In a study of 96 patients undergoing heart surgery, those who had music therapy had significantly improved mood and relaxation indicators (blood pressure, heart rate) than those who did not have music therapy [6].

MAGNETIC FIELD THERAPY
WHAT IT IS

Magnetic field therapy is the use of magnetism to aid healing of the body. Magnetic fields are everywhere and their effects on the human body are only beginning to be understood.

The use of the magnets varies widely. Generally, therapy can be divided into two categories: stationary and alternating. Stationary fields are generated by magnets, whereas alternating fields are generated by electrical devices. Stationary magnets can be placed in mattresses or pillows to act therapeutically during sleep, or they can be applied directly to acupuncture points or specific organs depending on the practitioner's approach. Alternating fields involve large machines that can be maneuvered in relation to the patient to generate the exact strength and positional attitude.

Therapy can involve treatment sessions of just a few minutes or prolonged at-home application, such as sleeping with specially placed magnets. Sometimes several treatments spread over weeks are indicated, depending on the disorder.

USES

Magnetic field therapy has been used to treat

- sleep disorders
- anxiety
- infections

CAUTION

Magnetic stimulation of the brain is experimental and regulated by the Food and Drug Administration. In response to some research that may link nonionizing low-frequency radiation, the American Cancer Society recently suggested that consumers may want to avoid too many electronic devices that function within the electromagnetic spectrum.

- chronic pain
- bone breaks
- ligament sprains
- tendon tears
- minor to severe bruises
- muscle strains and spasms
- inflammatory problems such as tendonitis, carpal tunnel syndrome, and arthritis

Researchers have also reported experiments with magnetism for

- hepatitis
- breast cancer
- diabetes
- epileptic seizures

How magnetism might affect human physiology remains unclear. Researchers announced in a preliminary study that they had found crystals of magnetite in human brain tissue, suggesting a possible mechanism by which magnets might affect the brain. But the research was at the early stages, and scientists were uncertain just what the finding might mean.

LIGHT THERAPY
WHAT IT IS

Although we don't often realize it, light has a profound effect on mental and physical health. We use light to set our internal clocks and give us cues as to when to sleep and wake. Our skin uses the ultraviolet light from the sun to help manufacture vitamin D—a vitamin that is key to building bone strength.

Light can be used therapeutically in several ways. It can be sent at specific frequencies and intervals into the eyes in a therapy known as syntonics, or it can be used to bathe the entire body in full-spectrum rays. In Scandinavia and Siberia—places where sunlight is hard to come by in the winter months—children often undergo full-spectrum light therapy to ensure that their skin produces enough vitamin D for healthy bone development. Light boxes, which slowly increase the amount of light in the room in an approximation of dawn, are often used to treat certain types of depression.

Rays from sunlight stimulate the pea-sized organ in the head known as the pineal gland. The light affects the gland's secretion of melatonin, a hormone that influences many bodily functions, including sleep, ovulation, and the secretion of other hormones. Light has been used to treat successfully a wide range of medical problems from seasonal affective disorder to psoriasis. The use of green or blue light is the standard medical treatment for neonatal jaundice.

Syntonics, the therapeutic application of light through the eyes, has been used clinically in the field of optometry for more than 60 years in the treatment of a range of visual dysfunctions affecting general performance, behavior, and academic achievement. The syntonic approach involves prescribing different frequencies (different colors) of light to stimulate and balance the autonomic nervous system.

The therapeutic approach of syntonics was conceived by Dr. Harry Riley Spitler based on his belief that the application of certain light frequencies by way of the eyes could restore balance within the body's regulatory centers. Clinical application of selected light frequencies in optometry began in the early 1920s. Now, the study of syntonics is available to all doctors of optometry postgraduate curricula.

USES

Light's well-documented effect on brain chemistry has opened the door for its use in a wide range of neurologic disorders. It is also a popular therapy for certain dermatologic disorders and may have an application in cases of lupus erythematosus.

Learning Disabilities—A study involving application of syntonics to 18 patients with reading difficulties resulted in unexpected substantial increases in visual fields. Most patients also reported greater release of emotions, less hyperactivity, less tension, and a greater ability to handle criticism and confrontation; 75 percent reported improved academic scores, 40 percent experienced significant improvement in handwriting, and 11 percent totally eliminated daily use of methylphenidate (Ritalin) [7].

Psoriasis—Psoriasis is a skin disease that involves the uncontrolled growth of skin cells. This growth produces thick red eruptions that cause itching and pain. A therapy called PUVA treatment—ultraviolet A (UVA) light after the administration of the drug psoralen, which heightens the body's sensitivity to ultraviolet light—may bring relief to some people with psoriasis. The benefits need to be weighed against the risks of prolonged exposure to ultraviolet radiation.

Seasonal Affective Disorder—One of the most common causes of depression, seasonal affective disorder (SAD), is directly caused by the seasonal lack of light experienced during the winter months by people who live in northern climates. SAD is one of light therapy's greatest successes. Many studies have shown that exposure to ambient light and its subsequent effects on the body's own melatonin production can ease the depressive symptoms of SAD [8].

RESOURCES
MUSIC AND SOUND

- Sound Healers Association
  P.O. Box 2240
  Boulder, CO 80306
  303-443-8181
  fax 303-443-6023
  Publishes an international directory and resource guide, containing articles and more than 250 listings, including sound healers, teachers, musicians, music therapists, centers and institutes, companies, and researchers in the field.

- Jeff Volk
  c/o Macromedia
  P.O. Box 279
  Epping, NH 03857
  Produces books, tapes, and videos on therapeutic use of sound and music and organizes an annual International Sound Colloquium.

- The Bonny Foundation
  2020 Simmons
  Salina, KS 67401
  913-827-1497
  Directed by Helen Bonny, the founder of the process of guided imagery and music (GIM); one of 11 centers specializing in GIM, accredited by the Association for Music and Imagery. Produces the *Journal of the Association for Music and Imagery*.

- The Institute for Music, Health and Education
  3010 Hennepin Ave. South, #269
  Minneapolis, MN 55408
  612-377-5700

Trains students to use toning to release stress, balance the mind and body, improve the ear's ability to listen, and improve the speaking and singing voice.

- The National Association of Music Therapy
  8455 Colesville Rd., Ste. 930
  Silver Spring, MD 20910
  301-589-3300
  Registers music therapists, accredits schools, publishes a journal, videotapes, and books on music therapy, and holds an annual conference. Recently joined with the American Association for Music Therapy, which treats mental illness and provides referrals to music therapists.

MAGNETIC FIELD THERAPY
- Bio-Electro-Magnetics Institute
  2490 West Moana Ln.
  Reno, NV 89509-3936
  702-827-9099

LIGHT THERAPY
- Society for Light Treatment and Biological Rhythms
  10200 W. 44th Ave., Ste. 304
  Wheat Ridge, CO 80033-2840
  303-424-3697
  e-mail sltbr@resourcenter.com
  International nonprofit association of more than 400 researchers and clinicians.

- Dinshah Health Society
  P.O. Box 707
  Malaga, NJ 08328
  609-692-4686
  A layperson's group that advocates the value of color therapy. Provides information about lighting equipment and other resources.

- The College of Synoptic Optometry
  c/o Bradford D. Smith
  15 Western Ave.
  Augusta, ME 04330
  207-623-3911

Yoga

IN SANSKRIT, THE WORD YOGA MEANS UNION OR JOINING. PRACTICED IN INDIA FOR THOUSANDS OF YEARS, YOGA HAS BECOME INCREASINGLY POPULAR IN THE WEST AS A MEANS OF PROMOTING HEALTH AND RELAXATION AND OF TREATING CHRONIC CONDITIONS SUCH AS BACK PAIN AND CORONARY ARTERY DISEASE.

HISTORY

Yoga has its origins in the ancient religion of Hinduism. It is described in the second century B.C. book of yoga sutras by Patanjali. These sutras (aphorisms or rules) are terse passages that embody yogic teaching.

WHAT IT IS

As practiced traditionally in India, yoga includes a set of ethical imperatives and moral precepts, including diet, exercise, and meditative aspects. In the West, yoga focuses primarily on postures (gentle stretching exercises), breathing exercises, and meditation. Yoga is frequently used in Western medicine to enhance health and treat chronic disease.

Practitioners of yoga have long known that they are able to affect mental and physical responses traditionally thought to be beyond the ability of the conscious mind to control. Recent scientific research in other areas, such as biofeedback (see page 188), confirm that many body functions (such as blood pressure and heart rate) once thought to be beyond conscious control can be changed through meditation and relaxation techniques.

Key elements of yoga include the following:

- *Asanas* (postures)—Postures are gentle stretching movements designed to help balance the mind and body.
- *Pranayama*—A combination of the Sanskrit words *prana* (vital energy) and *ayama* (to expand), *pranayamas* are specially developed breathing techniques.
- Concentration/Meditation practices— A variety of techniques are used, including imagery, visualization, focusing on objects, and sound.

A typical yoga session lasts 20 minutes to an hour and may be practiced at home alone or in a classroom with others and an instructor. Sessions usually begin with gentle postures to relax tense muscles and joints and then move on to more difficult postures. Movements are slow and gentle. Students are instructed to breathe slowly from deep in the abdomen and are taught specific breathing techniques known as *pranayamas*. Yoga sessions also involve relaxation and meditation and often end with chants, such as "Let there be peace," to help the mind and body relax.

TYPES OF YOGA

A variety of forms of yoga are practiced in the West. While these share common elements, some focus more on postures and breathing exercises, whereas others have a greater focus on spirituality. Yoga forms constitute a ladder of sorts, from the "lowest" form of Hatha yoga, with its focus on physical postures and breathing techniques, to the "highest" form known as Raja, or "union by mental mastery."

A few names you may hear include the following:

- Hatha yoga ("the yoga of vitality")—An easy-to-learn basic form of yoga very popular in the United States.
- Karma yoga ("the yoga of action")—This yoga emphasizes self-

less action and service, such as that practiced by Mahatma Ghandi.

- Mantra yoga ("union by voice or sound")—This form includes the rhythmic repetitions of specific sounds, or mantras, and has been popularized in the West by Transcendental Meditation founder Maharishi Mahesh Yogi.
- Laya or Kundalini yoga ("union by arousal of latent psychic nerve force")—This form emphasizes the awakening of psychic energy and the union of the male and female parts of the individual.
- Raja yoga—This highest form of yoga seeks to transcend the body and its senses and communicate with the universal spirit.

USES

Thousands of studies have confirmed that yoga can allow people to control a wide range of body functions, including

- blood pressure
- body temperature
- brain waves (as measured by electroencephalography [EEG])
- heart rate
- metabolic rate
- respiratory function
- skin resistance

Studies show that people who practice yoga have reduced anxiety, are more resistant to stress, and have lower blood pressure, more efficient heart function, better respiratory function, and improved physical fitness. Yoga may also be useful in helping people with addictions, cancer, heart disease, high blood pressure, and migraines.

Although yoga has been shown to be beneficial in a variety of conditions, it is not considered a therapy for specific illnesses. Rather, yoga employs a broad holistic approach that focuses on teaching people a new lifestyle, way of thinking, and way of being in the world.

ASTHMA

Studies conducted at yoga institutions in India have reported impressive success in improving asthma. For example, one study of 255 people with asthma found that yoga therapy resulted in improvement or cure in 74 percent of asthma patients. Another study of 114 patients treated over one year by yoga found a 76 percent rate of improvement or cure and that asthma attacks could usually be prevented by yoga methods without resorting to drugs [1].

Yet another Indian study of 15 people with asthma claims a 93 percent improvement rate over a 9-year period. That study found improvement was linked with improved concentration, and the addition of a meditative procedure made the treatment more effective than simple postures and *pranayama*. Yoga practice also resulted in greater reduction in anxiety scores than drug therapy. Its authors believe that yoga practice helps patients through enabling them to gain access to their own internal experience and increased self-awareness [1].

A study of 46 adolescents with asthma found that yoga practice resulted in a significant increase in pulmonary function and exercise capacity and led to fewer symptoms and medications. Patients were given daily training in yoga for 90 minutes in the morning and one hour in the evening for 40 days. Practice included yogic cleansing procedures (*kriyas*), maintenance of yogic body postures (*asanas*), and yogic breathing practices (*pranayama*) [2].

While these and other Indian studies were conducted within the context of a culture that embraces yoga and at institutions that center around the complete philosophy of yoga, scientific studies in the West have found a number of benefits from yoga practice as well.

HIGH BLOOD PRESSURE

The relaxation and exercise components of yoga have a major role to play in the treatment and prevention of high blood pressure (hypertension). A combination of biofeedback and yogic breathing and relaxation techniques has been found to lower blood pressure and reduce the need for high blood pressure medication in people suffering from high blood pressure. In 20 patients with high blood pressure who practiced biofeedback and yoga techniques, 5 were able to stop their blood pressure medication completely, 5 were able to reduce significantly the amount of medication they were taking, and another 4 had lower blood pressure than at the beginning of the three-month study.

PAIN MANAGEMENT

Yoga is believed to reduce pain by helping the brain's pain center regulate the gate-controlling mechanism located in the spinal cord and the secretion of naturally occurring painkillers in the body. Breathing exercises used in yoga can also reduce pain. Because muscles tend to relax when you exhale, length-ening the time of exhalation can help produce relaxation and reduce muscle tension. Awareness of breathing patterns helps to achieve calmer, slower respirations and aid in relaxation and pain management.

Yoga's inclusion of relaxation techniques and meditation can also help reduce pain. Part of the effectiveness of yoga in reducing pain is due to its focus on self-awareness. This self-awareness can have a protective effect and allow for early preventive action [4].

BACK PAIN

Back pain is the most common reason to seek medical attention. Yoga has consistently been used to cure and prevent back pain by enhancing strength and flexibility. Both acute and long-term stress can lead to muscle tension and exacerbate back problems. A number of components of yoga help to ease back pain:

- *Asanas (Postures)*—Practicing of postures provides gentle stretching and movements that increase flexibility and help correct bad posture.
- *Prasana (Breathing Exercises)*—Breathing patterns can affect the spinal cord in a variety of ways, such as movement of the ribs and changes in pressure within the chest and abdomen. The process of exhaling can help relax muscles.
- *Relaxation and Meditation*—Relaxation provides a physiologic antidote to stress. Imaging techniques may also be used. For example, imagining a movement before it is actually performed makes it easier to move the muscles that are being used.
- *Self-Awareness*—Yoga also strives to increase self-awareness on both a

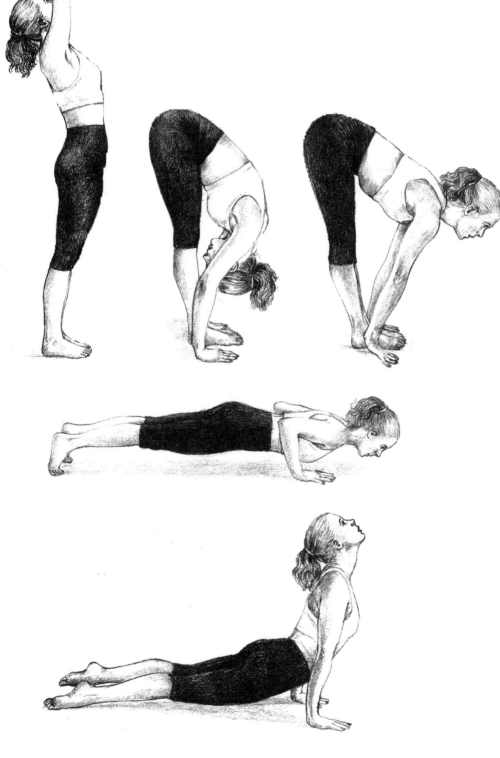

THE SALUTE TO THE SUN

1) Stand with your feet together and inhale while you raise your arms over head, palms touching. 2) Exhale and bend down, touching your palms to the floor. 3) Inhale and lift your head and chest as high as you can. 4) Walk your legs back until you reach a push-up position. 5) With the tops of your feet against the floor, push your upper body up and look upward. The exercise is completed by moving to the inverted V pose (pictured on page 140) followed by the first three poses in reverse order. Correct form is very important in yoga, but don't worry if you cannot do the poses perfectly the first time. Practice will improve your flexibility and strength and eventually improve your form.

physical and psychological level. This allows people to take early corrective action, such as adjusting their posture, when discomfort is first noticed.

Patients who study yoga learn to induce relaxation and then can use the technique whenever pain appears. Practicing yoga can provide chronic pain sufferers with useful tools to actively cope with their pain and help counter feelings of helplessness and depression.

MENTAL PERFORMANCE

A common technique used in yoga is breathing through one nostril at a time. Electroencephalogram (EEG) studies of the electrical impulses of the brain have shown that breathing through one nostril results in increased activity on the opposite side of the brain. Some experts suggest that the regular practice of breathing through one nostril may help improve communication between the right and left side of the brain [5].

Other studies show this increased brain activity is associated with better performance and suggest that yoga can enhance cognitive performance. For example, a study of 23 men found that breathing through one nostril resulted in better performance of tasks associated with the opposite side of the brain [6].

DIABETES

A study of 149 persons with non–insulin-dependent diabetes found that 104 had lowered blood sugar and needed less oral antidiabetes medication after regularly practicing yoga. Because the patients were placed on a vegetarian diet during the study, however, the effect of yoga practice alone on blood sugar levels cannot be determined [7].

MOOD CHANGE AND VITALITY

Mental health and physical energy are difficult to quantify, but virtually everyone who participates in yoga over a period of time reports a positive effect on outlook and energy level. A British study of 71 healthy volunteers aged 21 to 76 found that a 30-minute program of yogic stretch and breathing exercises was simple to learn and resulted in a "markedly invigorating" effect on perceptions of both mental and physical energy and improved mood.

The study compared relaxation, visualization, and yoga. It found that those who practiced yoga had a significantly greater increase in perceptions of mental and physical energy and feelings of alertness and enthusiasm than the other groups. Relaxation was found to make people more sleepy and sluggish after a session, and visualization made them more sluggish and less content than those who practiced yoga [8].

RESOURCES

Yoga classes are frequently offered at local schools and exercise and recreation centers. Check your local health food store, local alternative therapies publication, or even the yellow pages.
- Yoga Journal
  2054 University Ave.
  Berkeley, CA 94704-1082
  800-359-YOGA

The Yoga Journal publishes a national directory of yoga teachers and organizations.

Appendix 1: References

ACUPRESSURE

1. Dundee JW, et al. Non-invasive stimulation of the P6 (Neiguan) antiemetic acupuncture point in cancer chemotherapy. *Journal of the Royal Society of Medicine* 1991;84:210–212.
2. Dundee JW, et al. P6 acupressure reduces morning sickness. *Journal of the Royal Society of Medicine* 1988;81:456–457.
3. De Aloysio D, Penacchioni P. Morning sickness control in early pregnancy by Neiguan point acupressure. *Obstetrics & Gynecology* 1992;80:852–854.
4. Barsoum G, et al. Postoperative nausea is relieved by acupressure. *Journal of the Royal Society of Medicine* 1990;83:86–89.
5. Melzack R, Bentley KC, Relief of dental pain by ice massage of either hand or the contralateral arm. *Journal of the Canadian Dental Association* 1983;4:257–260.

ACUPUNCTURE

1. Bullock ML, et al. Controlled trial of acupuncture for severe recidivist alcoholism. *Lancet* 1989;ii:1435–1439.
2. Brewington V, et al. Acupuncture as a detoxification treatment: an analysis of controlled research. *Journal of Substance Abuse Treatment* 1994;11:289–307.
3. Christensen BV, et al. Acupuncture treatment of severe knee osteoarthrosis. a long-term study. *Acta Anaesthesiologica Scandinavica* 1992;36:519–525.
4. Dundee JW, et al. Effect of stimulation of the P6 antiemetic point on postoperative nausea and vomiting. *British Journal of Anaesthesia* 1989;63:612–618.
5. Dundee JW, et al. Acupuncture prophylaxis of cancer chemotherapy-induced sickness. *Journal of the Royal Society of Medicine* 1989;82:268–271.
6. Coan RM, et al. The acupuncture treatment of low back pain: a randomized controlled study. *American Journal of Chinese Medicine* 1980;VIII:181–189.
7. Helms JM. Acupuncture for the management of primary dysmenorrhea. *Obstetrics & Gynecology* 1987;69:51–56.
8. Vincent CA. A Controlled trial of the treatment of migraine by acupuncture. *Clinical Journal of Pain* 1989;5:305–312.
9. Coan RM, et al. The acupuncture treatment of neck pain: a randomized controlled study. *American Journal of Chinese Medicine* 1982;IX:326–332.
10. Lee Y-H, et al. Acupuncture in the treatment of renal colic. *Journal of Urology* 1992;147:16–18.

AROMATHERAPY

1. Buckle J. Aromatherapy. *Nursing Times* 1993;89:32–35.
2. Stevensen C. Measuring the effects of aromatherapy. *Nursing Times* 1992;88:62–63.
3. Gobel H, et al. Effect of peppermint and eucalyptus oil preparations on neurophysiological and experimental algesimetric headache parameters. *Cephalalgia* 1994;14:228–234.
4. Rose J, Behm F. Inhalation of vapor from black pepper extract reduces smoking withdrawal symptoms. *Drug & Alcohol Dependence* 1994;34:225–229.
5. Bassett IB, et al. A comparative study of tea-tree oil versus benzoyl peroxide in the treatment of acne. *Medical Journal of Austrailia* 1990;153:455–458.
6. Buck DS, et al. Comparison of two topical preparations for the treatment of onychomycosis: *Melaleuca alternifolia* (tea tree) oil and clotrimazole. *Journal of Family Practice* 1994;38:601–605.
7. Pena E. *Melaleuca alternifolia* oil: its use in trichomonal vaginitis and other vaginal infections. *Obstetric & Gynecology* 1962;19

AYURVEDIC MEDICINE

1. Jacob A, et al. Effect of the Indian gooseberry (AMLA) on serum cholesterol levels in men aged 35–55 years. *European Journal of Clinical Nutrition* 1988;42:939–944.
2. Thyagarajan SP. Effect of phyllanthus amarus on chronic carriers of hepatitis B virus. *Lancet* 1988;ii:764–766.
3. Charles V, Charles S. The use and efficacy of *Azadirachta indica* ADR ("Neem") and *Curcuma longa* ("Tumeric") in scabies. *Tropical Geographic Medicine* 1992;44:178–181.
4. Alexander CN, et al. Transcendental Meditation, mindfulness, and longevity: an experimental study with the elderly. *Journal of Personal and Social Psychology* 1989;57:950–964.
5. Schneider RH, et al. A randomised controlled trial of stress reduction for hypertension in older African Americans. *Hypertension* 1995;26:820–827.
6. Wallace RK, et al. Systolic blood pressure and long-term practice of the Transcendental Meditation and TM-Sidhi program: effects of TM on systolic blood pressure. *Psychosomatic Medicine* 1983;45:41–46.
7. Jevning R, et al. The physiology of meditation: a review: a wakeful hypometabolic integrated response. *Neuroscience and Biobehavior Review* 1992;16:415–424.

8. Werner OR, et al. Long-term endocrinologic changes in subjects practicing the Transcendental Meditation and TM-Sidha program. *Psychosomatic Medicine* 1986;48:59–66.

BIOFEEDBACK

1. Iwata G, et al. New biofeedback therapy in children with encopresis. *European Journal of Pediatric Surgery* 1995;5:231–234.
2. Keck JO, et al. Biofeedback training is useful in fecal incontinence but disappointing in constipation. *Dis Colon Rectum* 1994;37:1271–1276.
3. Sangwan YP, et al. Can manometric parameters predict response to biofeedback therapy in fecal incontinence? *Diseases of the Colon and Rectum* 1995;38:1021–1025.
4. Cox DJ, et al. Simple electromyographic biofeedback treatment for chronic pediatric constipation/encopresis:preliminary report. *Biofeedback and Self-Regulation* 1994;19:41–50.
5. Wauguier A, et al. Changes in cerebral blood flow velocity associated with biofeedback-assisted relaxation treatment of migraine headaches are specific for the middle cerebral artery. *Headache* 1995;35:358–362.
6. Grazzi L, Bussone G. Italian experience of electromyographic-biofeedback treatment of episodic common migraine: preliminary results. *Headache* 1993;33:439–441.
7. Labbe EE. Treatment of childhood migraine with autogenic training and skin temperature biofeedback: a component analysis. *Headache* 1995;35:10–13.
8. Gauthier J, et al. The role of home practice in the thermal biofeedback treatment of migraine headache. *Journal of Consulting and Clinical Psychology* 1994;62:180–184.
9. Arena JG, et al. A comparison of frontal electromyographic biofeedback training, trapezius electromyographic biofeedback training, and progressive muscle relaxation therapy in the treatment of tension headache. *Headache* 1995;35:411–419.
10. Hahn YB, et al. The effect of thermal biofeedback and progressive muscle relaxation training in reducing blood pressure of patients with essential hypertension. *Image—The Journal of Nursing Scholarship* 1993;25:204–207.
11. Flor H, Birbaumer N. Comparison of the efficacy of electromyographic biofeedback, cognitive-behavioral therapy, and conservative medical interventions in the treatment of chronic musculoskeletal pain. *Journal of Consulting and Clinical Psychol-*

ogy 1993;61:653–658.
12. Newton-John TR, et al. Cognitive-behavioral therapy versus EMG biofeedback in the treatment of chronic low back pain. *Behaviour Research and Therapy* 1995;33:691–697.
13. Intiso D, et al. Rehabilitation of walking with electromyographic biofeedback in foot-drop after stroke. *Stroke* 1994;25:1189–1192.
14. Schleenbaker RE, Mainous AG, III. Electromyographic biofeedback for neuromuscular reeducation in the hemiplegic stroke patient: a meta-analysis. *Archives of Physical Medicine and Rehabilitation* 1993;74:1301–1304.
15. Delk KK, et al. The effects of biofeedback assisted breathing retraining on lung functions in patients with cystic fibrosis. *Chest* 1994;105:23–28.
16. Susset J, et al. A predictive score index for the outcome of associated biofeedback and vaginal electrical stimulation in the treatment of female incontinence. *Journal of Urology* 1995;153:1567–1568.

BODYWORK

1. Heidt P. Effect of Therapeutic Touch on anxiety level of hospitalized patients. *Nursing Research* 1981;30:32–37.
2. Keller E, Bzdek VM. Effects of Therapeutic Touch on tension headache pain. *Nursing Research* 1986;35:101–105.
3. Meehan TC. Therapeutic Touch and postoperative pain: a Rogerian research study. *Nursing Science Quarterly* 1993;6:69–78.
4. National Institutes of Health. Alternative medicine: expanding medical horizons, a report to the National Institutes of Health on alternative medical systems and practices in the United States. December 1994;NIH Publication No. 94–066:p.143.
5. McKechnie AA, et al. Anxiety states: a preliminary report on the value of connective tissue massage. *Journal of Psychosomatic Research* 1983;27:125–129.
6. Field T, et al. Massage reduces anxiety in child and adolescent psychiatric patients. *Journal of the American Academy of Childhood and Adolescent Psychiatry* 1992;31:125–131.
7. Weintraub M. Shiatsu, Swedish muscle massage, and trigger point suppression in spinal pain syndrome. *American Journal of Pain Management* 1992;2:74–78.
8. Ferrell-Torry AT, Glick OJ. The use of therapeutic massage as a nursing intervention to modify anxiety and the perception of cancer pain. *Cancer Nursing*

1993;16:93–101.
9. Field T, et al. Tactile/kinesthetic stimulation effects on preterm neonates. *Pediatrics* 1986;77:654–658.
10. Wheeden A, et al. Massage effects on cocaine-exposed preterm neonates. *Developmental and Behavioral Pediatrics* 1993;14:318–322.
11.Lake B, Acute back pain: Treatment by the application of Feldenkrais principles. *Australian Family Physician* 1985;14:1175–1178.
12. Gutman G, et al. Feldenkrais versus conventional exercises for the elderly. *Journal of Gerontology* 1977;32:562–572.
13. Witt PL, MacKinnon J. Trager psychophysical integration: a method to improve chest mobility of patients with chronic lung disease. *Physical Therapy* 1986;66:214–217.
14. Oleson T, Flocco W. Randomized controlled study of premenstrual symptoms treated with ear, hand, and foot reflexology. *Obstetrics & Gynecology* 1993;83:906–911.
15. Weinberg RS, Hunt VV. Effects of structural integration on state-trait anxiety. *Journal of Clinical Psychology* 1979;35:319–322.
16. Wetzel W. Reiki healing: a physiologic perspective. *Journal of Holistic Nursing* 1989;7:1.

CHELATION THERAPY

1. Grier M, Meyers D. So much writing, so little science: a review of 37 years of literature on edetate sodium chelation therapy. *Annals of Pharmacotherapy* 1993;27:1504–1509.
2. Olszewer E, Carter JP. EDTA chelation therapy in chronic degenerative disease. *Med Hypotheses* 1988;27:41–49.

CHIROPRACTIC MEDICINE

1. Meade TW, et al. Randomised comparison of chiropractic and hospital outpatient management for low back pain: results from extended follow up. *British Medical Journal* 1995;311:349–351.
2. Hurwitz EL. The relative impact of chiropractic vs. medical management of low back pain on health status in a multispecialty group practice. *Journal of Manipulative and Physiological Therapeutics* 1994;17:74–82.
3. Lamm LC, et al. Chiropractic scope of practice: what the law allows—update 1993. *Journal of Manipulative and Physiological Therapeutics* 1995;18:16–20.
4. Tuchin PJ, Bonello R. Preliminary find-

ings of analysis of chiropractic utilization and cost in the workers' compensation system of New South Wales, Australia. *Journal of Manipulative and Physiological Therapeutics* 1995; 18:503–511.
5. Stano M. Further analysis of health care costs for chiropractic and medical patients. *Journal of Manipulative and Physiological Therapeutics* 1994;17:442–446.
6. Stano M. A comparison of health care costs for chiropractic and medical patients. *Journal of Manipulative and Physiological Therapeutics* 1993;16:291–299.
7. Sawyer CE, Kassak K. Patient satisfaction with chiropractic care. *Journal of Manipulative and Physiological Therapeutics* 1993;16:25–32.
8. Cox JM. Patient benefits of attending a chiropractic low back wellness clinic. *Journal of Manipulative and Physiological Therapeutics* 1994;17:25–28.

ENVIRONMENTAL MEDICINE

1. Buchwald D, Garrity D. Comparison of patients with chronic fatigue syndrome, fibromyalgia, and multiple chemical sensitivities. *Archives of Internal Medicine* 1994;154:2049–2053.
2. Jaffe RM. A novel treatment for fibromyalgia improves clinical outcomes in a community-based study. *American Association for the Advancement of Science (AAAS)*, Feb. 9, 1996.
3. Monro J, et al. Food allergy in migraine: a study of dietary exclusion and RAST. *Lancet* 1980;ii:1–4.
4. Egger J, et al. Is migraine food allergy? a double-blind controlled trial of oligoantigenic diet treatment. *Lancet* 1983;ii:865–869.
5. Rea WJ, et al. Recurrent environmentally triggered thrombophlebitis: a five-year follow-up. *Annals of Allergy* 1981; 47: 338–344.
Guided Imagery and Creative Visualization
1. Manyande A, et al. Preoperative rehearsal of active coping imagery influences subjective and hormonal responses to abdominal surgery. *Psychosomatic Medicine* 1995;57:177–182.
2. Thompson, MB, Coppens NM. The effects of guided imagery on anxiety levels and movement of clients undergoing magnetic resonance imaging. *Holistic Nursing Practice* 1994;8:59–69.
3. Pederson C. Effect of imagery on children's pain and anxiety during cardiac catheterization. *Journal of Pediatric Nursing* 1995;10:365–374.
4. Feher SD, et al. Increasing breast milk

production for premature infants with a relaxation/imagery audiotape. *Pediatrics* 1989;83:57–60.

5. Post-White J. The effects of imagery on emotions, immune function, and cancer outcome. *MAINlines* 1993;14:18–20.

6. Bridge LR, et al. Relaxation and imagery in the treatment of breast cancer. *British Medical Journal* 1988;297:1169–1172.

7. Troesch LM, et al. The influence of guided imagery on chemotherapy-related nausea and vomiting. *Oncology Nursing Forum* 1993; 20:1179–1185.

8. Rider MS, et al. Effect of immune system imagery on secretory IgA, *Biofeedback and Self-Regulation* 1990;15:317–333.

9. Porretta DL, Surburg PR. Imagery and physical practice in the acquisition of gross motor timing of coincidence by adolescents with mild mental retardation. *Perception & Motor Skills* 1995;80:1171–1183.

10. Rees BL. Effect of relaxation with guided imagery on anxiety, depression, and self-esteem in primiparas. *Journal of Holistic Nursing* 1995;13:255–267.

11. Wynd CA. Relaxation imagery used for stress reduction in the prevention of smoking relapse. *Journal of Advanced Nursing* 1992;17:294–302.

HERBAL MEDICINE

1. Shida T, et al. Effect of aloe extract on peripheral phagocytosis in adult bronchial asthma. *Planta Medica* 1985; 51:273–275.

2. Kahlon JB, et al. In vitro evaluation of the synergistic antiviral effects of acemanna in combination with azidothymidine and acyclovir. *Molecular Biotherapy* 1991;3:214–223.

3. McCarthy GM, et al. Effect of topical capsaicin in the therapy of painful osteoarthritis of the hands. *Journal of Rheumatology* 1992;19:604–607.

4. McCarty DJ, et al. Treatment of pain due to fibromyalgia with topical capsaicin: a pilot study. *Seminars in Arthritis and Rheumatism* 1994;23:41–47.

5. The Capsaicin Study Group. Treatment of painful diabetic neuropathy with topical capsaicin: a multicenter, double-blind, vehicle-controlled study. *Archives of Internal Medicine* 1991;151:2225–2229.

6. Watson CP, et al. Post-herpetic neuralgia and topical capsaicin. *Pain* 1988;33:333–340.

7. Bernstein JE, et al. Topical capsaicin treatment of chronic postherpetic neuralgia. *Journal of the American Academy of Dermatology* 1989;21:265–270.

8. Watson CP, Evans RJ. The postmastec-

tomy pain syndrome and topical capsaicin: a randomized trial. *Pain* 1992;51:375–379.

9. Sobota AE. Inhibition of bacterial adherence by cranberry juice: potential use for the treatment of urinary tract infections. *Journal of Urology* 1984;131:1013–1016.

10. Avorn J, et al. Reduction of bacteriuria and pyuria after ingestion of cranberry juice. *Journal of the American Medical Association* 1994;271:751–754.

11. Murphy JJ, et al. Randomized double-blind placebo-controlled trial of feverfew in migraine prevention. *Lancet* 1988;ii:189–192.

12. Neil A, Silagy C. Garlic: its cardio-protective properties. *Current Opinion in Lipidology* 1994;5:6–10.

13. Jain AK, et al. Can garlic reduce levels of serum lipids? A controlled clinical study. *American Journal of Medicine* 1993;94:632–635.

14. Vorberg C, Schneider B. Therapy with garlic: results of a placebo-controlled double-blind study. *British Journal of Clinical Practice* 1990;69(suppl):7–11.

15. Bordia A. Effect of garlic on blood lipids in patients with coronary heart disease. *American Journal of Clinical Nutrition* 1981;34:2100–2103.

16. Warshafsky S, et al. Effect of garlic on total serum cholesterol: a meta-analysis. *Annals of Internal Medicine* 1993;119:599–605.

17. Bordia A. Effect of garlic on human platelet aggregation in vitro. *Atherosclerosis* 1979;30:355–360.

18. Auer W, et al. Hypertension and hyperlipidaemia: garlic helps in mild cases. *British Journal of Clinical Practice* 1990;69(suppl):3–6.

19. Ghannoum MA. Studies on the anticandidal mode of action of allium sativum (garlic). *Journal of General Microbiolology* 1988;134:2917–2924.

20. Johnson MG, Vaughn RH. Death of *Salmonella typhimurium* and *Escherichia coli* in the presence of freshly reconstituted dehydrated garlic and onion. *Applied Microbiology* 1969;17:903–905.

21. Wargovich MJ. Diallyl sulfide, a flavor component of garlic (*Allium sativum*), inhibits dimethyl hydrazine-induced colon cancer. *Carcinogensis* 1987;8:487–489.

22. Nishino N, et al. Antitumor-promoting activity of garlic extracts. *Oncology* 1989;46:277–280.

23. Lin XY, et al. Dietary garlic suppresses DNA adducts caused by N-nitroso compounds. *Carcinogenesis* 1994;15:349–352.

24. Srivastava KC, Mustafa T. Ginger [*Zin-*

giber officinale] in rheumatism and musculoskeletal disorders. *Medical Hypotheses* 1992;39:342–348.

25. Fischer-Rasmussen W, et al. Ginger treatment of hyperemesis gravidarum. *European Journal of Obstetrics, Gynecology, and Reproductive Biology* 1990;38:19–24.

26. Grontved A, et al. Gingerroot against seasickness: a controlled trial on the open sea. *Acta Oto-laryngologica* 1988;105:45–49.

27. Mowrey DB, Clayson DE. Motion sickness, ginger, and psychophysics. *Lancet* 1982;i:655–657.

28. Bone ME, et al. Gingerroot—a new antiemetic: the effect of gingerroot on postoperative nausea and vomiting after major gynecological surgery. *Anesthesia* 1990;45:669–671.

29. Kleijnen J, Knipschild P. *Ginkgo biloba* for cerebral insufficiency. *British Journal of Clinical Pharmacology* 1992;34:352–358.

30. Hofferberth B. The efficacy of EGb 761 in patients with senile dementia of the Alzheimer type: a double-blind, placebo-controlled study on different levels of investigation. *Human Psychopharmacology* 1994;9:215–222.

31. Yun TK, Choi SY. A case-control study of ginseng intake and cancer. *International Journal of Epidemiology* 1990;19:871–876.

32. D'Angelo L, et al. A double-blind, placebo-controlled clinical study on the effect of a standardized ginseng extract on psychomotor performance in healthy volunteers. *Journal of Ethnopharmacology* 1986;16:15–22.

33. Khosla PK, et al. Berberine, a potential drug for trachoma. *Revue Internationale du Trachome et de Pathologie Oculaire Tropicale et Subtropicale et de Sante Publique* 1992;69:147–165.

34. Rabbani GH, et al. Randomized controlled trial of berberine sulfate therapy for diarrhea due to enterotoxigenic *Escherichia coli* and *Vibrio cholerae*. *Journal of Infectious Diseases*1987;155:979–984.

35. Morgan AG, et al. Comparison between cimetidine and Caved-S in the treatment of gastric ulceration, and subsequent maintenance therapy. *Gut* 1982;23:545–551.

36. WD Rees, et al. Effect of deglycerrhizinated liquorice on gastric mucosal damage by aspirin. *Scandinavian Journal of Gastroenterology* 1979;14:605–607.

37. Salmi HA, Sarna S. Effect of silymarin on chemical, functional, and morphological alterations of the liver: a double-blind controlled study. *Scandinavian Journal of Gastroenterology* 1982;17:517–520.

38. Ferenci P, et al. Randomized controlled trial of silymarin treatment in patients with cirrhosis of the liver. *Journal of Hepatology* 1989;9:105–113.

39. Ernst E. St.-John's-wort, an antidepressant? a systematic, criteria-based review. *Phytomedicine* 1995;2:67–71.

HOMEOPATHY

1. Reilly D, et al. Is evidence for homeopathy reproducible? *Lancet* 1994;ii:1601–1606.

2. Jacobs J, et al. Treatment of acute childhood diarrhea with homeopathic medicine: a randomized clinical trial in Nicaragua. *Pediatrics* 1994;93:719–725.

3. Reilly DT, et al. Is homeopathy a placebo response? Controlled trial of homeopathic potency, with pollen in hay fever as model. *Lancet* 1986;ii:881–886.

HYPERTHERMIA

1. Standish L, et al. One-year open trial of naturopathic trewatment of HIV infection class IV-A in men. *Journal of Naturopathic Medicine* 1992;3:42–64.

2. Spire B, et al. Inactivation of lymphadenopathy-associated virus by heat, gamma rays and ultraviolet light. *Lancet* 1985;ii:400–403.

3. Cole HM, ed. Diagnostic and therapeutic technology assessment: hyperthermia as an adjuvant treatment for recurrent breast cancer and primary malignant melanoma. *Journal of the American Medical Association* 1994;271:797–802.

4. Seegenschmeidt MH, et al. Superficial Chest wall recurrences of breast cancer : prognostic treatment factors for combined radiation therapy and hyperthermia. *Radiology* 1989;173:551–558.

5. Overgaard J, et al. Randomised trial of hyperthermia as adjuvant to radiotherapy for recurrent or metastatic malignant melanoma. *Lancet* 1995;i:540–543.

HYPNOTHERAPY

1. Manusov EG. Clinical applications of hypnotherapy. *Journal of Family Practice* 1990;31:180–184.

2. Johnson JM. Teaching self-hypnosis in pregnancy, labor and delivery. *Medical Care Nurse* 1980;5:98–101.

3. Mehl LE. Hypnosis and conversion of the breech to the vertex presentation. *Archives of Family Medicine* 1994;3:881–887

4. Rabkin, et al. A randomized trial comparing smoking cessation programs utilizing behavior modification, health education or hypnosis. *Addictive Behaviors* 1984;9:157–173.

MEDITATION

1. Kabat-Zinn J. An outpatient program in behavioral medicine for chronic pain patients based on the practice of mindfulness meditation: theoretical considerations and preliminary results. *General Hospital Psychiatry* 1982;4:33–47.

2. Miller JJ, et al. Three-year follow-up and clinical implications of a mindfulness meditation-based stress reduction intervention in the treatment of anxiety disorders. *General Hospital Psychiatry* 1995;17:192–200.

3. Schneider RH, et al. A randomised controlled trial of stress reduction for hypertension in older African Americans. *Hypertension* 1995;26:820–827.

4. Harte JL, et al. The effects of running and mediation on beta-endorphin, corticotropin- releasing hormone and cortisol in plasma, and on mood. *Biological Psychology* 1995;40:251–265.

5. Kaplan KH, et al. The impact of a meditation-based stress reduction program on fibromyalgia. *General Hospital Psychiatry* 1993;15:284–289.

6. Deepak KK, et al. Meditation improves clinicoelectroencephalographic measures in drug- resistant epileptics. *Biofeedback and Self Regulation* 1994;19:25–40.

MIND/BODY MEDICINE

1. Bowers JJ. Therapy through art: facilitating treatment of sexual abuse. *Journal of Psychosocial Nursing and Mental Health Services* 1992;30:15–24.

2. Bonner G. [Art therapy—an additional possibility in group psychotherapy with adolescents] *Praxis der Kinderpsychologie und Kinderpsychiatrie* 1991;40:177–184.

3. Frye B. Art and multiple personality disorder: an expressive framework for occupational therapy. *American Journal of Occupational Therapy* 1990;44:1013–1022.

4. Hines-Martin VP, Ising M. Use of art therapy with post-traumatic stress disordered veteran clients. *Journal of Psychosocial Nursing and Mental Health Services* 1993;31:29–36.

5. Fassino S. Ferrero A. [Art therapy and chronic schizophrenia: reflections on various aspects of social feelings and the creative self]. *Minerva Psichiatrica* 1992;33:73–77.

6. Tyszkiewicz M. Art therapy as a stimulation in the process of social adjustment of schizophrenia patients. *Psychiatria Polska* 1994;28:183–190.

7. Leste A, Rust J. Effects of dance on anxiety. *American Journal of Dance Therapy* 1990;12:19–25.

8. Emdon T. Memory aid: treatment of trauma patients. *Nursing Times* 1992;88:50–52.

9. Hossack A, Standige K. Using an imaginary scrapbook for neurolinguistic programming in the aftermath of a clinical depression: a case study. *The Gerontologist* 1993;33:265–268.

10. Friedmann E, et al. Animal companions and one-year survival of patients after discharge from a coronary care unit. *Public Health Reports* 1980;95:307–312.

11. Byrd R. Positive therapeutic effects of intercessory prayer in a coronary care unit population. *Southern Medical Journal* 1988;81:826–829.

12. Levin JS, Vanderpool HY. Is religion therapeutically significant for hypertension? *Social Science and Medicine* 1989;29:69–78.

13. Trojan A. Benefits of self help groups: a survey of 232 members from 65 disease related groups. *Social Science and Medicine* 1989;29:225–232.

14. Kiecolt-Glaser JK, et al. Marital quality, marital disruption, and immune function. *Pscyhosomatic Medicine* 1987;49:13–34.

15. Berkman LF, Syme SL. Social networks, host resistance, and mortality: a nine-year follow-up study of Alameda County residents. *American Journal of Epidemiology* 1979;109:186–204.

16. House J, et al. Social relationships and health. *Science* 1988;241:540–545.

17. Bruhn J, Wolf S. Update on Roseto, PA: testing a prediction. *Pscyhosomatic Medicine* 1978;40:86.

NATUROPATHIC MEDICINE

1. Bergner P. Safety, effectiveness, and cost effectiveness in naturopathic medicine. American Association of Naturopathic Physicians 1991.

NUTRITIONAL THERAPY

1. Shintani TT, et al. Obesity and cardiovascular risk intervention through the ad libitum feeding of traditional Hawaiian diet. *American Journal of Clinical Nutrition* 1991;53:1647S-1651S.

2. Schaefer EJ, et al. Changes in plasma lipoprotein concentrations and composition in response to a low-fat, high-fiber diet are associated with changes in serum estrogen concentrations in premenopausal women. *Metabolism* 1995;44:749–756.

3. Willett WC, et al. Relation of meat, fat, and fiber intake to the risk of colon cancer in a prospective study among women. *New England Journal of Medicine* 1990;323:1664–1672.

4. Ziegler RG. Vegetables, fruits, and carotenoids and the risk of cancer. *American Journal of Clinical Nutrition* 1991;53:251S-259S.

5. Barnard RJ, et al. Diet and exercise in the treatment of non-insulin-dependent diabetes mellitus: the need for early emphasis. *Diabetes Care* 1994;17:1469–1472.

6. Snowdon DA, et al. Meat consumption and fatal ischemic heart disease. *Preventive Medicine* 1984;13:490–500.

7. Ornish D, et al. Can lifestyle changes reverse coronary heart disease? the lifestyle heart trial. *Lancet* 1990;ii:129–133.

8. Barnard ND, et al. Factors that facilitate compliance to lower fat intake. *Archives of Family Medicine* 1995;4:153–158.

9. Barnard N, et al. The medical costs attributable to meat consumption. *Preventive Medicine* 1995;24:646–655.

10. Chiu BC-H, et al. Diet and risk of non-Hodgkin Lymphoma in older women. *Journal of the American Medical Association* 1996;275:1315–1321.

11. Robertson WG, et al. Prevalence of urinary stone disease in vegetarians. *European Urology* 1982;8:334–339.

12. Haugen MA, et al. Changes in plasma phospholipid fatty acids and their relationship to disease activity in rheumatoid arthritis patients treated with a vegetarian diet. *British Journal of Nutrition* 1994;72:555–566.

13. Siscovick DS, et al. Dietary intake and cell membrane levels of long-chain n-3 polyunsaturated fatty acids and the risk of primary cardiac arrest. *Journal of the American Medical Association* 1995;274:1363–1367.

14. Burr ML, et al. Effects of changes in fat, fish, and fibre intakes on death and myocardial reinfarction: diet and reinfarction trial (DART). *Lancet* 1989;ii:757–761.

15. Kremer JM, et al. Effects of high-dose fish oil on rheumatoid arthritis after stopping nonsteroidal anti-inflammatory drugs: clinical and immune correlates. *Arthritis and Rheumatism* 1995;38:1107–1114.

16. Carter JP, et al. Hypothesis: dietary management may improve survival from nutritionally linked cancers based on analysis of representative cases. *Journal of the American College of Nutrition* 1993;12:209–226.

17. Griffin SM, et al. Acid resistant lipase as replacement therapy in chronic exocrine insufficiency. *Gut* 1989;30:1012–1015.

18. Barillas C, Solomons NW. Effective reduction of lactose maldigestion in preschool children by direct addition of beta-galactosidase to milk at meal time. *Gastroenterology* 1987;79:766–772.

19. Phelan JJ, et al. Coeliac disease: the abolition of gliadin toxicity by enzymes from *Aspergillus niger*. *Clinical Science* 1977;53:35–43.

20. Fitzgerald DE, et al. Relief of chronic arterial obstruction using intravenous brinase. *Scandinavian Journal of Thoracic and Cardiovascular Surgery* 1979;13:327–332.

21. Chandra RK. Effect of vitamin and trace-element supplementation on immune responses and infection in elderly subjects. *Lancet* 1992;340:1124–1127.

22. Dragan AM, et al. Studies concerning acute biological changes after exogenous administration of 1 gram of L-carnitine in elite athletes. *Physiologie* 1987;24:231–234.

23. Huertas R, et al. Respiratory chain enzymes in muscle of endurance athletes:efficacy of L-carnitine. *Biochemical and Biophysical Research Communications* 1992;188:102–107.

24. National Cancer Institute. *CancerNet News* Jan 1996.

25. Meyskens FL Jr, et al. Enhancement of regression of cervical intraepithelial neoplasia II (moderate dysplasia) with topically applied all-*trans*-retinoic acid: a randomized trial. *JNCI: Journal of the National Cancer Institute* 1994;86:539–543.

26. Giovannuci E, et al. Folate, methionine, and alcohol intake and risk of colorectal adenoma. *JNCI: Journal of the National Cancer Institute* 1993;85:875–884.

27. Poydock ME. Effect of combined ascorbic acid and B-12 on survival of mice with implanted Ehrlich carcinoma and L1210 leukemia. *American Journal of Clinical Nutrition* 1991;54:1261S-1265S.

28. Bielory L, Gandhi R. Asthma and vitamin C. *Annals of Allergy* 1994;73:89–96.

29. Jacques PF, et al. Nutritional status in persons with and without senile cataract: blood vitamin and mineral levels. *American Journal of Clinical Nutrition* 1988;48:152–158.

30. Gridley G, et al. Vitamin supplement use and reduced risk of oral and pharyngeal cancer. *American Journal of Epidemiology* 1992;135:1083–1092.

31. Stampfer MJ, Rimm EB. Epidemiologic evidence for vitamin E in prevention of cardiovascular disease. *American Journal of Clinical Nutrition* 1995;62:1365S-1369S.

32. Robertson JM, et al. Vitamin E intake and risk of cataracts in humans. *Annals of the New York Academy of Sciences* 1989;570:372–382.

33. Lefavi R. Report to the Federation of American Societies for Experimental Biology [FASEB] 1991.

34. Anderson RA, Polansky MM. Report to the Federation of American Societies for Experimental Biology [FASEB] 1990.

35. Singh RB, et al. Can dietary magnesium modulate lipoprotein metabolism? *Magnesium and Trace Elements* 1990;9:255–264.

36. Woods KL, et al. Intravenous magnesium sulphate in suspected acute myocardial infarction: results of the second Leicester Intravenous Magnesium Intervention Trial (LIMIT-2). *Lancet* 1992;i:1553–1558.

37. Woods KL, Fletcher S. Long-term outcome after intravenous magnesium sulfate in suspected acute myocardial infarction: the second Leicester Intravenous Magnesium Intervention Trial (LIMIT- 2). *Lancet* 1994;ii:816–819

38. Patki PS, et al. Efficacy of potassium and magnesium in essential hypertension: a double-blind, placebo-controlled, crossover study. *British Medical Journal* 1990;301:521–523.

39. Siani A, et al. Increasing the dietary potassium intake reduces the need for anti-hypertensive medication. *Annals of Internal Medicine* 1991;115:753–759.

40. Benton D, Cook R. The impact of selenium supplementation on mood. *Biological Psychiatry* 1991;29:1092–1098.

41. Shamberger RJ, Frost DV. Possible protective effect of selenium against cancer. *Canadian Medical Association Journal* 1969;100:682.

42. Virtamo J, et al. Serum selenium and the risk of coronary heart disease and stroke. *American Journal of Epidemiology* 1985;122:276–282.

43. Pauling L. Orthomolecular psychiatry: varying the concentrations of substances normally present in the human body may control mental disease. *Science* 1968;160:265–271.

OSTEOPATHY

1. Hoehler FK, Tobis JS, Buerger AA. Spinal manipulation for low back pain. *Journal of the American Medical Association* 1981;245:1835–1839.

2. Levine DZ. Burning pain in an extremity. *Postgraduate Medicine* 1991;90:175–178, 183–185.

3. Sucher BM. Myofascial release of carpal tunnel syndrome. *Journal of the American Osteopathic Assocociation* 1993;93:92–94,100–101.
4. Sucher BM. Myofascial manipulative release of carpal tunnel syndrome: documentation with magnetic resonance imaging. *Journal of the American Osteopathic Assocociation* 1993;93:1273–1278.
5. Frymann VM, Carney RE, Springall P. Effect of osteopathic medical management on neurological development in children. *Journal of the American Osteopathic Assocociation* 1992;92:729–744.
6. Johnston WL, et al. Palpatory findings in the cervicothoracic region: variations in normotensive and hypertensive subjects: a preliminary report. *Journal of the American Osteopathic Assocociation* 1980;79:300–308.

OXYGEN THERAPY
1. Reillo MR. Hyperbaric oxygen therapy for the management of associated symptoms of HIV/AIDS. *AIDS Weekly* 1994;28:29–30.
2. Myers RA, et al. Value of hyperbaric oxygen in suspected carbon monoxide poisoning. *Journal of the American Medical Association* 1981;246:2478–2480.
3. Hart GB, et al. Gas gangrene II: a 15–year experience with hyperbaric oxygen. *Journal of Trauma* 1983;23:995–1000.
4. Grim PS, et al. Hyperbaric oxygen therapy. *Journal of the American Medical Association* 1990;263:2216–2220.
5. Carpendale M, et al. Does ozone alleviate AIDS diarrhea? *Journal of Clinical Gastroenterology* 1993;17:142–145.

QIGONG
1. Sancier K. Scientific reports on medical qigong. *Qigong Magazine* Summer 1992.
2. Sancier K. Scientific reports on medical qigong. *Qigong Magazine* Spring 1992.
3. Sancier K, Hu B. Medical applications of qigong and emitted qi on humans, animals, cell cultures and plants: review of selected scientific research. *American Journal of Acupuncture* 1991;19:367–367.
4. Ryu H, et al. Effect of qigong training on proportions of T lymphocyte subsets in human peripheral blood. *American Journal of Chinese Medicine* 1995;23:27–36.
5. Ryu H, et al. Delayed cutaneous hypersensitivity reactions in qigong (chun do sun bup) trainees by multitest cell-mediated immunity. *American Journal of Chinese Medicine* 1995;23:139–144.

TRADITIONAL CHINESE MEDICINE
1. Gao YT, et al. Reduced risk of esophageal cancer associated with green tea consumption. *Journal of the National Cancer Institiue* 1994;86:855–858.
2. Imai K, Nakachi K. Cross-sectional study of effects of drinking green tea on cardiovascular and liver diseases, *British Medical Journal* 1995;310:693–695.
3. Yongshun B. Clinical observations on the treatment of 98 cases of peptic ulcer by massage. *Journal of Traditional Chinese Medicine* 1993;13:50–51.
4. Guosheng H, et al. A study on the clinical effect and immunological mechanism in the treatment of Hashimoto's thyroiditis by moxibustion. *Journal of Traditional Chinese Medicine* 1993;13:14–18.
5. Yongnian Y. Therapeutic effects of the blood-activating and stasis-reducing method in 80 cases of coronary heart disease. *Journal of Traditional Chinese Medicine* 1995;15:10–13.
6. Yingming G, Shufen Z. Yi shou jiang zhi (de-blood-lipid) tablets in the treatment of hyperlipemia. *Journal of Traditional Chinese Medicine* 1995;15:178–179.
7. Sun Y, et al. Clinical observation and treatment of hyperkinesia in children by traditional Chinese medicine. *Journal of Traditional Chinese Medicine* 1994;14:105–109.
8. Kong XT, et al. Treatment of acute bronchiolitis with Chinese herbs. *Archives of Disease in Childhood* 1993;68:468–471.
9. Ziqi K, et al. Observation of therapeutic effect in 50 cases of chronic renal failure treated with rhubarb and adjuvant drugs. *Journal of Traditional Chinese Medicine* 1993;13:249–252.
10. Suting L, et al. Clinical observation on 80 children with peptic ulcer treated primarily by traditional Chinese medicine. *Journal of Traditional Chinese Medicine* 1995;15:14–17.
11. Ding Y, Xiaoxin H. Traditional Chinese herbs in treatment of neurological and neurosurgical disorders. *Canadian Journal of Neurologic Science* 1986;13:210–213.

WAVE THERAPY
1. Aldridge D. Alzheimer's disease: rhythm, timing and music as therapy. *Biomedical Pharmacotherapy* 1994;48:275–281.
2. Hanser SB, Thompson LW. Effects of a music therapy strategy on depressed older adults. *Journal of the American Medical Association* 1995;273:1318.
3. Mornhinweg GC, Voignier RR. Music for sleep disturbance in the elderly. *Journal of Holistic Nursing* 1995;13:248–254.
4. Tang W, Yao X, Zheng Z. Rehabilitative effect of music therapy for residual schizophrenia: a one-month randomised controlled trial in Shanghai. *British Journal of Psychiatry* 1994;24(suppl):38–44.
5. Menegazzi JJ, et al. A randomized, controlled trial of the use of music during laceration repair. *Annals of Emergency Medicine* 1991;20:348–350.
6. Barnason S, Zimmerman L, Nieveen J. The effects of music interventions on anxiety in the patient after coronary artery bypass grafting. *Heart and Lung* 1995;24:124–132.
7. Liberman J. The effect of syntonic (colored light) stimulation on certain visual and cognitive functions. *Journal of Optometry and Vision Development* 1986;17
8. Oren DA, et al. Exposure to ambient light in patients with winter seasonal affective disorder. *American Journal Psychiatry* 1994;151:591–593;
9. Thompson C, Stinson D, Smith A. Seasonal affective disorder and season-dependant abnormalities of melatonin suppression by light. *Lancet* 1990;ii:703–706.

YOGA
1. Goyeche J. Asthma: the yoga perspective part II: yoga therapy in the treatment of asthma. *Journal of Asthma* 1982;19:189–201.
2. Jain SC, et al. Effect of yoga training on exercise tolerance in adolescents with childhood asthma. *Journal of Asthma* 1991;28:437–442.
3. Patel CH. Yoga and biofeedback in the management of hypertension. *Lancet* 1973;ii:1053–1055.
4. Nespor K. Pain management and yoga. *International Journal of Psychosomatics* 1991;38:76–81.
5. Werntz DA, et al. Selective hemispheric stimulation by unilateral forced nostril breathing. *Human Neurobiology* 1987;6:165–171.
6. Shannahoff-Khalsa DS, et al. The effects of unilateral forced nostril breathing on cognition, *International Journal of Neuromedicine* 1991;57:239–249.
7. Jain SC, et al. A study of response patterns of non-insulin-dependent diabetes to yoga therapy. *Diabetes Research and Clinical Practice* 1993;19:69–74.
8. Wood C. Mood change and perceptions of vitality: a comparison of the effects of relaxation, visualization and yoga. *Journal of the Royal Society of Medicine* 1993;86:254–258.

Many couples opt for natural childbirth for any of several reasons:

- They want to approach childbirth as a normal life process, not a medical condition.
- They want to eliminate or reduce drug exposure to mother and child during labor and delivery.
- They want to feel they are active participants while giving birth, not just patients expected to "follow doctor's orders."
- They want to limit the recovery time often required after conventional childbirth.
- They want to be at home.

Natural childbirth doesn't mean just one thing. There are choices to make after the initial decision to give birth naturally. The following are some of the options available.

HOME BIRTH

Birth at home offers parents the advantage of maintaining the most control over birthing circumstances. The ambient comfort of home can ease anxiety and provide access to belongings that can further induce feelings of calm and well-being. At home, the mother can set her own "policies" on who attends the birth, what can be and can't be done during labor and delivery, and so on. Some couples choose to have a physician in attendance; others have a midwife. And after the birth, the mother and child don't have to "pack up and go home"; they're already there where the family can be supportive.

SAFETY

In the early 20th century, 95 percent of births in the United States took place at home. But with the advent of obstetrics as a field of medicine, the hospital came to be viewed as the only safe place to have a baby. Over the years, that attitude became firmly ingrained in the American psyche, with home births being viewed as a risky option. By 1990, 95 percent of American babies were born in hospitals. Still, giving birth at home remains a prevalent practice in many developed countries. For example, in the Netherlands (which has a lower infant mortality rate than the United States), 40 percent of births are at home.

One of the largest studies comparing hospital births and out-of-hospital births (which included home and birthing-center births) in the United States was done by the Centers for Disease Control and Prevention in the mid-1970s. Results showed that the infant death rate in hospitals was 12 per 1,000 live births, whereas for planned, attended home births the death rate dropped to 4 per 1,000 live births.

PREPARATION

Educate yourself thoroughly about childbirth (as you should no matter what setting you choose for birthing). Find a physician or midwife who will attend your birth. Interview several if necessary to find the right match for you. Finally, have a contingency plan set up in advance for going to the hospital should complications arise.

BIRTHING CENTERS

Birthing centers focus their facilities and policies around the mother and family. For instance, the woman in labor can wear her own clothing, shower, walk, and have visitors as she wishes. The key appeal of birthing centers is that they offer a homelike setting plus the benefits of professional medical care. Some birthing centers are referred to as freestanding, meaning they are completely unconnected with any hospital. Many hospitals also have now opened birthing centers, in response to consumer demand for an alternative to the "high-tech, low-touch" hospital birth setting.

SAFETY

The National Birth Center Study, published in the New England Journal of Medicine in 1989, found an infant mortality rate of 1.3 deaths per 1,000 live births, well within safe limits. Also, in these births, the rate of cesarean sections (carried out in backup hospitals) was 4.4 percent, compared with a U.S. national average of 25 percent.

PREPARATION

Visit the center, meet the staff, and find out if their policies match your preferences. What medical equipment is on site, and what is the center's plan for using hospital backup?

HOSPITAL BIRTH

Many hospitals have dramatically changed their approaches to respond to what parents want. You can have a natural birth in the hospital. Some hospitals now employ midwives who give the mother close, personal attention.

SAFETY

People assume hospitals are the safest birthing setting, although no scientific study has proved hospital birth to be more safe than a planned home or birthing-center birth.

PREPARATION

Choose a health professional who's sympathetic to your birth preferences. Visit the birthing facilities, meet staff, and check out policies on medical interventions, who can be with you during labor, and so on.

RESOURCES

- American College of Nurse-Midwives
  818 Connecticut Ave. NW, Ste. 900
  Washington, DC 20006
  202-728-9860
  fax 202-728-9897
  http://www.acnm.org
  A professional organization of nurse-midwives. Provides information on birthing alternatives and finding a nurse-midwife in your area.

- National Association of Childbearing Centers
  3123 Gottschall Rd.
  Perkiomenville, PA 18074
  215-234-8068
  Holds workshops throughout the United Sates on opening a birthing center. Packet of guidelines and referrals to centers in your area available by sending $1.

Appendix 3: Common Remedies

CASTOR OIL PACKS

- Fold a 20×20–inch piece of wool flannel in half and then in half again.
- Fill a shallow basin with several inches of cold-pressed castor oil.
- Soak the flannel in the oil and then remove, squeezing out only enough oil so the cloth isn't dripping.
- Put the folded flannel on the body (the location depends on the ailment).
- Cover with plastic (such as from a shopping bag) to prevent staining. Then cover with a heating pad or hot-water bottle.
- Set the heating pad to medium-high, or as high as tolerable.
- Leave on for about 1 hour.
- Afterward, clean the skin with bicarbonate of soda.

The soaked cloth can be kept in the covered basin for about 15 more uses.

ROBERT'S FORMULA

Robert's Formula is a classic naturopathic remedy. It calls for mixing together the following dried herbs and other ingredients:

- 8 parts American cranesbill (*Geranium maculatum*)
- 8 parts cabbage (*Brassica oleracea*)
- 2 parts duodenal substance
- 8 parts goldenseal (*Hydrastis canadensis*)
- 8 parts marshmallow root (*Althaea officinalis*)
- 1 part niacinamide (related to niacin, or vitamin B_3)
- 2 parts pancreatin
- 8 parts pokeroot (*Phytolacca americana*)
- 8 parts purple coneflower (*Echinacea angustifolia*)
- 8 parts slippery elm (*Ulmus fulva*)
- 4 parts wild indigo (*Baptisia tinctoria*)

A typical prescription for Robert's Formula is to take about ½ teaspoon 3 times a day. If used in capsule form, take 2 capsules before each meal.

ECHINACEA BASICS

Purple coneflower, also known as echinacea, is a powerful infection fighter and booster of the immune system. Here are some of the ways the herb may be prescribed:

- Mix 2 dropperfuls of commercially prepared tincture to 1 cup of warm water. Drink 3 to 4 times daily.
- Take three 200-mg capsules of the freeze-dried herb 3 times a day.
- Drink a half cup of tea made from the dried herb 3 times daily.

This herb should not be taken continuously for long periods of time because it may lose its effectiveness.